A Pleasing Birth

Midwives and Maternity Care in the Netherlands

A Pleasing Birth

Midwives and Maternity Care in the Netherlands

RAYMOND DE VRIES

TEMPLE UNIVERSITY PRESS
Philadelphia

Temple University Press
1601 North Broad Street
Philadelphia, PA 19122
www.temple.edu/tempress

⊗The paper used in this publication meets the requirements of the
American National Standard for Information Sciences—Permanence
of Paper for Printed Library Materials, ANSI Z39.48-1992

Library of Congress Cataloging-in-Publication Data

De Vries, Raymond G.
  A pleasing birth : midwives and maternity care in the Netherlands /
Raymond De Vries.
    p. cm.
  Includes bibliographical references and index.
  ISBN 1-59213-102-6 (cl. : alk. paper) – ISBN 1-59213-103-4 (pbk. : alk. paper)
    1. Maternal health services—Netherlands. 2. Midwifery—Netherlands.
    I. Title

RG964.N4D4 2004
618.2'0233'09492–dc22   2004044034

2 4 6 8 9 7 5 3 1

Contents

Preface

My CHILDREN and I arrived in the Netherlands on a cold, clear January day. I had come to study how Dutch babies get born. My children, mildly intrigued by the idea of living in Europe, agreed to come along, making my sabbatical a family affair.

We spent those first few mid-winter days exploring our new surroundings. We bicycled through the Dutch countryside along canals and past cows, farmhouses, and cafes. We visited the schools my children would be attending and became familiar with the bus routes we would travel to and from work and school. We rode the trains from Hilversum—the nearest city to our new home—to Amsterdam and back, learning how to negotiate the stations, schedules, and conductors. We tasted a variety of new and exotic foods, cuisines that found their way to the Netherlands from Indonesia, Turkey, and Morocco.

All the while I watched my children closely, eager to see their response to their new home. I had been to the Netherlands before and expected that they, like most tourists from the United States, would be impressed by the canals, the windmills, and the church towers. But these children, aged 11, 14, and 16, were no tourists: They were well aware that they would be living here for the next 12 months. For them, the most remarkable feature of the Netherlands was its smallness. In this tiny country everything seemed to be half-sized: the roads, the cars, the street signs, the grocery stores. They were most impressed (perhaps I should say *depressed*) by the size of our new living quarters. We had rented a typical Dutch home, a row-house, referred to in Dutch as an *eengezinswoning* (literally, "one-family living place") a label that caused my children, as it would most Americans, to scoff. By American standards, these houses are, at best, large enough for only half a family: The bedrooms are tiny and lack closets, the kitchen has the feel of a galley on a sloop, the single toilet is squeezed into a room so small one cannot turn around when the door is closed, and the living room serves also as the dining room.

Impossibly small for Americans, the architecture of Dutch homes makes sense in a small country with many people. Interior design is the art of efficiency, maximizing space and light. Not one square centimeter is wasted: Front-loading washing machines are tucked under kitchen counters; stairways appear from ceilings; clotheslines are stretched in hallways. Windows are used liberally. Nearly every home in the Netherlands has a large window in the front and in the rear, allowing a flood of natural light, giving small spaces a more open feel.

To the casual observer these cute Dutch homes are nothing more than practical adaptations to limited space. Had we not lived in the Netherlands, I would have been satisfied by that simple syllogism: tiny country = tiny homes. However, after a few months in our Lilliputian house, I came to understand that Dutch homes are not just about economizing on space; they also reflect and reinforce peculiarly Dutch ideas about the importance of the nuclear family. In accommodating to our new home we discovered we were spending more time together than we did in our much larger house in Minnesota. Small homes force families to live together in a way inhabitants of large American houses can avoid. The combined living and dining room of the *eengezinswoning* becomes the hub of family life. Here the children do their homework, parents read and chat, and the family plays games or watches television. Bedrooms are sleeping rooms (*slaapkamers*), and living rooms are really rooms where life is actually *lived*. Stroll down the street in the Netherlands at dusk, just before the curtains are drawn, and you will see framed in each large front window the Dutch family living together.

Our deeper understanding of the meaning of Dutch architecture was hard won: It took some time for us middle-class Americans to find ways to share bedrooms, bathrooms, and living rooms. American teenagers are used to having separate bedrooms, places of refuge from annoying siblings and parents. American parents are *not* used to having to wait in line for the toilet and the shower.

The shortage of space weighed heavily on me. My research was generating expanding piles of notes, documents, language tapes and books, and I had nowhere to work. Lacking room elsewhere, it became my habit to colonize the dining area after we had finished our dinner. My books and papers began in neat, organized piles, but somehow they would slowly march out to occupy not only the table, but also the seats of the encircling chairs. One evening, a few months after our arrival, I was hard at work amidst these piles, complete with frazzled hair and perplexed look, when my 14-year-old son wandered over to marvel at the chaos. He looked over the tangle of government reports and graphs describing Dutch maternity care, and, after a few minutes, he shook his head, slapped me on the back, and walking away, said—with the candor of youth—"Dad, I hate to tell you this, but no one cares about birth in the Netherlands."

Of course he was right. *I* was fascinated with the way the Dutch organize maternity care, but who else aside from a few birth activists, a handful of midwives, and an occasional obstetrician would be? This tiny country with its tiny houses, tucked in the swampland north of France and west of Germany, is little noticed on the world stage. News from the Netherlands rarely finds it way into newspapers in other countries. Every once in a great while you might find a story about Dutch drug policy or euthanasia on the third page, or perhaps some quaint personal interest story in the B-section. Not atypical is a report from the Associated Press that appeared in my local paper: "Marijuana Now Legal in Dutch Pharmacies" (*Minneapolis Star Tribune*, 18 March 2003, A7), or this piece from the *New York Times*: "The New Reefer Madness [in the Netherlands]: Drive-Through Shops" (*New York Times*, 28 May 2001, A4). When the Dutch Prime Minister visits the White House in Washington, it is not front-page news. Who in the United States can even *name* the Dutch Prime Minister?

Who, indeed, cares about birth in the Netherlands?

But social research often proves the wisdom of the biblical aphorism, "the foolish things of the world . . . confound the wise" (1 Corinthians 1:27). Thus a political scientist can go bowling (who cares about *bowling*?) and discover important truths about American social life (Putnam 2000). Similarly, we will see that birth in the Netherlands has a resonance that reaches far beyond the borders of this small country. In studying the peculiarities of the Dutch way of birth, we will learn how health systems are formed and how they can be successfully reformed.

I had come to the Netherlands for both personal and professional reasons. My name, De Vries, betrays my personal interest. Impossible for most Americans to spell, let alone pronounce, De Vries is perhaps the most common name in the Netherlands, the Jones of the lowlands. I am, in fact, a third generation Dutch-American. My grandparents, all four, were immigrants from the Netherlands, part of the flood of

Europeans that arrived at Ellis Island at the beginning of the twentieth century. They settled in the Dutch neighborhoods of northern New Jersey, from whence their descendants, in good American fashion, spread out to the corners of the continent.

I grew up hearing a very funny language traded back and forth among aunts and uncles, a secret code for communicating above the heads of us monolingual children. My knowledge of Dutch was limited to the names of certain household items: I was six or seven years old before I learned that not everyone called a dustpan and brush, the "fayghee and blek." I was, as my parents wished me to be, 100 percent American. And yet I remained curious about my roots in a different land, interested in the practices and ideas that made the De Vries and Greydanus families distinctive. I had been to the Netherlands a number of times—first as part of the backpacking tour of Europe that was nearly obligatory for American college students in the early 1970s, and thereafter for a few professional meetings. But I longed for a chance to live there, to become familiar with the language and the everyday life of the land where my ancestors had lived for countless generations.

Had my interest in the Netherlands been *only* personal, the book you hold in your hands would be a travelogue or a personal history rather than a piece of social and cultural analysis. My *professional* interest in the Netherlands grew out of my graduate school research on the sociological dimensions of birth practices. I began this work unaware of any connection it might have to my family history. To my delight, while digging through references on midwifery and obstetrics, I kept finding articles that described the Netherlands as "unique," "the exception," "a system worthy of emulation."

What caused this commentary? What made Dutch maternity care so peculiar? One simple fact: Unlike women in every other country in western Europe, unlike women in the United States, Canada, and the developed nations of Asia, women in the Netherlands continued to have their babies at home. According to some accounts I read, Dutch women were actually *encouraged* to have their babies at home. This was, and remains, very unusual. It is true that in the middle and late 1980s some women in developed countries were choosing to give birth at home, but data from the Dutch government showed a home birth rate of more than 30 percent through the 1980s and into the 1990s. At that time no other country with a sophisticated, highly technological medical system had more than 2 *percent* of births occurring outside the hospital,[1] and most of those births were precipitous deliveries, births that occur so fast that the laboring mother is unable to make it to the hospital.

To outsiders Dutch birth practices seemed to be caught in a nineteenth century time warp. In the late 1970s obstetricians in the United States had dismissed home birth as child abuse. Could birth at home be safe for babies and mothers? Here was a second curious fact about birth in the Netherlands: This seemingly archaic system was producing some of the lowest morbidity and mortality rates in the world.

What was going on over there? Why hadn't the Dutch conformed to the standards that dictated that modern women give birth in the hospital surrounded by the safety of high technology and the comfort of pain-relieving anesthesiology? And why did the Dutch system work so well?

No one seemed to be able to explain the Dutch difference. Several had tried. The journalists, physicians, historians, and social scientists who wrote about Dutch obstetrics felt obliged to offer reasons for the persistence of home birth there, but their explanations were unconvincing. Some believed it was Dutch stubbornness; others saw it as backwardness. Some credited the geography of the lowlands; others associated Dutch birth with Calvinism. Still others suggested that Dutch women were better suited to birth at home because they were bigger and healthier than women elsewhere. Interesting explanations all, but most were conjectural, based on scant, or no, evidence.

One *might* argue that the peculiarity of Dutch maternity care is nothing more than a cultural flourish. It is well-known that there are cultural variations in the way societies treat disease, so should we be surprised to discover that different countries treat birth differently? Well, no and yes. For if we look closely at the different forms of medical treatment offered in different modern nations, we find that they are, in fact, all mere variations on the theme of allopathic medicine. Yes, rates of surgery and patterns of prescription drug use vary between countries. Underlying these treatments (and nearly all treatments in modern nations), however, is the single, unvarying allopathic principle that the proper response to disease is medication and surgery. Modern medicine is active and interventionist. Obstetrical practice in the

---

1. The home birth rate in the United Kingdom went above 2 percent in 1997. See Declercq, De Vries, Salvesen, and Viisainen (2001).

Netherlands is especially odd because it is *watchful and reactive,* violating the fundamental premise of modern medicine.

The more I read about Dutch maternity care, the more I saw that it was an *exceptional* exception and not just a quaint custom practiced by people with wooden shoes. While the rest of the modern world was captivated by the wonders of new technology and eagerly applied this technology to the "problems" of birth, this small country, which is otherwise sympathetic to technology, continued to insist that birth is a healthy process best accomplished free from drugs and machinery in the comfort and safety (!) of the mother's home. Something was going on over there that promised to teach us, not just about the way we do birth, but more generally, about the way we think about and organize health care.

I had to get to the Netherlands. Finishing my studies of birth in the United States, which issued in several articles and a monograph on making midwives legal (see De Vries 1985, 1996), I began to seek the means for an extended stay in the land of my ancestors. I was naively optimistic about getting funded: After all, maternity care in the Netherlands was extremely interesting, and it had not been carefully described in the English language literature. The few reports of the system that existed were broadly descriptive, based on a one- or two-week fact-finding tour: just enough time to gather some (not always reliable) statistics. Furthermore, granting agencies would surely notice that the distinctiveness of Dutch obstetrics offered a perfect opportunity to do a quasi-experiment. Here was one country among a number of like-situated countries that had a different outcome. By comparing these countries and working backwards from the present systems to the conditions that generated them, I would be able to isolate the cultural and social variables that explained birth care in the Netherlands.

My early attempts to get funding failed. Perhaps it was because my proposals were poorly conceived, perhaps it was because of the perceived insignificance of the Netherlands. I persisted, applying to a wide range of private foundations and public agencies. Finally, in 1993, reviewers for the Senior International Fellows program of the Fogarty Center of the National Institutes of Health agreed there might be something to learn in the Netherlands, and I was awarded the funds necessary to begin my research.

My family and I left America for the Netherlands in early 1994, a temporary and comparatively advantaged reversal of the immigration story played out by my grandparents nearly one century ago. The Netherlands proved to be richer ground for sociological research than I had imagined: another way of saying that I soon realized my tidy little study would remain neither tidy nor little. I started with a simple question: Why is the Dutch way of birthing children so different? But this simple question led, ineluctably and almost immediately, to larger questions. What is the place of maternity care in the larger health care system? How is government policy on health care made? How does the political system influence health care? Who pays for health care and who profits from health care services? What elements of Dutch culture (for example, ideas about the body, about gender, about families) support their particular health care system?

As I pursued these unanticipated questions, I gradually understood that I had *two* stories to tell. The first is the obvious one, about the way children are born in the Netherlands. This story—the story of Dutch maternity care—is a fascinating one, complete with a colorful cast of heroes and villains, political intrigue, and competing professional and scientific interests. The second story is an account of the way health care systems operate. At every step of my research, the facts of Dutch maternity care forced me to rethink and revise the widely accepted stories academics tell about the way health care systems work and develop. This second story is more abstract than the first, but no less interesting and—because it forces us to revise much of the knowledge of health policy and medical sociology that is taken for granted—it is, perhaps, the more important.

This book is my effort to tell these two stories. Taken together, the stories suggest a new way of thinking about health policy. Health care systems are unwieldy beasts. Their size and complexity frustrate individuals who need health services and stymie the most well-intended reform efforts, turning would-be improvements into new inefficiencies. With the constant change wrought by new technologies, new financing schemes, and new political alliances, policy researchers and social scientists are hard-pressed simply to *describe* how these large systems work. If we cannot describe the forces that shape the delivery of health services, we have no hope of improving the quality or reducing the inefficiency of health care. But how can we gain this much-needed understanding? In the following pages I demonstrate that the best way to learn about the operation of complex health care systems is to look at one small slice of health care in one small country. I argue that a rich description of maternity care in the Netherlands allows us to see the many factors at work in the creation and evolution of health care services, and helps us avoid the problems that plague those who wish to explain the organization of medical care.

When I began my research I was well aware of its policy implications for obstetrics in the United States: We Americans needed to learn how to make birth less medical, using fewer drugs, less technology, and less intervention. But, as you will see, I learned far more than this. Lessons learned from Dutch maternity care have broader application and can help us to find new ways to reform health care and to respond to the high cost and limited accessibility of modern medicine.

The tortured evolution of American health care over the last decade—highlighted by government-sponsored incremental change and unmanageable managed care—has made two things evident: (1) The system must be changed, and (2) we know very little about how to bring about the changes that are needed. If we are to succeed in the reform of health care, we must have a better understanding of the many forces that *form* medical systems. We need to know more than medical sociologists, economists, and health policy analysts have told us: We need to know how medical systems come to take the shapes they do. Study of maternity care in the Netherlands will close gaps in our knowledge of the social and cultural foundations of health care. In turn, this knowledge will serve as the first step in effective reform, not just of maternity care, but also of health systems.

My description and analysis of Dutch midwifery is based on 16 months of research done from 1994 to 1995. During that period, I interviewed midwives, clients, gynecologists, midwife educators, government officials, policymakers, researchers, staff of the association of health insurers, and staff of the professional associations of midwives, general practitioners, and gynecologists.[2] I visited several midwife practices and three schools of midwifery. I read all major government reports on midwifery published since 1940 and read uncounted articles in the professional journals of Dutch midwives, general practitioners, and specialists. I also read popular literature related to birth and midwifery, including articles in newspapers, magazines, and how-to books for new mothers and fathers. Since leaving the field in 1995, I have visited the Netherlands several times, both

---

2. I draw on these interviews extensively in my analysis. Some of these interviews were done in English and some were done in Dutch. In many instances my interviewees, regardless of the language we were using, would use a Dutch word or expression that is not easily translated. In those cases you will find the words and phrases remain in Dutch, followed by an English approximation.

virtually and physically, updating my data and following developments in health care and midwifery.

*   *   *   *   *

Part I of *A Pleasing Birth* sets the stage for the two stories of Dutch maternity care. After a brief meditation on what makes for a pleasing birth, I go on in Chapter 1 to describe the opportunities afforded by the study of birth in the Netherlands, showing how a careful look at the specific features that make Dutch birth different enhances our understanding of health care systems in general. In Chapter 2, I offer a thorough description of the Dutch system, describing its uniqueness in the modern world.

In Part II, I begin my explanation of how Dutch maternity care avoided the turn toward technology that characterizes all other modern obstetric systems. In providing this explanation I look to the unique *structural* features of Dutch society. Chapter 3 examines how the infrastructure of Dutch society—including its health insurance system, its health policy process, its educational and professional institutions, and its system of hospitals and roads—sustain the unique Dutch way of birth. In Chapter 4, I explore the political arrangements, both outside and inside of health care, that protect the existing maternity system.

These structural explanations are an important first step in helping us understand the form of Dutch maternity care, but they can take us only so far. In Part III I ask, "Why did the Dutch (and not their neighbors in surrounding countries) *create* and *maintain* the structures that lend support to midwife-assisted birth at home?" Chapter 5 answers this question by looking at the critical role cultural ideas and values played in the creation of the Dutch way of birth. In Chapter 6, I examine the science that informs health policy. Bringing together the themes of Parts II and III, I offer a sociology of obstetric science, an analysis that shows the footprints of structure and culture in the science that has been used to both support and to criticize Dutch obstetrics.

In Part IV, I move to the second story, using what we have learned about Dutch maternity care to explain the way health care systems are *formed* and *re-formed*. In Chapter 7, I look at how changes that are occurring in Dutch society and medicine are threatening Dutch obstetrics, and I discuss the steps the government is taking to protect their unique way of birth. After summarizing the cultural and structural forces that created (and continue to create) Dutch maternity care, I go on, in Chapter 8, to consider how my research can be used by health activists, medical sociologists, and health policy makers.

*   *   *   *   *

Although I was unaware of it, my lessons about the Dutch difference began during those first days in our tiny home in the Netherlands. We could not help but notice that the Dutch see the world with different eyes. Blessed with boundless space, we in the United States see ourselves as a country without limits. Many of us live in large houses with large rooms, and large yards. The Dutch have spent centuries fighting the sea and rising rivers. Hemmed in by canals and dikes, they have a keener appreciation of limits. As we begin life in the third millennium, we Americans are beginning to discover our limits: Our large houses cost too much to heat, to cool, and to light. And our limitless health care system has created a crisis of cost and confidence. There are better ways to build homes *and* to organize health care. Looking to maternity care in the Netherlands, we can find a way to live within our limits and to create a more just and effective health care system.

A NOTE ON LANGUAGE

In order to tell the story of health care and childbirth in the Netherlands, I must put Dutch terms into words that are understandable to an English-speaking audience. In some cases the obvious word is not the best word. For example, use of the word *Dutch* itself. Residents of the Netherlands have grown accustomed to this adjective, but if pressed, most will admit they are not fond of the word. It is a derivative of *deutsch*, or German. In their language the national adjective is *Nederlands(e)*, better translated as Netherlandish (as in Finnish, Swedish, Danish) rather than Dutch. In an effort to respect the language and to avoid all the connotations of the word Dutch—"dutch treat," "dutch uncle," wooden shoes, and windmills—I tried using the word *Netherlandish* in this book. In the end it sounded too pretentious; it might work for those in the art world, but it seemed to clutter up this book. Please note, however, that although the use of the word *Dutch* makes for smoother reading, it confuses the translation of many abbreviations of organizations and government agencies: All those Ns become Ds. For example, the Royal Dutch Organization of Midwives

(RDOM) is in fact the *Koninklijke Nederlandse Organisatie van Verlos-kundigen* (KNOV).

As with all moves from one language to another, it is easy to misrepresent meaning. For example, the Dutch word *welzijn* is most often and easily translated as *welfare*. But the word literally means "well-being," and the Dutch sense of the word is closer to that translation than it is to the heavily loaded (American) English word *welfare*. Because my goal is to get the reader to understand the *concept* represented by the word and not just the word itself, and because one of the central arguments of this book is that health systems must be understood as cultural products, I will ask you, the reader, to become familiar with certain Dutch words and phrases. I do this only when no suitable English word exists or when the common English translation of a Dutch word is misleading. To assist you in gaining a working knowledge of these Dutch words I have prepared a glossary to which you can refer. Because language is an important carrier of culture, it is important for you to become familiar with a few Dutch words and the distinctive meanings they carry. In several places in the text, I include the Dutch word along with the English translation of the word. I do this out of respect for language and to remind you, the reader, that the English translation is only an approximation of the meaning of that word in Dutch. In each chapter the first use of a Dutch word is italicized; thereafter it appears in nonitalicized type.

Perhaps the best example of how meaning can be lost in translation is found in the Dutch words for midwife. The Dutch use two different words for midwife. *Vroedvrouw*, literally "wise woman," is the more traditional term; *verloskundige*—"expert in delivery" or "expert in obstetrics"—is the more modern word. In the mid-1970s the official term was switched from *vroedvrouw* to *verloskundige;*[3] but in the common language of the streets both words are used. Generally, the practitioners who favor the term vroedvrouw are those who are actively advocating for home birth and autonomous midwifery, whereas those who prefer verloskundige are midwives seeking to fit their occupation in the modern professional structure. If I simply translated both terms as *midwife*, the nuance that separates activist midwives

---

3. In 1975, the two existing professional associations of midwives merged and the new association was named the *Nederlandse Organsatie van Verloskundigen*. In 1978, the government replaced vroedvrouw with verloskundige in all laws referring to midwives (Drenth 1998, 81).

from other midwives would be lost (see van der Hulst 1989). Consider this exchange with a midwife educator:

I noticed that you use the word vroedvrouw, *and not* verloskundige. *So you feel that's an unfortunate change of names?*

Ja.

That happened before you became a vroedvrouw?

Yes, I think in 1975. It happened in the period when I was in training. Op mijn diploma staat nog *Vroedvrouw.* [On my diploma it still says "Vroedvrouw."] So afterwards, a year later it said *Verloskundige* on the diplomas. And it started about 1974, when men came in the profession, that they decided to change the word.

Who's they? Is that the government again?

The government, ja.

I've noticed also on the elevator downstairs it says Vroedvrouwenopleiding, *[Vroedvrouw education] not verloskundige. Has that just stayed the same here, in Amsterdam? Or did you change it? Or . . .*

No. Officially the name of our school is *Kweekschool voor vroedvrouwen* (Vocational school for *vroedvrouwen*). And then people would say, "It's a very old-fashioned name; you should change it. You should change it; you should make it *Akademie voor verloskundigen,* or *Hogeschool voor verloskundigen.*" And we discussed a lot about it, and then we said "No, we have to use that name, because it's a very old name, and it's good to have that old name, *Kweekschool voor vroedvrouwen.*"

Is it still used by other schools, Kweekschool?

No.

It's not used in any other . . .?

The school in Kerkrade is called *Vroedvrouwenschool,* and Rotterdam is called *Rotterdamse opleiding tot verloskundige.* So they changed it. And we are still the *Kweekschool voor vroedvrouwen.* And we are not discussing that any more. That's our name, and that's what it is.

Acknowledgments

Doing the research for this book was great fun: There was the excitement of moving back to the land of my ancestors, of learning the language, of traveling the length and breadth of the Netherlands, of meeting interesting people and hearing them talk about their work and lives. All this would have been impossible without the help of others.

Lacking financial support I would have remained a tourist. Funds from the Fogarty Center of the National Institutes of Health (Grant number F06-TW01954), the NIVEL (Netherlands Institute for Health Care Research), the Catharina Schrader Stichting, and the faculty development fund of St. Olaf College made this work possible. I am grateful.

Money only gets you so far; if not for the hospitality of colleagues and friends in the Netherlands, my sojourn would have been far less pleasant and far less productive. Koos and Els van der Velden (*en jongens*), Wouter and Mariken Meijer, Sjoerd Kooiker and Martha van der Pijl (and René), Lea Jabaaij and Loek Stokx (and Co), Sandra and Thomas Krelage, Ton Zondervan, Wilma Elferink, Annemiek Cuppen, and Frederika and Sean Charles introduced me (and my family) to Dutch culture and kindly provided food and shelter, collected me at the airport, allowed me to use their bicycles, and gently corrected my Dutch.

Colleagues at the NIVEL were extremely patient and supportive, and on occasion even paid for my beer at *de Steeg*. Among others, Harald Abrahamse, Rudi Bakker, Koos van der Velden, Sjoerd Kooiker, Loek Stokx, Lea Jabaaij, Jack Hutten, Wouter Meijer, and Peter Groenewegen offered helpful advice and comments on my work. Trees Wiegers and Lammert Hingtsman, who are the experts on maternity care in the Netherlands, have been most kind in sharing their knowledge and their work with me. Lieneke Notenboom, my first, unofficial instructor in Dutch, spent untold time transcribing my interviews and allowed me to stay in her home during one summer visit. Her careful transcriptions and suggestions for further reading enriched my work. And Jouke van der Zee, the director of the NIVEL, was an unfailing supporter of my research.

The shaping of research findings into a book—with its countless hours of writing and rewriting—does not provide the same rush as being in the field, but it has its own rewards. Here, too, I was helped by generous friends and colleagues on both sides of the Atlantic. Hilary Marland, Ina May Gaskin, Robbie Davis-Floyd, Barbara Katz-Rothman, and Gene Declercq read drafts of the manuscript; their comments greatly improved the quality of this book. The "Birth by Design" folks, including Edwin van Teijlingen, Sirpa Wrede, Cecilia Benoit, Ivy Bourgeault, Jane Sandall, Bernike Pasveer, and Beate Schücking, were a constant source of ideas and encouragement. Marilyn Curl shared articles from her archives on the mistreatment of American women during labor and birth. Steve Polansky and Alvin Handelman are two of the world's finest editors. My colleagues at the Institute for Advanced Study in Princeton, New Jersey, listened to my half-baked ideas and helped me find a way to make them more fully baked.

The move from a collection of chapters in a little yellow folder on a computer screen to a published book also requires help. Jonathan Matson, agent *extraordinaire*, has literally given me his time. Jessica Mesman and Carl Elliott listened to me whine about the difficulty of finding the right publisher and never tired in their encouragement. Mike Mihelich helped out with questions of design. Micah Kleit at Temple University Press went to bat for this project and calmed me when I was overwrought. Jennifer French deserves far more than this simple acknowledgment for her patience in dealing with one pain-in-the-neck author.

Most deserving of thanks, of course, are those who subjected themselves to this research. Included here are all the good and patient people in the Netherlands who gave me their time, and the members of my family, who were willing to be uprooted for the sake of my curiosity. Among those who were especially helpful to my work in the field were Annemiek Cuppen—who died in 1998—Drs. Kloosterman, Bleker, Kierse, and Klomp, Aya Crebas, Beatrijs Smulders, and Wilma Elferink. My family—Jesse, Rocky, Anna, and Charlotte—not only agreed to join me in this adventure; they actually came to enjoy many of the things I like about the Netherlands: *hagelslag, dropjes, lunetta, brood, fritjes, witbier, cafés, voetbal, treinen,* and the *Efteling.*

This book is dedicated to all the women and men who have helped, and are helping, to preserve the sane and humane way of birth found in the Netherlands. Long may they, and the Dutch way of birth, survive.

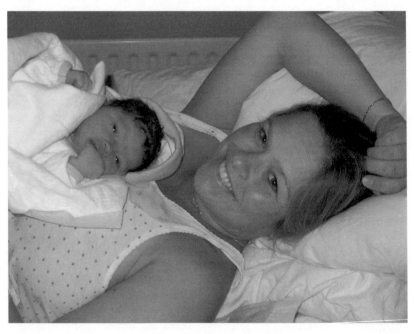

Een bevalling dat bevalt (a pleasing birth) in the Netherlands. Reproduced with permission from Marcel Wessels.

I. BIRTH CARE/HEALTH CARE

AMONG THE many interesting things I discovered while studying the Dutch language, none was more fascinating than learning that the verb *bevallen*, means both "to give birth" and "to please." *Een bevalling dat bevalt* is, literally, "a birth that pleases," or, translated more fluently, "a pleasing birth." Given what I knew of birth in the Netherlands, it seemed fitting that in Dutch, "a pleasing birth" would be a redundancy. Of course, not all women agree on the features of a pleasing birth. For some women the ideal birth is one that takes place in the company of family and friends. Other women prefer to be alone. Some women desire analgesia and anesthesia to relieve the pain of labor, others choose to give birth without the assistance of drugs. For some, the most satisfying birth occurs in the security and familiarity of their own home, although others find the hospital the most reassuring place to bring their child into the world. Some birthing women are happiest when attended by an obstetrician-gynecologist; some favor the services of a midwife.

The following birth story-told in Dutch and translated into English- is an account of a pleasing birth in the Netherlands.

> *Mijn tweede zwangerschap was niet zo stralend en vitaal als mijn eerste; vaak verkouden en vermoeid. Wilde graag dat deze tweede op 1 mei geboren zou worden, zo'n mooie datum. Maar op 26 April, na mijn laatste afspraak met de vroedvrouw, voelde ik een kleine wee en een tijdje later weer een kleintje.*

My second pregnancy was not as exciting as my first, I was often tired and had many colds. I was hoping that this child would be born on the first of May, it is such a perfect date. But on the 26th of April, after my last appointment with the midwife, my contractions began. I felt a weak contraction, and then a while later, another small one.

> *Besloot om lekker vroeg naar bed te gaan. Als ik kan slapen, misschien gingen de weeën dan wel weg. Dat lukt niet. Ik had nu duidelijk weeën en ging met mijn blote dikke buik bij de warme kachel staan. Wat lekker was. De weeën werden duidelijker en regelmatiger en we belden de vroedvrouw.*

I decided to go to bed nice and early. If I could get to sleep, maybe the contractions would stop. That did not work. I was definitely having contractions, so I went with my big bare belly and stood in front of the gas heater. That felt great! The contractions became stronger and more regular, and we called the midwife.

Eerste kwam de co-assistent en daarna de vroedvrouw. Ook Jetske, mijn vriendin, kwam met een grote bos sterk geurende lelies. Buurman Otto kwam to-evallig binnen en vroeg of hij mocht blijven. Dat mocht. Tussen de weeën kon ik me nog heel goed ontspannen en als er weer een op kwam zetten, ving ik hem/haar behendig op. Voelde me een bedreven baarster. Ze namen intussen in hoeveelheid en intensiteit toe en binnen de kortste tijd herinnerde ik me weer haarscherp hoe venijnig sommige weeën kunnen zijn.

First came the assistant and then the midwife. My friend Jetske came with a big bouquet of fragrant lilies. My neighbor Otto happened to come by and asked if he could stay. Sure, why not? Between contractions I was able to relax, and when another came, I was able to handle it easily. I felt like an old hand at this. Gradually the contractions became more frequent and intense, and I suddenly recalled how vicious some contractions can be.

Ik raakte geïrriteerd en ongeduldig. Ik had er echt genoeg van, ik wilde dit nooit meer. Snel kwamen toen de persweeën en ik moest ze nog even op een afstand houden, wegblazen. Maar ze waren zo machtig dat ik mee moest en tegelijk genoot ik daarvan. De vroedvrouw brak de vliezen. En toen kwam als een enorme opluchting mijn tweede kind naar buiten, een prachtig meisje met donker haar, Rosa.

I began to feel irritated and impatient. I had had enough of this, I wanted no more. Soon came the urge to push, but I had to keep these strong contractions at a distance, I had to puff them away. But they were so powerful I had to go along with them, and when I did I found that I enjoyed them. The midwife broke the membranes. And then, an enormous relief, my second child arrived, a beautiful little girl with dark hair, Rosa.

Zij lag veilig en warm naast me, met tussenpozen zachtjes kreunend alsof ze bij moest komen van de tocht naar buiten. Toen iedereen weg was en Frans, mijn man, lag te slapen op de bank en Swaan, mijn dochtertje, in haar bed, en Rosa in mijn arm, veranderde de kamer in een eiland van rust, het middelpunt van het universum.

She lay next to me safe and warm, softly groaning as if gradually recovering from her journey. When everyone had gone and Frans, my husband, was sleeping on the sofa and Swaan, my little daughter, was in her bed, and Rosa in my arms, the room changed into an island of rest, the center of the universe.

—"The Birth of Rosa"[1]

---

1. From *Bevallen and Opstaan,* Spanjer et al. 1994, 366–367.

When we hear stories of labor and delivery it is easy to conclude that every woman has her own idea of a pleasing birth. But is the definition of, or the agenda for, a pleasing birth an individual creation? Can we assume that the decisions we make about how we want our birth to proceed—or the decisions we make about *any* health care service we use—are based on nothing more than our individual preferences? When we look closely at women's preferences for care at birth we find a pattern beneath the variation. The hospital, with its bright lights, gleaming stainless steel, and state-of-the-art machinery, comforts an American mother but terrorizes a birthing woman newly arrived in the United States from rural Laos. A laboring woman from Paris would panic if placed in the simple hut and birthing hammock that reassure mothers-to-be in the Yucatan. The home birth described above—quite common in the Netherlands—seems outlandish and risky to a pregnant woman in nearby Berlin.

No one is surprised to find that women in rural Laos have a definition of a good birth that differs from the definition shared by women who live in the suburbs of the United States. It *is* surprising, however, to find widely disparate conceptions of a pleasing birth in societies that are quite similar. Dutch society is not unlike other European or North American societies, and yet women there have an anomalous conception of a pleasing birth: More than 75 percent of pregnant women in the Netherlands choose midwife care at the beginning of their pregnancy, and more than 40 percent choose to have their babies at home (Wiegers 2002).[2] These numbers stand in stark contrast to the rest of the modern world: In the United States fewer than 10 percent of pregnant woman seek the care of a midwife, and home birth is exceedingly rare in countries with modern medical systems.

This is odd. Medical science and clinical practice are no less sophisticated in the Netherlands than they are in the United States or Europe. Why has midwife-assisted home birth persisted there? The bright light of science is supposed to dispel the mists of folklore and superstition. Medical science put an end to the elixirs, potions, and ointments of traveling medicine men, but in the Netherlands the science of obstetrics has been unable to eliminate old-fashioned birth at home or to standardize the procedures used to accomplish birth.

---

2. As we will see in Chapter 2, not all the women who choose birth at home actually deliver there.

If we were to embark on an international study of heart bypass procedures in the countries of Europe and North America, the only variation
we would discover would be in the language used in the operating
theaters. The setting, the actors, and the techniques are so similar it
would be difficult to know if we were watching Finnish or French
physicians at work were it *not* for the language. A tour of birthing
rooms in these same countries would yield no such confusion. Not
only do the *settings* vary—from delivery rooms, to birthing rooms, to
bedrooms—but so do the *practices*, which range from very low technology (using only a fetoscope and a blood-pressure cuff) to very high
technology (complete with electronic monitoring equipment, surgical
tools, infant warmers, and the like). There are also differences in those
who attend birth—midwives, general practitioners, gynecologists,
obstetricians. More than any other branch of medicine, maternity care
is marked by the culture and society in which it is found.[3]

The marks of culture and society on birth care extend beyond clinical procedures to the science of obstetrics. If we were to continue the
comparative study of birth practices that we began with our tour of
birthing rooms, we would find several distinct "sciences of birth."
There is scientific literature that supports maternity care in the
Netherlands, with its high rate of home births and low rate of cesarean
sections (13.7 percent in 2002), *and* scientific literature that supports obstetric practice in the United States, where less than 1 percent of births
take place at home and, in 2002, more than 26 percent of women were
delivered by cesarean section.[4] The co-existence of separate and often
contradictory sciences of birth forces us to conclude that in the world
of maternity care the relationship between science and practice is
turned upside down: Rather than science generating medical practice,
practice generates science.

Most citizens of the early twenty-first century are aware that science
does not exist in some culture-free vacuum: The once revolutionary
ideas of Thomas Kuhn (1962)—demonstrating that science proceeds

---

3. These marks are visible both *between* and *within* societies. The modal Dutch birth
is radically different from the modal birth in the United States, and the modal birth to an
upper-class, well-educated woman in the Netherlands will look different from the modal
birth for a working-class Dutch woman. For the most part, my concern in this book is
with the variation *between* societies.

4. In 2002, the cesarean section rate in the United States was 26.1 percent.

not by the gradual accretion of knowledge, but by leaps between paradigms—are now standard fare in business schools and motivational seminars. But the science of obstetrics is a special case, exceeding what most laypersons, and even social scientists, believe to be the influence of culture on medical knowledge and practice. Obstetrics is best thought of as a "cultured science," a science that is thoroughly embedded in its host culture.

1 Dutch Birth and the Shape of Health Care

ON THE second of June 1994, an extraordinary meeting took place in the Dutch town of Ede. The Netherlands Organization of Midwives (NOV),[1] with the support of the Ministry of Welfare, Health, and Culture (WVC),[2] sponsored a one-day conference to inaugurate a public campaign to promote birth at home. Under the title "Een Goede Keuze Bevalt Beter" ("A Good Choice Means a Better Birth"[3]), the purpose of the symposium was to consider ways to halt a decrease in the number of Dutch women choosing to have their babies at home, a decrease that many members of the health care community found worrisome. Included on the program were representatives of physician organizations (both general practitioners and gynecologists),[4] government officials, researchers, policymakers, and representatives of consumer organizations.

---

1. The NOV is the *Nederlandse Organisatie van Verloskundigen*. In June 1998, in recognition of the 100-year existence of the NOV, the organization was crowned with the title *Koninklijk* (Royal); the NOV is now known as the KNOV (see Croon 1998). See also note 4.

2. The WVC is the *Ministerie van Welzijn, Volksgezondheid, en Cultuur*, literally, "Ministry of Well-Being, People's Health, and Culture." As noted in the preface, *welzijn* is often translated as *welfare*, but, in America, the word welfare has come to mean "payments from the government to the poor and the disadvantaged." The Dutch word retains the broader meaning of well-being or health. In 1994, a new government was formed, and it made some adjustments in the different ministries. Beginning on October 1994, the ministry responsible for the people's health became the VWS, *Ministerie van Volksgezondheid, Welzijn, en Sport*.

3. The title of the campaign is a play on words. Because the verb *bevallen* means both "to give birth" and "to please," the title can be interpreted, "A good choice means a better birth" or "A good choice is more pleasing."

4. In the United States we refer to the physician specialist who provides care at birth as an obstetrician or an obstetrician/gynecologist. In the Netherlands this person is typically called a gynecologist. Several words in the Dutch language can be used to denote an obstetrician: *obstetricus*, *vrouwenarts*, and *gynecoloog*, but the last is most common. Interestingly, the Dutch word for obstetrics, *verloskunde* (literally "expertise in delivery"), is now more commonly associated with midwifery. When referring to the Dutch physician-specialist in childbirth I will follow the Dutch convention and use the term gynecologist or gynecoloog.

Those who attended the symposium heard reports of government-financed research on midwives' attitudes toward the place of birth (midwives find home birth both more satisfying and more intense) and on the safety of birth at home for properly screened women (birth at home is at least as safe as hospital birth for women having their first child; for women who already have had one child, home birth brings better results). They heard Mevrouw Netelenbos, chairperson of the Dutch parliament's Committee for Health (*Commissee voor de Volksgezondheid*) proclaim the government's respect for the autonomy of midwives and its willingness to support them, "The midwife can do much on her own, but she must be protected. The government cannot stand at a distance." And they heard the executive director of the NOV, Mevrouw Zwart, reflect on the *weeën* of the campaign. Weeën is the Dutch word for the contractions of labor, but it can also be translated as the W's, as in who (*wie*), what (*wat*), where (*waar*), when (*wanneer*), and why (*waarom*). She described the audience targeted by the campaign (pregnant women, their partners, and other influential relatives as well as midwives and other caregivers), the means of the campaign (brochures, press releases, a nationwide telephone information line, and visits to groups of midwives, nurses, and physicians), and the why of the campaign: the preservation of the possibility of choice in the place of birth, giving special emphasis to birth at home.[5]

To the Dutch this meeting did not seem unusual. It is not uncommon for the government and professional associations to join together in campaigns in the interest of public health. But those of us who know a bit about maternity care, and who are *not* Dutch, find it difficult to believe a conference like this could take place. Public promotion of home birth? With the full support of the government?[6] In other nations with modern health systems, home birth is thought to belong to the dark ages of medicine; in the United States, those choosing home birth have been identified as members of the "lunatic fringe." Physicians (including specialists!) joining together with midwives to promote home

---

5. Amelink and van Leent (1994) summarize the proceedings of the conference.

6. The government remains strong in its support of birth at home: In describing the budgetary measures meant to help midwives, the Ministry of Health noted: "The starting point in the search for solutions for problems in midwifery is that it *must remain possible to give birth at home*" (Ministerie van Volksgezondheid, Welzijn, en Sport 2001, 63, emphasis added).

birth? Midwives in the United States have become accustomed to physician resistance to their practicing even *in hospitals*: To have a physician publicly support midwife-assisted birth at home is nearly unthinkable.

This meeting was, for me, the first inkling that study of Dutch maternity care would shed new light, not just on birth practices, but on well-established understandings of how health systems operate. The events that occurred in Ede on that June day flew in the face of much of what I had learned as a medical sociologist. Something different was going on here, something that would force me to rethink most of the work social scientists had done on the development of the professions and on the influence of technology on medicine.

According to the conventional logic of professions, an occupational group with more power—for instance, medicine—will always control the turf of groups with less power, say, midwives and nurses. In the United States and the United Kingdom there is good evidence to support this theory. Several histories of midwives and medical men in those countries suggest that the structural and cultural power of physicians conspired to suppress, if not eliminate, midwifery. Midwives were not only chased from practice by doctors who did not appreciate the competition, but the polished image of American medicine created a situation that caused immigrant women to abandon their midwives and seek the care of "modern" medical men (see Borst 1995). But in the Netherlands, this medical hegemony explanation does not work. If we want to save the theory and use it to explain the situation of Dutch midwives, we need to come up with a new, more flexible definition of hegemony, or we must create a tortured explanation that shows how physician support of a competing occupation serves the long-term interest of the medical profession—neither of which is, finally, practicable.

Similarly, the "technological imperative"—the notion that if the technology exists, it will be used—is widely accepted by those who study the relationship between society and technology and the larger public. We need not look far for proof of the technological imperative: Experts and nonexperts alike see the rapid proliferation of the sometimes useful, sometimes annoying, cellular phone as ample evidence that technology always makes a way for itself, even if it violates established rules of etiquette. In the world of medicine and maternity care there are numerous examples of technology forcing its way into, and sometimes disrupting, the relationship between clients and practitioners. Magnetic resonance imaging (MRI) replaces consultations about migraines, and electronic fetal monitoring (EFM) takes the place of regular and reassuring visits from the obstetric nurse. Most studies of care at birth, even those done in remote societies, regard complete hospitalization and increased technological intervention as the logical and unavoidable result of the application of modern science to the "problem" of birth. But here again the facts of Dutch maternity care subvert cherished theory. The Netherlands is as technologically sophisticated as any modern nation, and yet midwives and general practitioners[7]— who together attend approximately half of all births in the Netherlands—use very few modern technologies. Midwives do not encourage prenatal testing (see Rothman 2001), and they eschew the use of EFM, using fetoscopes instead.[8]

The meeting in Ede underscored the simple fact that birth in the Netherlands is accomplished much differently than it is elsewhere. For most who found themselves in Ede on that day, this was not earth-shattering news; I am sure, in fact, that many participants found the meeting a bit boring. Seen from the perspective of a foreigner, however, this mundane event reveals larger truths. When we begin to explain the simple facts of Dutch maternity care, we must discard ideas that we have long taken for granted. Everything I learned in graduate school taught me that the Dutch system of birth could not possibly survive into the twenty-first century: The advancement of medical technology and the development of medical specialties lead, inevitably, to the hospitalization of birth and the diminishment of midwifery. But wait. Those people on the platform are saying that the government of the Netherlands and medical specialists are working hard to make sure midwife-assisted birth at home continues and thrives. The Dutch, then, were not just reviewing the details of a public health campaign; they were, it must be said, falsifying important truths about the way health systems work. They were suggesting it was possible to see a different

---

7. The statistics of birth in the Netherlands are presented in Chapter 2.

8. Many midwives use *toeters* to listen to fetal heart tones. Carved from wood, in the shape of a small trumpet (about 6–7 inches in length) these "primitive" fetoscopes put the midwife in very close contact with her client, allowing her to use not just her sense of hearing but also her senses of touch, smell, and sight, in prenatal assessment.

future for health care: a future where powerful professions did not always insist on more complete and more costly control, a future where new and complex technology does not always prevail. As I listened, I realized that our old theories about health systems were being challenged, if not consigned to the trash bin. The facts of this meeting called for a new approach to describing and analyzing health care, an approach that promised a more hopeful future for the organization of health services.

Understanding Health Care Systems

How does one begin to revise long-held theories of how health care systems operate? It is tempting to limit our revisions to the *content* of these theories. The meeting in Ede makes it clear that our content is lacking—we learned that patterns we thought universal are in fact bound by culture[9]—but it also calls into question the way we go about building our theories. Faulty content suggests faulty methods. It is not all that difficult to tweak a theory and make it fit a new situation. But at some point we must stop and assess the methods we use to generate our ideas about health systems. Where do our theories come from? How do we test them? What causes us to decide they no longer work?

It is not surprising to find flaws in the ways we have studied and theorized about the organization of health care. Those who wish to make accurate generalizations about health systems must come to

---

9. Some might be surprised to find the taint of ethnocentricity in the work of social scientists. Remember, we too are creatures of culture, and in the areas of science and medicine we often assume high levels of abstraction give culture very little room to operate. I recently completed a project on maternity care that brought together social scientists from several countries in Europe and North America (see De Vries et al. 2001). We fancied ourselves quite cosmopolitan and open to cultural variations, but, as we proceeded with our collaborative work, we discovered that our ideas, our theories, and our methods were culturally bound. One example illustrates: At our first meeting, our group got into a frustrating debate about what should be included in a chapter examining the role of the state in maternity care. The more we talked, the more confused and frustrated we became. In an effort to clear the air, someone asked: "What is the main task of the state?" The Americans in the group replied: "To ensure that individual women have freedom of choice" and "to make choices available for childbearing women." The Europeans in the group had a different response: "To ensure that the poorest women in society have access to a reasonable quality of maternity care" and "to ensure that all women have access to good maternity care." We thought we were all being good, open-minded scholars, but in fact, we were talking from our own culturally colored perspectives.

terms with their daunting size, complexity, and ever-changing natures. In an effort to make sense of a structure that is overwhelmingly complex, health systems analysts typically choose one of two paths: the path of the "detailer" or the path of the "tourist."

The first path, that of the detailer, leads through a jungle of information; awash in facts and figures, dates, and names, we see health care systems as the product of tens of thousands of events, each influencing the ones that follow. Caught in this flood, we become fatalists. Having no hope of identifying larger trends or patterns, the best we can do is to provide a faithful inventory of the many details that contribute to the present state of health care in one society.

The second path is the way of the tourist. Analysts who choose this path blithely skip from one health system to the next, building theories on the differences they see between the forests, but failing to notice the trees. Health care tourists bring back some interesting pictures, but they leave us wondering about the details they have overlooked.

These approaches are clearly illustrated in two well-known books, books that have influenced popular and professional attitudes about health care and health care reform: Paul Starr's (1982) prodigious analysis of the social transformation of American medicine and Lynn Payer's (1985) comparative study of medicine in four western countries. Starr's historical research provides us with a meticulous account of the critical events in the formation of American medicine, but in the end we are left with mere description of the structure of health care: physician organizations, insurance companies, medical institutions (schools and hospitals), and political alliances. As with much sociology of medicine, we are given an elaborate account of the structures of health care, but we learn little of the larger forces that gave shape to the current system and lead to its widespread acceptance. In sociological terms, we see again and again how medical and political structures shaped the way health services are delivered, but we are told almost nothing of the way these structures came to be.[10] Overwhelmed by detail, we are convinced that the best we can do is to describe what has already occurred.

---

10. Starr's opening essay on the cultural authority of medicine is not matched by an analysis of the influence of American culture on health care practice.

Payer is more of a health systems tourist. She gives us an interesting picture of how culture, in the form of national character, influences patterns of medical treatment. An American journalist working in several European nations, she noticed significant differences in the response to illness in various countries. This led her to correlate data on the use of medical services, including the consumption of drugs (and other remedies), with descriptions of "well-known" traits of national culture. Her conclusions are credible but simplistic: Fascinated by machinery, Americans are inclined to rely on technology when ill; true to the romantic tradition of their past, Germans pay undue attention to the heart, blaming a whole assortment of conditions on "heart insufficiency"; the fine aesthetic tastes of the French lead them to respond to breast cancer with lumpectomies rather than mastectomies; and the British have an odd preoccupation with the bowels. Payer's findings are interesting *and* challenging—for example, she notes that the survival rates for breast cancer in France are no different from those in the United States, where more women must live with the disfiguration of radical surgery—but in the end, her book reads like a tour guide of European and American medicine. She tells us very little about the structure of health care in each nation and how it supports (or fails to support) cultural ideas about health and illness.

There is a "third way" to build theory about health systems, a way that avoids the deficiencies of the detailer and the tourist. This new approach is suggested by what one must do to explain why Dutch maternity care, described on that June morning in Ede, is so different from obstetrics elsewhere. If we are to find an explanation for the peculiarities of birth in the Netherlands, we need historical detail, not a sweeping history of an *entire* health system (á la Starr). We need to understand the cultural background that animates birth care in the lowlands; we do not need global comparisons between health services in several countries (á la Payer). In order to explain the Dutch difference we must *limit* ourselves to *one* branch of medicine (verloskunde) in *one* small country. In so doing we are able to isolate a smaller set of details and events that formed, and now maintain, this health service, facts that would be lost in the flood of information presented by detailers and ignored in the macro studies of tourists.

Interestingly, a more focused and modest approach to health care analysis allows us to better understand the forces that organize *large* health care delivery systems. Lessons learned in the study of a small slice of one health system in its social and cultural context can show us how health systems are built. When our analysis of birth in the Netherlands is complete, we will have a firm grasp on the way social structures—political, professional, educational, scientific, governmental, corporate, and medical—shape the way health care is delivered, and we will better appreciate how medical services are supported by the cultural ideas of a society.

Will the study of *any* branch of medicine in *any* country yield equal success in explaining the operation of larger health care systems? Perhaps. There are, however, distinctive features of *birth,* of the *Netherlands,* and of birth in the Netherlands, that make Dutch verloskunde an ideal and particularly resonant site for study of how health systems are put together.

Why Birth?

Several years ago, the distinguished Dutch gynecologist/obstetrician, Professor Gerrit-Jan Kloosterman, was invited to London to give a lecture to an international association of obstetricians and gynecologists. Kloosterman, Chair of Obstetrics at the University of Amsterdam at the time, was well-respected and well-known for his support of the Dutch practice of midwife-assisted births at home. He was in the middle of his lecture—an analysis of the Dutch system, which showed that the continued use of midwife-attended home birth posed no danger to mothers and babies—when a strange thing happened. While he was talking, several members of the audience got up and left the room, noisily, in an obvious display of displeasure with his presentation.

After he finished the lecture, Kloosterman and the president of the association discussed the small protest. They asked themselves, "Why doesn't this happen in other specialties?" They agreed it would be unheard of for physicians to walk out in the middle of a lecture about cardiology, even if they thought the data were suspect. Protocol in the science of medicine dictates that disagreements about data be hashed out in collegial exchanges: One does not protest against data, one challenges the data on the basis of methodology or analytic technique. Kloosterman and the president concluded that obstetrics does not really belong in the field of medicine. Perhaps, they conjectured, obstetrics would be better located in the field of physiology. After all, it is the only discipline in medicine where something happens by itself, and, in most cases, everything ends well with no intervention. Thinking about this incident, Kloosterman concluded:

> Obstetrics is wider and broader than pure medicine. It has to do with the whole of life, the way you look at life, making objective discussion difficult. You are almost unable to split the problem off into pure science; always your outlook on life is involved.[11]

Kloosterman has it right. One need not look too far into the world of maternity care to find the wide gap between scientific evidence and clinical practice. For example, consider this: In May 1998 the U.S. National Center for Health Statistics released a report on the comparative infant mortality rates for midwives and physicians in the United States. The study included all single, vaginal births in the United States in 1991 delivered between 35 and 43 weeks gestation. Controlling for risk factors,[12] midwives were found to have significantly lower rates of infant mortality and better outcomes with regard to birthweight:

- 19 percent lower infant mortality (death of the child in the first year after birth)
- 33 percent lower neonatal mortality (death of the child in the first 28 days after birth)
- 31 percent lower risk of low birthweight
- 37 grams heavier mean birthweight

The report notes that, in general, midwives' practices include higher numbers of poor and minority women who are at greater risk of poor birth outcome. The report concludes:

> The differences in birth outcomes between certified nurse midwife and physician attended births may be explained in part by difference in prenatal, labor and delivery care practices. Other studies have shown certified nurse midwives generally spend more time with patients during

---

11. Unless otherwise noted, all quotes are from field notes and interviews.

12. Controlling for risk eliminates the argument that poorer outcomes for physicians are a consequence of the fact that they see patients at higher risk. It *is* true that higher-risk women are referred to physician care, but these comparisons are made *within* risk categories, so we are looking at outcomes when physicians and midwives care for women at the *same level* of risk.

prenatal visits and put more emphasis on patient counseling and education, and providing emotional support. Most certified nurse midwives are with their patients on a one-to-one basis during the entire labor and delivery process providing patient care and emotional support, in contrast with physicians' care which is more episodic. (NCHS 1998)

The data are persuasive, but, consistent with Kloosterman's observations, six years after its publication this study has had almost *no* effect on health policy and the delivery of care in the United States. Although they apparently provide less expensive, more satisfying, and more effective care, certified nurse midwives attended 8 percent of all births in the United States in 2001 (Martin et al. 2002).

Taken together, these two stories highlight the fact that, more than any other area of medical practice, the organization and provision of maternity care is a highly charged mix of medical science, cultural ideas, and structural forces. Other medical specialties are marked by a technical uniformity that crosses national borders, but the design of care at birth varies widely and clearly bears the marks of the society in which it is found (see De Vries et al. 2001). This complicates clinical practice, but affords us a wonderful opportunity to examine the many factors that shape the delivery of care at birth and other medical services. In important ways, birth is to the study of health care as chromosome 22 was to the study of the human genome. Scientists chose chromosome 22— the smallest and simplest of human chromosomes—as the first to be mapped in its entirety. Scientists were convinced that the lessons learned here could be applied to the other, more complex chromosomes. Maternity care plays the same role for researchers interested in health care systems—not because it is simple but because, unlike other medical specialties, the influence of culture and society is not masked by uniformity in technology and practice. Maternity care is different from other forms of medical care for these reasons:

- What is at stake in care at birth is not the survival of one patient, but the reproduction of society.
- Embedded in the care given to women at birth are ideas about sexuality, about women, and about families.
- All other medical specialties (with the possible exception of pediatrics) begin with a focus on disease, but the essential task here is the supervision of normal, healthy, physical growth.

- The quality of maternity care in both senses of that word—its nature and its outcomes—often is used as a measure for the quality of an entire health care system.
- Infant mortality rates have become a shorthand measure for the adequacy of a society's health system and its overall quality of life.

Recognizing these distinctive features of birth, social scientists and historians have given much attention to the development of maternity care, particularly in the United States and England (see, for example, Arney 1982; Wertz and Wertz 1977; Sullivan and Weitz 1988; Leavitt 1986; Rothman 1982; Litoff 1978, 1986; Donegan 1978; Donnison 1977; Oakley 1980, 1984). But with few exceptions, these studies suffer from too narrow a focus. Done for the most part in the late seventies and early eighties—when interest in the role of women in society was at its peak—these studies used maternity care as an occasion to observe the struggle between the sexes. The titles of many of the studies reflect the emphasis on struggle, power, and domination. We read about "captured wombs," about "women confined," about "misogyny." Often the labor of childbirth becomes a metaphor for a larger struggle: Consider *In Labor: Women and Power in the Birthplace* (Rothman 1982) or *Labor Pains: Modern Midwives and Home Birth* (Sullivan and Weitz 1988). We are left with the impression that the history of childbirth care can be reduced to a study in interprofessional, intergender rivalry. We are told much about the place and treatment of women in society, but left unstudied is the way the structure of obstetric care imports societal views of the body and its abilities, ideas about health and illness and about the role of medical treatment in the course of life.

My study of birth in the Netherlands broadens this work, showing that the shape of obstetric care is the result of far more than gender wars. The relationship among caregivers and clients at birth is constantly being renegotiated; it is the product of changing social conditions (costs of health care, policy decisions, etc.) and cultural beliefs (faith in technology, religious ideas, ideas about gender, etc.).

WHY THE NETHERLANDS?

As does birth, the Netherlands offers distinct advantages for those who would understand the delivery of medical care. Two characteristics of this country—its relatively small size (approximately twice the size of New Jersey in land area and population) and its language (rarely spoken or taught outside its borders)—make it ideal for the study of health systems. Small size improves accessibility: Statistics are easy to keep and readily available; occupational groups involved are a manageable size (there are approximately 1,700 practicing midwives and 675 practicing *gynecologen*[13]); and geographic smallness allows one researcher to cover the territory. The *vreemde taal* (strange language), on the other hand, provides an advantage by *reducing* accessibility. The Dutch language is spoken only in the Netherlands, part of Belgium, and in a few small former colonies. This makes the conversation over maternity care a mostly in-house affair. This is less true in a small country like, say, New Zealand, where the use of English extends the obstetric conversation to the United States, the United Kingdom, Australia, and Canada, if not the entire world.

The very things that make the Netherlands an attractive location for my study explain why Americans seldom choose it as a site for medical or social scientific research. Because it is small, the country is seen as unimportant and unrepresentative. Few are willing to invest the time required to learn a language spoken in such a small corner of the world. The Netherlands is more likely to be a tourist destination than a research site; consequently, events there are often explained with a simple reference to Dutch quaintness. In this land of canals and drawbridges, wooden shoes and windmills, tulips, and cheese markets, who is surprised by home birth?

The progressive nature of Dutch social policy—in the areas of euthanasia, prostitution, drugs, and childbirth—does attract the attention of *buitenlanders* (foreigners). But these progressive policies are seen only as interesting experiments, not as opportunities to see how policy is formed in a social and cultural context. Outside interest has a polemical, not an analytical, cast. Government officials from other countries wage arguments about the wisdom of the policy in question. Some insist (often after a one-week fact-finding trip) that the Netherlands offers a model to be emulated, while others declare the policy to be a curious, quaint, or dangerous anomaly (certainly, given enough time,

---

13. Gynecologen is the plural of gynecoloog. See van der Velden et al. (2001) and Hingstman and Kenens (2002).

the Dutch will follow the example of other Western countries). With very few exceptions, all studies of Dutch obstetrics published in other languages are reduced to polemics, to arguments for or against the system.

CHANGING HEALTH CARE: THE URGE TO REFORM

My analysis of birth in the Netherlands illustrates how cultural factors and social structures come together to produce health care systems. My goal is to provide a better understanding of how health systems work, but the explanations I offer can be used by those who aspire to the more practical goal of changing health systems. There can be no *re-forming* of a health care system until the initial *forming* of the system is understood. The mess that is American health care, and our continued failed efforts to improve the situation, are ample evidence of our lack of knowledge about the formation and operation of health care systems. Typically, our attempts at reform are based on the notion that economic models can predict health care behaviors. We invite failure when the reforms we propose do not pay attention to the social and cultural context of caregiving. The attempt of the Clintons to change American health care in the early 1990s failed, not just because of political insensitivity, but also because of a poor understanding of the forces that created American health care and now hold it together. Like the failed Clinton plan, the de facto economic reforms ushered in by the rise of health maintenance organizations (HMOs) and other managed care organizations (MCOs) are proving unpopular, suffering much criticism, and generating calls for a new health care bill of rights.

Unfortunately, knowledge alone cannot eliminate the difficulties of implementing change. There are many who would like to see the Dutch obstetric system transplanted to the United States, and there are many who would like to see the United States adopt a Canadian-style system of health care financing. But, as this study shows, it is unreasonable to expect a system that works in one society to work in another; effective transplantation of a health care idea from one society to another is extremely difficult. To assume that health care ideas can be transplanted like kidneys is to assume that health care is nothing more than clinical or administrative technique. Will the Dutch system of maternity care work elsewhere? Can it work among women and health care providers with a different view of their bodies, their families, and their homes? Can a Canadian-style system of health care finance work among a people with a different view of solidarity, the shared responsibility of members of a society for each other? The transplantation of health policy requires sensitivity to these types of questions. Brilliant policy ideas will not succeed unless they take into account the culture we all carry inside us. An example from the world of maternity care illustrates this point.

Anita discovers she is pregnant. She and her partner are delighted. What Anita does next will seem, to her, to be completely natural, matter-of-fact: "This is what one does when she is pregnant." But the matter-of-factness of "what one does when she is pregnant" is, in fact, not so simple. What Anita does if she is living in Oaxaca, Mexico, will be quite different from what Anita does if she is a lifelong resident of Oslo, Norway. Anita in Harlem (New York) will respond differently to her pregnancy than Anita in Haarlem (the Netherlands).

The choices Anita can imagine are constrained by what she knows, what she has experienced, what she has seen around her, and what she has heard. Anita in New York might have heard, of course, about women in Africa giving birth in their huts, squatting with tight grip on two cords, but she "knows" the "proper" way to give birth is in the "clean comfort of a modern hospital," close to the "safety" of monitors and obstetric "experts." Anita in the Netherlands will wonder about the preference of American women for hospitalized, medicated birth because she "knows" that birth at home is the safest and most comfortable choice. This comment from a Dutch woman reflects that particular, culturally contingent matter-of-factness, the feeling that "of course this is the right way to give birth": "At home you are free to give birth as you like, and your child is not born into the merry-go-round of the medical world. The mother can give birth without all the medical equipment and, besides, a hospital is a breeding ground for bacteria." It is a happy fact of social life that, for most of us, what seems the right and proper way of doing things is exactly what our society offers us. As Peter Berger (1963) says, *we desire the very things society limits us to.*

For American women, hospital birth seems right and home birth seems frightening, but for many Dutch women home birth is the only appropriate option:

It was a very special experience to give birth at home with my husband and children on one side of my bed and the midwife on the other. My sister was at the foot of the bed holding a mirror; just before the birth she and I had done all the shopping. My boys were especially interested in the technical details: how the head comes out, the clamping of the cord, the birth of the placenta. The midwife had told them what to expect so they were completely unafraid. I was struck by how calm the boys were through the whole thing; they asked few questions. For them this was the most normal business in the world.

When I interviewed ordinary clients of Dutch midwives—that is, women not otherwise active in issues related to birth or Dutch obstetrics—they would always express absolute disbelief that women in the United States could not arrange a birth at home as easily as they could a birth in the hospital. How can that be? Why would a healthy woman choose to give birth in a hospital attended by a specialist?

What looks like "choice," then, is actually a decision constrained by culture and by structure. Anita in New York will "choose" among epidural, cesarean section, and paracervical block. Anita in the Netherlands will "choose" among birth at home or in a policlinic, with a midwife or with a general practitioner.

Legislatures and ministries of health can change health policy, but how can we change what everyone *knows* to be the proper way to give and receive care? When you or I call on the services of the health care system (be it for supervision of an essentially healthy process, like pregnancy and childbirth, or the treatment of an illness) we have certain ideas about proper and improper forms of caregiving, ideas that cannot be changed by a simple change in health policy. Embedded in what everyone "knows" about medical care are cultural notions about the body, about healing and the healing professions, about religion, and about countless other aspects of our lives together.

The cultural dimension of health care systems complicates change, but it does not make it impossible. Would-be reformers have two choices: They must find ways to implement change that fit with cultural ideas, or they must create a credible challenge to the cultural ideas that inhibit reform. Analysts who are detailers or tourists have little to offer in this regard. The detailers do not notice the cultural foundation of care, and the tourists, who have given us so many pretty pictures of the influence of culture, cannot speak to the way culture and structure interact. In the following pages I present a completed picture of the way health services come to be, allowing us to understand and, if we so desire, to change the way care is delivered.

*   *   *   *   *

A day in June. A symposium on home birth in the Netherlands. For the participants perhaps a little boring. But this mundane event conceals the complicated process that gives form to health care services. The maternity care system in the Netherlands, taken for granted by most Dutch citizens, gives us the window we need to understand the forming and reforming of health care; it offers us the knowledge we need to promote much needed change in our own health care system.

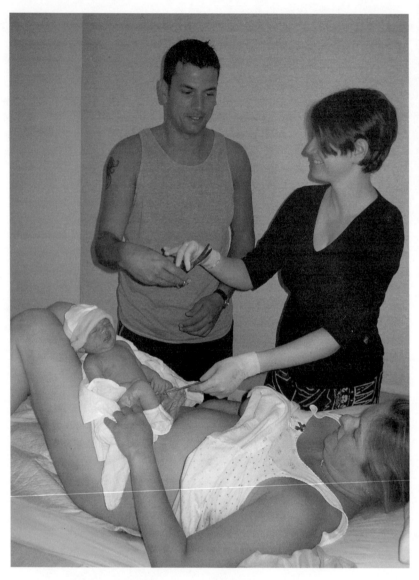

A home birth in the Netherlands: Midwife and father prepare to cut the umbilical cord. Reproduced with permission from Marcel Wessels.

2 *Uniek, Bewonderd, en Verguisd* (Unique, Admired, and Reviled)

NEARLY ALL reports and research articles on Dutch obstetrics begin with a comment on the stunning peculiarity of the way birth is accomplished in the Netherlands. In her foreword to the anthology, *Successful Home Birth and Midwifery: The Dutch Model*, Jordan (1993, iv) identifies Dutch maternity care as a "most anomalous phenomenon" that "has always been an inspiration." Akrich and Pasveer open their book-length study of maternity care in the Netherlands and France by noting, "the differences between the two countries are striking [*les différences entre les deux pays sont frappantes*] . . . more than a third of births occur at home in the Netherlands, as opposed to France, where 99.5% occur in the hospital. . . . Epidural analgesia is used in 70% of births in France and only 15% of Dutch births" (1996, 21–22).

In her article on Dutch obstetrics, Hiddinga says the midwifery care system in the Netherlands "may rejoice [*zich verheugen*] in the routine attention of a broad public, both national and international . . . This has everything to do with the extraordinary [*bijzonder*] character of the Dutch system of care around pregnancy and birth" (1998, 189). The singularity of the Dutch system in modern obstetrics makes it difficult to avoid this exclamatory language. As you have no doubt noticed, I, too, have resorted to the use of superlatives in my opening chapters. In an effort to emphasize the special character of Dutch maternity care I refer to it as *unusual* and *especially odd.*

The peculiar obstetric habits of the Dutch often find their way into the professional literature as a foil for more ordinary (i.e., medical) maternity care practices, a way of promoting alternative approaches to birth. Analyses of the Dutch system have been used to encourage less interventive obstetrics (Van Alten et al. 1989; Treffers et al. 1990; Tew and Damstra-Wijmenga 1991; Treffers and Pel 1993; Oppenheimer 1993; Hingstman 1994) and to describe how features of the system might be profitably exported to other countries (Mehl-Madrona and

Mehl-Madrona 1993; Rothman 1993; Treffers 1993; Mander 1995; Wilson 1998; Van Teijlingen 2003). Oppenheimer's reflection on what the United Kingdom might learn from the Dutch is a typical example of the admiration expressed for the Dutch way of birth:

> The major features and philosophies of the Dutch system . . . have some-
> thing to teach us—nationally agreed criteria of risk, training and support
> of midwives in more independent methods, and good communication
> and confidence between providers of primary and secondary care.
> Perhaps we can achieve not only low perinatal and maternal mortality
> and morbidity but also less dissatisfaction among consumers, more job
> satisfaction among midwives, and more rational working for obstetric
> staff. (1993, 1402)

The recent recognition and regulation of midwifery in the provinces of Canada also drew inspiration from the Netherlands: "One of the most important strategies and ultimate influences on the development of Canadian midwifery was the connections made with the broader International Confederation of Midwives and the ultimate pursuit of a Dutch-like model of midwifery care . . . midwifery in the Netherlands was always a source of inspiration" (Bourgeault, Benoit, and Davis-Floyd 2004, 8): Given the reputation of the Netherlands as the home of nontechnological birth, it is no surprise that when the World Health Organization (WHO) was looking to create a practical guide for care in normal birth they called on the services of a Dutch gynecologist and a Dutch midwife (see World Health Organization 1999).

The Dutch response to this attention ranges from pride to embarrassment. It is not unusual for the national newspapers to carry stories that celebrate the fact that Dutch women, unlike their sisters in the rest of the industrialized world, are free to have their babies at home. In a full-page story contrasting the different ways maternity care is delivered in the countries of Europe, the editors of *De Telegraaf*, the most widely read newspaper in the country, observed that "in England, France, Belgium, and Germany birthing is treated more warily; it is not possible to have a baby at home and every detail of pregnancy is treated medically." The article goes on to say "the continued possibility to give birth at home [in the Netherlands] is the result of a well-organized system [where] midwives are trained to be more independent [and] have a high level of competence (*De Telegraaf* 1995, TA1). The *NRC Handelsblad* described the peculiarities of Dutch birth in one of its weekly *Profiel* sections. One of the articles in the section acknowledged that the continued discussion of the relative advantages and disadvantages of home and hospital birth in the Netherlands is a bit out of date (*achterhaald*): Elsewhere in the Western world, the preference for hospital birth long ago carried the day. But, evincing their pride, the writers go on to note: "Unlike all other Western, industrialized countries, where the vast majority of women give birth in the hospital, women in the Netherlands . . . can choose to have their babies at home. Because of an infrastructure of well educated midwives and maternity aides, about 30 percent of Dutch women give birth at home" (*NRC Weekeditie* 1996, 29).

Perhaps the best evidence of public pride in the Dutch way of birth is found in a short item published by *De Telegraaf* while I was living in the Netherlands. The article described a new British initiative to allow more births at home; it was titled, "Home birth possible in England" and carried the subtitle, "Unnecessarily many mistakes in hospitals." The author explained that English gynecologists, who had long opposed home birth, had had a change of heart and would now cooperate with women who choose to have their babies at home. The piece ended with this editorial comment: "[Midwives in England] have long been jealous of the circumstances that make home birth possible in the Netherlands" (*De Telegraaf* 1994). As far as the Dutch people are concerned, the seeming anachronism of birth at home is a cause for celebration, not shame.

Pride in the system is also visible in the great patience maternity care providers in the Netherlands show toward the many international visitors who want a first-hand look at Dutch obstetrics. Dutch gynecologists, Dutch midwives, Dutch health policy analysts, and Dutch researchers are regularly beset with requests from foreigners who are planning a short visit to the Netherlands and would like to gather information on how the Dutch obstetric system works. In response to a deluge of these requests, the Royal Dutch Organization of Midwives (the *Koninklijke Nederlandse Organisatie van Verloskundigen*, or KNOV) created a *Buitenlands Bureau* (Foreign Office)—staffed by volunteers—to whom all international visitors are directed. A midwife who volunteers in the *Bureau* explains her work:

> What we mostly do is receive midwives from other countries, and organize placements for a few weeks with [Dutch] midwives, so they can

watch them working. We send material when people are asking for information, and we are gathering material and then sending copies . . . [We also see] gynecologists, [general practitioners] . . . physiotherapists . . . [for them] we organize [meetings so] that they can talk to gynecologists, to a pediatrician, to a midwife [and] they can see a hospital, the midwifery school. . . . . For the groups of student midwives that are coming we organize a different program. Mostly a group like that I receive for twelve hours or [thereabouts]. I show them the school, the practice, and I tell them lots and lots about how the Dutch system is working. I tell them about how we are working with the home delivery and maternity assistants.

Most of the health care professionals I interviewed had stories of international visitors who arrived in varying states of incredulity with notebooks full of questions. Even *I*, after a few months at my host institution, the NIVEL,[1] was called upon to meet with the many visitors coming to learn more about birth in the Netherlands. The long lists of complicated questions they sent ahead took me aback. Did they know how much work would be required to gather the detailed statistics they were seeking or to answer their queries about the institutions and professionals that provided care? After all, I had spent months gathering this same information. How could I convey all this in one afternoon? Although these visits became tiring, I noticed my Dutch colleagues remained patient, seeing foreign interest as an opportunity to defend and promote this special feature of medical care in the Netherlands.

Among professionals, pride in Dutch obstetrics is slightly tempered by a realization that many outside of the Netherlands do not fully understand how their system works and regard it as a bit "irresponsible or even barbaric" (*De Telegraaf* 1995, TA1). This feeling is captured in the response of one of my colleagues at the NIVEL to a letter of inquiry about Dutch obstetrics from a German physician. The physician worked for the German Agency for Technical Cooperation, and he expressed the desire to learn how Dutch ideas could be used to strengthen the position of community-oriented midwives in Germany.

---

1. NIVEL was an acronym for *Nederlands Instituut voor Onderzoek van de Eerstelijnsgezondheidszorg* (Dutch Institute for Research on First Line Health Care). In 1996 the mission of the NIVEL was broadened to include research on all sectors of the health care system. The organization changed its name to *Nederlands Instituut voor Onderzoek van de Gezondheidszorg* (Dutch Institute for Research on Health Care), but held on to the acronym.

My colleague replied, "We thank you very much for your interest in the Dutch primary care obstetric system; it is an exception in the Western world and we are still very satisfied with it and even proud of it in Holland, but it is difficult to maintain a community-oriented obstetric system when all the surrounding countries look quite suspiciously at this primitive way of putting children into the world."

On the occasion of his appointment to the chair in obstetrics at the University of Leiden, Professor Keirse expressed a similar sentiment. In the oration that newly appointed professors are obliged to deliver, Keirse (1980, 13–14) claimed the most important characteristic of Dutch obstetrics is not home birth, or the unique organization of midwifery, or (even) its studied avoidance of intervention; rather, Keirse insisted, the most distinguishing characteristic of maternity care in the Netherlands "is and remains, that, in translation, *verloskunde* is too often understood not as 'Dutch obstetrics' but as 'double-Dutch'" (i.e., gibberish). Seventeen years later, Professor Bleker (1997, 409), chair of obstetrics at the University of Amsterdam, detected a similar attitude among his international colleagues: "In Canada, the US, England, France, Germany, Denmark, Sweden, and Russia . . . home birth is considered to be an anachronism and is dismissed as folklore, 'alternative perinatal service,' or even 'unwise domiciliary delivery.'"

The title of this chapter, *"Uniek, Bewonderd, en Verguisd,"* reflects the mixture of pride and doubt felt by those who provide maternity care in the Netherlands: It is borrowed from a 1987 report made by a committee of midwives, general practitioners, and gynecologists appointed by the government for the purpose of recommending steps to safeguard and promote the unique Dutch way of birth.

I must also note that there are those who find the Dutch system something of an embarrassment. Some members of the medical community in the Netherlands believe the "old-fashioned" approach of Dutch obstetrics is, in fact, dangerous. There is a healthy skepticism about Dutch obstetrics outside of the Netherlands, but nearly all of the published critiques of Dutch maternity care come from within, from gynecologists practicing in the Dutch system (see, e.g., T. Eskes 1980; 1992; T. Eskes et al. 1981; Lievaart and de Jong 1982; Hoogedoorn 1986).

What is the reality behind all this talk, all this attention, all these debates? What are the facts of Dutch obstetrics? Because the system is so odd and because most fact-finding trips are so short, many articles about birth in the Netherlands written by non-Netherlanders contain errors of fact and tone. For example, Mehl-Madrona and Mehl-Madrona, writing in 1993, claim, "over 70% of births [in the Netherlands] are still attended by midwives." *In fact*, midwives accompany about half of all births in the Netherlands (some of which are completed in cooperation with a gynecologist). As far back as 1910, the first year a breakdown by caregiver is available, midwives in the Netherlands attended 57.7 percent of *all* births, and at no point in the twentieth century did they attend more than 60 percent of Dutch births. Midwives *do* attend more than 70 percent of the births that occur at home. It is likely the authors heard this and somehow assumed that the 70 percent figure applied to *all* births. In her ethnographically based discussion of the lessons of Dutch obstetrics for Americans, Rothman (1993, 201) sets the scene by discussing windmills, tulips, bicycles, and Rembrandt, giving her readers over-romanticized pictures of Dutch midwifery and Dutch society. Her description of the Netherlands as a "Mecca for Midwives" and the home of noninterventive obstetrics makes it difficult to believe that Dutch midwives once argued for the right to wield forceps (see Marland 1995, 328) or that Dutch midwives are beginning to outfit their offices with the apparatus for sonograms (see Akrich and Pasveer 2001).

Even the Dutch misrepresent their obstetric system. In *Expecting*, its yearly special issue on pregnancy and birth, *Ouders Van Nú* (Parents of Today), a Dutch parenting magazine, reports, "Pregnancy in the Netherlands is not seen as an illness—requiring a great deal of medical help—but as a natural event that can be supervised well by a midwife. This leads to the following statistic: in the Netherlands about 70% of babies are born at home, without complication or unusual interventions" (Schiet 1994, 112). In the early 1960s this was the case—in 1960 72.6 percent of births occurred at home, in 1961 the number was 71.2 percent, and in 1962 it was 70.5 percent—but through the last decades of the twentieth century the percent of births at home continued to decline. By 1994, the date of the article in *Expecting*, the number of births at home represented slightly more than 30 percent of all births.

How can we cut through the hype, misstatements, and mischaracterizations? After sorting through dozens and dozens of descriptions of Dutch obstetrics, I am convinced that an accurate view of the system requires three things, presented in this order:

1. A brief description of the important players and places in Dutch obstetrics;
2. A selection of narrative accounts of what Dutch women do, and have done to them, when they are pregnant; and
3. A statistical summary of the how the system is (and has been) working.

A chronicle of the places and persons encountered by Dutch women as they travel through their pregnancies serves as an introduction for those who know little of maternity care in the Netherlands and brings life and meaning to the otherwise sterile statistical descriptions of Dutch obstetrics. The following three-part description of maternity care in the Netherlands clears up the many misconceptions about the Dutch difference. In setting the record straight, we begin to see the Dutch system as something more than just a curious anomaly; we begin to sort out the factors that led to the creation of a method of providing care at birth that is *uniek, bewonderd, en verguisd.*

GETTING A BABY IN THE NETHERLANDS

The first response of a woman who suspects she will be "getting"[2] a baby will be either a self-test with an over-the-counter pregnancy test kit or a trip to the general practitioner (*huisarts,* the plural form is *huisartsen*) for a pregnancy test. Those choosing the home test route will inform their huisarts if the results are positive. The huisarts is the hub of the health care system of the Netherlands: Nearly everyone in the country is registered with a huisarts in their neighborhood who serves as a family doctor and a gatekeeper to other medical services.[3] Only in exceptional cases would a Dutch woman go directly to a gynecologist when she believes she is pregnant, and in almost all of those cases she would do this on the advice of her huisarts.

Having confirmed her pregnancy and (perhaps) shared the happy news with relatives and friends, a Dutch woman can now contemplate how she will bring this child into the world. Will it be at home or in a

---

2. Women in the Netherlands do not *have* babies, they *get* (or *receive—krijgen*) babies. This is a small but significant difference in language—if one *gets,* rather than *has,* a baby, the child is regarded more as a gift than as a possession.

3. For more information about the role of the huisarts in the Dutch medical system see van der Velden (1999) and de Melker (1997).

hospital? What kind of practitioner will see to her prenatal care and attend the event? And what sort of care will be used after the birth?[4]

Dutch social policy directs women expecting a healthy birth into the first line (*eerstelijn*), or primary care, system. In the eerstelijn either a midwife or a huisarts will provide all prenatal care and will *begeleiden* (accompany)[5] a woman at birth. Women under the care of the eerstelijn are free to choose a birth at home or in the hospital. If they prefer a hospital birth, they will have what is known as *poliklinische bevalling* (polyclinic birth) under the supervision of their primary caregiver. The term polyclinic suggests a separate birthing center, but in fact, there are only a few birth clinics in the Netherlands; a poliklinische bevalling refers to an uncomplicated short stay (i.e., less than 24 hours) hospital birth.

If complications arise during pregnancy or birth, the primary caregiver will refer a woman to the second line (*tweedelijn*), or specialist, care. After assessing the complication, the specialist—in this case a gynecologist—may send the woman back to the eerstelijn or may keep the woman under his or her care in the tweedelijn for the duration of her prenatal care and for birth. Only women with complications of pregnancy or labor come under the care of a specialist, and all births supervised by a gynecologist take place in a hospital. Some of these births will require complete clinical care, others will take place in the polyclinic, and, if all goes well, mother and baby will return home within 24 hours.

More than 75 percent of Dutch women begin their prenatal care with a midwife, and an additional 7 percent begin with a huisarts (Wiegers and Coffie 2002, 64). As a result of referrals made to the tweedelijn during the course of prenatal care and labor, midwives are independently caring for slightly more than 36 percent of women at the time of birth, huisartsen an additional 3.5 percent, and gynecologists about 60 percent (some of which are in fact accompanied by midwives[6]). Of the women remaining in the care of the first line, the majority give birth at home, resulting in a total home birth rate of just over 30 percent.

---

4. In the following section I explain how these choices are constrained by social policies.

5. The use of this verb, which also describes the work of a conductor of an orchestra and an accompanist for musical performances, suggests a less dominating role for the caregiver.

6. Since 1995 midwife-accompanied births under the supervision of a gynecologist are recorded as births under the care of the specialist. See notes to Table 2.1.

A Dutch woman who wishes to prepare for childbirth may choose from at least five different approaches: *Zwangerschaps-gymnastiek, Zwangerschaps-yoga,* the *Mensendieck* method, *Psycho-profylaxe,* and *Haptonomie.* Each has a slightly different emphasis, and each suggests different roles for the mother's partner. The standard health insurance policy does *not* reimburse for the cost of these childbirth preparation classes.

Finally, there is the choice of postpartum caregiver. A much-discussed feature of Dutch obstetrics is the provision of postpartum care by specially trained providers: *kraamverzorgenden.*[7] These caregivers come to the home of the new parents and perform a variety of tasks, including household chores, marketing, cooking, watching the condition of mom and baby, offering instruction in baby care, and feeding. Because of a shortage of kraamverzorgenden in recent years, expectant parents must register for these services early in the pregnancy; parents also may choose how much or how little care they wish (see van Teijlingen 1990).

BIRTH STORIES

Having reviewed the basic details associated with getting a baby in the Netherlands, we can deepen and enrich our understanding of the different ways birth is accomplished there by listening to the stories of mothers. Of course, every one of the 200,000 births that occurs in the Netherlands each year has its unique elements, but the four short narratives that follow give us a sense of the tone and the feel of birth, of how birth is experienced in different settings and under different circumstances. The first two of these accounts describe home births, the third is the story of a polyclinic birth, and the last is a report of a planned home birth that was transferred to the hospital and the care of a gynecologist.

Birth at Home (1)

I was able to become pregnant thanks to artificial insemination done at the hospital. At first, the doctor wanted me to continue my care at the

---

7. These caregivers used to be known as *kraamverzorgsters,* a feminine term. The new name is gender neutral.

hospital, but he was not able to give me a convincing reason, because once I was pregnant I no longer had any reason to have problems. I went to a midwife practice not far from where I live; I was advised to go there by a doctor that I know.

At our first visit, around the twelfth week of my pregnancy, we were asked a lot of questions about the medical history of our family. I was weighed, the midwife took my blood pressure, she took a blood sample to see if I had anemia, and she examined my belly. She tried to listen to the heartbeat of my baby with a Doppler, but it didn't work. I also brought some urine that she didn't use, she told me that she would search for albumin only if there were other symptoms of toxemia. When I talked about this with my girlfriends they were surprised, because not all midwives do the same thing.

The midwife told me that everything was going well, very well, and moreover, she repeated it to me at every visit, and she asked me whether we had decided on a home birth or a polyclinic birth. We chose to do it at home: I don't like the hospital, and the contacts that I had during the insemination did not encourage me to return there.

We went back every month and after 30 weeks of pregnancy, every two weeks, and at the end, every week. In the practice there were four midwives. I saw each one of them during my prenatal visits to be sure that I knew the four of them before the birth, because it is the one on duty at the moment of the birth who will come. At one point I asked if it was required to do a sonogram. The midwife answered that she did not see any particular reason to do one, but if I absolutely insisted, it would not be a problem for her to send me to a hospital to have one done. I said no, because she thought it was not useful and because the stressful atmosphere I experienced at the hospital did not encourage me to return.

At about 26 weeks of pregnancy I began a preparatory course with a teacher recommended to me by the midwives. It was the *Mensendieck* method: this method is based on postures, it is pretty physical. The idea pleased me because there are many different kinds of courses but I found that in general they are too "soft" and psychological, etc. We were a group of 16 women at about the same stage of pregnancy, which was nice, because we could discuss. The majority of the women had chosen to give birth at home; one was leaning toward the polyclinic, but when the teacher explained to her that most of the labor would occur at home and she wouldn't go to the polyclinic until the end, she finally chose to have a home birth. In fact, she chose the polyclinic because she was scared to make too much noise for the neighbors.

We did a lot of breathing exercises and exercises for the perineum. Carita, the teacher, explained how the birth was going to happen. She said that we would be in a lot of pain, not a little, but really a lot, a lot, of pain and we needed to learn to work with it, to plunge ourselves into the suffering. Towards the end there was a class with the husbands to explain to them what was going to happen, what they would have to do, massage, etc. She insisted on the fact that the husband had to absolutely stay, no matter what happened, even if his wife screamed at him that she wanted him to leave.

At about 8 months the midwife explained how to get ready for the beginning of the birth and at what moment it was necessary to call her. We began to prepare ourselves a little bit: we bought a package at a maternity center with different accessories, including the things we needed to avoid making the bed and floor dirty. I made contact with an organization in order to arrange a postpartum caregiver for five hours per day.

One night I woke up at about 4:00 and I felt that there was something unusual going on. The midwives had said to me, if you are wondering if you are having contractions that means you are *not* having them. But I was sure that I was having them. It was not very painful; I strolled around the apartment then I woke up G. so that he could help me measure the frequency of the contractions. We listened to music and we had breakfast. At about 7:00 we called the midwife, who asked to speak to me. She said, "Given the way you are speaking to me, I do not think your labor is very advanced. If you want I can come right now, but in my opinion it can wait." So we took a turn in the park next door, and there, I began to experience a lot more pain; I was a little bit panicked. We called the midwife again and she came. She saw me huddled up in the corner of the room and she said to G., "Okay that's perfect. I really like to see this." She examined me and said that I was already at seven centimeters; she also listened to the baby's heartbeat with a special stethoscope and told me it was perfect. I was in a lot of pain. I was no longer capable of doing anything else, except to let myself be submerged in the suffering. I had a lot of pain in my back, which I did not really expect. I asked her if we couldn't just go to the hospital so that someone could do something for the pain, because I could no longer take it. She said, "Are you sure that is what you want? You are almost at compete dilation and you're going to be able to push really soon. I'm willing to, if you insist, but if we leave right now you won't even have the time to get pain relief before your baby is born." I didn't answer, but G. said that we would stay at the house; I must say that, in retrospect, I realize he made the decision.

They encouraged me beautifully; they told me all was going well. I was in pain and could no longer remember the things I learned to avoid suffering and that had been useful to me at the start of the birth; it was more like panic and I was not managing it well. Then my water broke and it was even more violent. I began to feel the need to push. The midwife helped me on to her special stool with G. seated behind me holding my back. When we were in that position it felt a bit different, it was still painful, but I could see the end of the tunnel. But in fact, my labor went on for a rather long time, and I became discouraged, probably because I was tired and I had the feeling that it would never end. I began to say incredible things to G. That he had to take me out of there, that I would never do this again, that I didn't want the baby anymore. He was a bit shocked, but he didn't react. Next the midwife told me that head was just there, she took out a mirror so that I could see the head. That scared me more than anything else. She continued to encourage me and finally I felt that the baby was coming out. I began to shiver with exhaustion. The midwife put our baby on my belly but I did not really know what to do with him. After a minute she said that I could try to feed him, and she gave a pair of scissors to G. so that he could cut the cord. Next the placenta came out and the midwife asked if we wanted to keep it.

Our son Joel was born at 2:00 in the afternoon: the midwife stayed for another hour and the postpartum caregiver was there for the afternoon. We were very tired but very excited and we spent the afternoon calling everyone to announce the news. We also drank champagne, I was really happy to be at home. (*"Récit néerlandais,"* in Akrich and Pasveer 1996, 7–12)

Birth at Home (2)

In the early morning of July 4 I woke up at five o'clock with a hard belly and a "contractiony" feeling deep in my stomach. For weeks I had been having hard bellies and often I had the feeling that this was the beginning. I thought this was probably another false alarm. But this time it wasn't. At 5:30 I woke up Dik: "The birth has begun, but you can go back to sleep." But like I, he could not get back to sleep. We were as excited about this birth as we were about the birth of our first son. In around fifteen minutes another contraction came, but I handled it well by concentrating on my belly.

We got our bedroom ready for the birth. The bed prepared, a small table arranged with the things the midwife would need. The cradle was already made up. At 7:30 Wouter woke up. He could feel something was in the air, saw the bed that we had prepared, and laid all his stuffed animals on it. Dik got him dressed and took him to the neighbor's. I called my friend in Amsterdam, the one who had agreed to take photos, and told her that she should begin to make her way to Alkmaar. Dik called the midwife who was busy with her office hours and she agreed to stop by at 11:30, unless she was needed earlier.

I gave all my plants water. At around 9:00 I felt the need to lie down in bed. The contractions came one after the other and I handled them well with fast breathing. When my waters broke there was blood mixed in with the amniotic fluid; Dik called the midwife and she said that she would come immediately. Dik sat behind me and I lay—half sitting—on my side in his arms. I felt very close to him.

Then came the desire to push. An overwhelming feeling. After blowing the contractions away two times, I had to push, whether I wished to or not. The midwife had not yet arrived. I grabbed my legs and gave in to the need to push. When Dik looked between my legs he saw the head was already there. He ran downstairs (between two contractions) and opened the front door. When he came back up, we heard the footsteps of the midwife.

At the moment that she came into our bedroom the head was completely out. "Sigh, sigh," she said, in order to prevent a tear. When I again felt the need to push, our David was born, at 10:24. I picked him up and wanted to bring him next to me, but his umbilical cord was very short and he had to stay lying on my belly. When the cord was cut I could look at him and feel him.

For two and a half hours he lay next to me with a warm blanket and a warm water bottle against his back, while the midwife, my late-arriving friend, and the postpartum caregiver sat chatting below. After such a fast birth it felt great to sit occupied with our child. After a while we dressed him and I washed up. Dik picked up Wouter. Impressed by all he saw, he began to get acquainted with his little brother.

He came next to me on the bed and immediately asked to hold his brother. Watching him getting to know his brother was very moving. "Eyes, ears, mouth, nose, hands, feet," he said, while he touched David in those places. David stared back at him quietly.

Suddenly Wouter said that I should hold the baby and he turned to Dik and demanded his full attention. They went for a walk and David fell asleep in my arms. ("Birth of David," in Spanjer et al. 1994, 342–343)

Polyclinic Birth

In the morning at 7:00 I hoisted myself out of our low bed in order to pee in a bucket we kept close by (I do not use the steep stairway to the WC more often than necessary). Nothing suggested that this day would be any different from the other days of my now forty-week long pregnancy, until I looked . . .something pink and fluffy floated in the pail, that gave the beginning of this day, unexpectedly, a whole different feeling. Is the mucus plug in the pail the sign for our departure? Shall we on Wednesday June 6 hold the "little mover" in our hands with no skin between us?

Standing up I felt a real contraction. It was like the contractions I had already felt from time to time, that left me with a rock hard belly; but those were just a kind of stiffness, with this contraction I had an overwhelming feeling that something was trying to get loose and begin moving.

The contractions began to come more often, slowly but surely, more forceful, stronger. The perspective of the day was narrowed to what was now happening, and we could see how things must go. In the evening at 7:00, in between contractions that were now coming every five minutes, we called our midwife. She would get on her motor scooter and meet us at the hospital. We would come in the car of some friends who were eating with the folks we shared our house with.

It is only ten minutes to the *Prinsengracht*, but I had to work hard to keep myself together. Every contraction left me like the wrinkled sand of the sea. When we got to the hospital I found it difficult to explain to the receptionist why I was there—my words and thoughts were wandering—but eventually we were taken to a room with a high bed, a chair and a childish picture on the wall. The nurse said it would still be some time and Wouter made himself comfortable in the chair with his book. I pulled on my pajamas and was just getting into the bed, when the dike broke and a warm stream soaked them through . . . I had the feeling that something was coming when I was putting them on.

The amniotic fluid had a spectacular effect on the nurse. The midwife had not yet arrived (difficulty starting her motor scooter we heard later) and it was clear things were now going fast. The contractions came very quickly one after the other and there was a new feeling, very low, as if the contraction was being condensed. The first "pushing contraction," came but I couldn't push because the midwife was still not there. I had to "blow" these contractions away. Wouter blew with me and I held his hands tightly. It seemed we were sabotaging a machine that was running perfectly.

Luckily the midwife was suddenly there, calm and alert, her always cold hands now warm. She said I was fully dilated and could begin pushing. I grabbed my knees and added all my own pushing power to the power of the contraction. It went well, and a bit of the head was visible. Wouter was excited, I was given a small mirror in order to get a first glimpse of our child: a thick wrinkle with black, wet hair.

The contractions became more painful, and a few times I had to breathe through them without pushing in order to prevent a tear. Then, suddenly, something slid through and I saw a blue-pink head and almost immediately shoulder, body, legs: our daughter laid there covered with a rich layer of white vernix. Mirre was born at eight minutes past ten with a flattened Maya-nose, long black hair and wide-open eyes. ("Birth of Mirre," in Spanjer et al. 1994, 360–361)

A Home Birth Transferred to the Care of a Gynecologist

Rothman describes a Dutch birth from an American's point of view. She had gone to the Netherlands to witness one (or two) of their storied home births, much discussed among birth activists in the United States. As she says, "It is kind of a rite of passage for the childbirth aficionado." But instead of witnessing a calm and cozy affair, she got to see what happens when a home birth mom is transferred to the care of a gynecologist.

> The labor was not progressing, and the midwife became concerned. Perhaps bladder pressure was a problem. She tried a catheter, change of position, more time, more changes. Then the decision to move to the hospital: helping the woman slip some clothes on, all of us helping her maneuver down [the] stairs, placing her in the car next to her boyfriend, waving goodbye to the worried grandmother-to-be, jumping in the car with the midwife, and the two cars going off to the hospital. I remember holding the hospital door open for the midwife, carrying one of her bags while she carried another, with the birth stool tucked under her arm. There was a friendly welcome at the entrance, and a warmer welcome from the nurse on duty. A brief exchange of information, and the nurse set things up the way the midwife liked them—an experienced team comfortably working together. More time, more changes of position. I found myself alone with the laboring woman, who was stretched out on a padded table, crying in a Dutch that even I could understand, "I want to go to sleep, let me sleep." Reassuring her (in English—who knows what a laboring woman understands of a language she studied in high school?), but aiming for the right tone of compassion and assurance, I said the midwife would be right back, "She's coming, she'll be right here." Then finally the consultation, . . . the obstetrician coming in, conferring with the midwife, briefly examining the woman, and agreeing to do a Caesarean section . . . the goodbyes, and the midwife assuring the woman and the boyfriend that things were now okay. She said she would see them tomorrow and off we went. (Rothman 1993, 206)

These stories of getting a baby in the Netherlands give us a feeling for the various settings of birth and the way different practitioners "accompany" those births; they allow us to stand in the *verloskamer* (delivery room) and to see and hear what happens there. No doubt some staunch supporters of home birth in other countries will find the attitudes of Dutch midwives and their clients a bit surprising. Unlike home birthers in countries where birth at home is the exception, Dutch women and men are under no strong compulsion to learn all they can about the birth process; rather, they trust the midwife to tell them what they need to know and do. Dutch midwives do not come early and stay late at births. They are busy professionals who must organize their work lives efficiently, and they do not hesitate to turn over care of a birthing woman to a gynecologist.

How They Are Born: Statistical Patterns in Dutch Obstetrics

Having gained an appreciation for the players, places, and stories of maternity care in the Netherlands, we look at society-wide trends: How many babies are born? Where do these births occur? Who attends these births? How many midwives, huisartsen, and gynecologists are offering their services to pregnant women? How large a role do midwives play in maternity care, and how is that role changing? What are the medical outcomes for mothers and babies? In doing my research in the Netherlands, I discovered that those who are a part of the maternity care system, both providers and clients, often are unaware of the big picture—of the larger patterns of care and the changes that are occurring in the way care is given. Participants encounter the system as individuals and often have no idea of what is going on at the national level. In the next few pages we raise our gaze to this higher level, adding a quantitative perspective to our qualitative understanding of Dutch birth. At this point I am interested in *describing* the Dutch situation; in later chapters I will revisit these numbers and examine how the structural and cultural features of Dutch society helped to create, and now maintain, this maternity care system.

I begin with the most general information related to births, namely, the number of births per year, the fertility rate, and the average number of children per woman. Figure 2-1 shows relatively high fertility rates for Dutch women extending from the after-war years on through the early 1970s. Notice, too, that the average number of children per woman—that is, the number of children a woman would be expected to have if the age-specific fertility rates for that year were applied to her lifetime—remain high from the 1940s through the early 1970s, when they drop sharply.

How are these babies getting born? Table 2-1 presents the most sought-after information about Dutch maternity care, statistics that describe the place of birth and the professional in attendance. It is these numbers that paint the stark contrast between birth in the Netherlands and birth elsewhere. In order to highlight the peculiarity of the Dutch system, Table 2-1 contrasts the situation in the Netherlands with that in

FIGURE 2-1

Birth Statistics, 1940–2000, the Netherlands

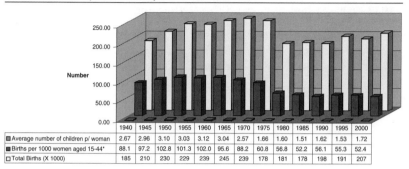

	1940	1945	1950	1955	1960	1965	1970	1975	1980	1985	1990	1995	2000
▣ Average number of children p/ woman	2.67	2.96	3.10	3.03	3.12	3.04	2.57	1.66	1.60	1.51	1.62	1.53	1.72
■ Births per 1000 women aged 15-44*	88.1	97.2	102.8	101.3	102.0	95.6	88.2	60.8	56.8	52.2	56.1	55.3	52.4
☐ Total Births (X 1000)	185	210	230	229	239	245	239	178	181	178	198	191	207

Source: CBS *(Central Bureau voor de Statistiek).*

the United States, where home birth and midwife-assisted births are much rarer.

Figures 2-2 and 2-3 offer a graphical representation of these data; Figure 2-2 highlights the great disparity between the rates of home birth in the Netherlands and the United States. Figure 2-3 shows the stark difference between the role of midwives in the Netherlands and the United States.

For those who know little about the way birth occurs in industrialized countries, Figure 2-3 will underscore the notion that the Netherlands is a "Mecca for Midwives." Birth activists, however, will find these data alarming. If the Netherlands is the Mecca for midwives, why are they attending less than half of all births? Why is the percentage of births accompanied by midwives shrinking in recent years? In Sweden and Norway midwives attend nearly all births. In fact, because midwives monopolize birth in Sweden, the government does not even *record* the distribution of deliveries. After failing to find "percent of births attended by midwives" in an exhaustive search of the Web site of the Swedish Statistics Bureau *(Statistika Centralbryån,* www.scb.se), I asked a colleague in Sweden to track down this number. After *her* search she reported, "The kind of statistics you are looking for may not exist as such in Sweden. Since the medical regulations state that the normal delivery is always the responsibility of the midwife, there is really no direct reason for checking the numbers [of] midwives/doctors. Of course

TABLE 2-1

Distribution of Live Births by Place of Delivery and Attendant, 1940–2000, United States and the Netherlands (in Percent)

| | UNITED STATES | | | | | NETHERLANDS | | | |
| | Place of Delivery | | Attendant | | | Place of Delivery | | Attendant** | |
Year	Hospital	Not in Hosp.*	M.D.	Midwife	Other	Hosp.***	Home	M.D.	Midwife
1940	55.8	44.2	90.8	8.7	0.6	n/a	n/a	51.3	47.7
1945	78.8	21.1	93.5	6.1	0.3	n/a	n/a	62.8	36.1
1950	88.0	12.0	95.1	4.5	0.4	n/a	n/a	58.1	41.1
1955	94.4	5.6	96.9	2.9	0.3	23.9	76.1	58.5	40.9
1960	96.6	3.4	97.8	2.0	0.2	27.4	72.6	63.0	36.6
1965	97.4	2.6	98.3	1.5	0.3	31.5	68.5	64.2	35.3
1970	99.4	0.6	99.5	0.4	0.1	46.7	57.3	62.7	36.7
1975	99.1	0.9	98.8	0.9	0.3	55.6	44.4	59.9	38.6
1980	99.0	1.0	97.4	1.7	0.8	64.6	35.4	59.7	39.4
1985	99.0	1.0	96.7	2.7	0.6	63.4	36.6	57.8	41.7
1990	98.9	1.1	95.3	3.9	0.8	67.9	32.1	53.9	44.1
1991	98.9	1.1	94.8	4.4	0.8	69.3	31.0	53.6	45.0
1992	98.9	1.1	94.5	4.9	0.6	68.5	31.5	53.1	45.8
1993	99.0	1.0	94.0	5.3	0.7	69.3	30.7	52.9	46.4
1994##	99.0	1.0	93.8	5.5	0.6	65.7	33.8	n/a	n/a
1995#	99.0	1.0	93.3	5.9	0.6	68.4	31.6	63.7	36.3
1996#	99.0	1.0	92.8	6.5	0.6	69.7	30.3	63.9	36.1
1997#	99.0	1.0	92.4	7.0	0.6	70.4	29.6	64.7	35.3
1998#	99.0	1.0	92.0	7.4	0.6	70.9	29.1	63.7	36.3
1999#	99.1	0.9	91.8	7.7	0.5	69.2	30.8	65.5	34.5
2000#	99.0	1.0	91.7	7.7	0.5	69.7	30.3	66.1	33.9
2001	99.1	0.9	91.4	8.0	0.5				

Note: n/a: not available.

*Includes free-standing birth centers in 2000; 23,843 (0.6 percent of all births) were at home.

**Excludes births with shared responsibility and cases where attendant is unknown.

***Includes, starting in 1970, "polyclinic" (i.e., short-stay) hospital births.

##Data for the Netherlands in 1994 are from the "Health Survey," as reported in *Vademecum of Health Statistics of the Netherlands*, Centraal Bureau voor de Statistiek, 1998 (p. 98).

#Data for the Netherlands in 1995, 1996, 1997 1998, 1999, and 2000 are from *De Thuisbevalling in Nederland. Eindrapportage: 1995–2000* (Home birth in the Netherlands. End report: 1995–2000). *TNO-Preventie en Gezondheid*, January 2002. Leiden. See footnote for Table 2-2 for an explanation of the change in data collection techniques and the effect of that change on the meaning of the data.

there are deliveries finished by doctors in emergency cases, but there has always been a midwife at [the] start so it may be hard to define what is a doctor's delivery [or a] midwife's delivery."[8]

Norway has a similar maternity care system, and its extensive Medical Birth Registry (1997)—complete with facts about *every* aspect of birth—has no entry for "attendant at birth." Recall, however, that unlike the Netherlands, almost no births take place at home in these countries.

Distribution of the responsibility for attending births between midwives and physicians can be understood as a result of differences in the numbers of each type of practitioner. Figure 2-4 gives us a picture of the different numbers of midwives, huisartsen, and gynecologists practicing in the Netherlands. Of course, not all huisartsen include maternity care in their practice; a recent survey indicates that 16 percent of huisartsen provide care during pregnancy and birth, and an additional 22 percent offer care only during pregnancy (Wiegers and Hingstman 1999a); in 2000, huisartsen accompanied 6.7 percent of births in the Netherlands (TNO 2002). Like most European nations, the Netherlands has far more midwives than gynecologists. Once again, the United States is on the opposite end of the continuum: In the United States the ratio is reversed—there are about 40,000 practicing obstetrician-gynecologists and approximately 8,000 practicing midwives.[9]

Sources for Table 2-1:

For the United States: U.S. Department of Health and Human Service *Vital Statistics of the United States, Vol. 1—Natality*, Hyattsville, MD, U.S. Department of Health and Human Services, 1993; National Center for Health Statistics, Hyattsville, MD, "Live births by place of delivery and attendant, according to race and Hispanic origin: United States, selected years 1975–99," (available at http://www.cdc.gov/nchs/datawh/statab/unpubd/natality/natab99.htm); National Center for Health Statistics, "Births, Final Data for 2002." *National Vital Statistics Reports*, Vol. 52, No. 10.

For the Netherlands: Centraal Bureau voor de Statistiek, *1899–1989: Negentig jaren statistiek in tijdreeksen*, 's-Gravenhage, CBS Publikaties, 1989; Centraal Bureau voor de Statistiek, *Geborenen naar aard verloskundige hulp en plaats van geboorte*, Voorburg, CBS, 1990, 1992; TNO, *De Thuisbevalling in Nederland. Eindrapportage: 1995–2000* (Home birth in the Netherlands. End report: 1995–2000). *TNO-Preventie en Gezondheid*, January 2002. Leiden.

---

8. Lena Milton, personal communication, September 2000.

9. The numbers of obstetrician-gynecologists and midwives are not well-monitored in the United States. These estimates are taken from the American College of Gynecologists (www.acog.org), Rooks (1997), and DeVries (1996, 165–166). The number of midwives includes both Certified Nurse Midwives and nonnurse midwives.

FIGURE 2-2

Home Births in the United States and the Netherlands, 1955–2000 (as a Percentage of All Births)

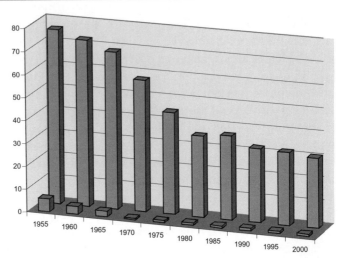

	1955	1960	1965	1970	1975	1980	1985	1990	1995	2000
United States	5.6	3.4	2.6	0.6	0.9	1	1	1.1	1	1
Netherlands	76.1	72.6	68.5	57.3	44.4	35.4	36.6	32.1	31.6	30.3

Source: See Table 2-1.

Tallies of practitioners tell only part of the story. We also need to see what these practitioners are doing. Table 2-2 gives us this information by describing the work of midwives in the Netherlands between 1965 and 2000. Several trends in this table deserve further comment. Note that in the second half of the twentieth century midwives gradually assumed responsibility for a larger share of *all* births and moved from a minority to a majority position in attending home births. Midwives also increased their role as attendants at birth in institutions. But perhaps the most dramatic change in this time period is the change in the place of work for midwives: In 1965, 82 percent of all midwife-attended births occurred at home, but by 1993 this number had dropped to less than 50 percent.[10]

---

10. Beginning in 1995 the government collected data on birth in a different way, making it impossible to compare these numbers with those from earlier years. See note to Table 2-2.

FIGURE 2-3

Midwife-Attended Births as a Percentage of All Births: Netherlands and the United States, 1940–2000

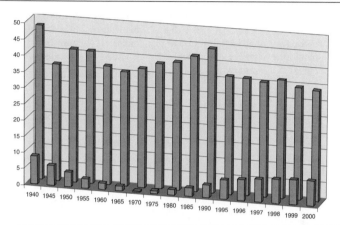

	1940	1945	1950	1955	1960	1965	1970	1975	1980	1985	1990	1995	1996	1997	1998	1999	2000
United States	8.7	6.1	4.5	2.9	2	1.5	0.4	0.9	1.7	2.7	3.9	5.9	6.5	7	7.4	7.7	7.7
Netherlands	47.7	36.1	41.1	40.9	36.6	35.3	36.7	38.6	39.4	41.7	44.4	36.3	36.1	35.3	36.3	34.5	33.9

Source: See Table 2-1.

FIGURE 2-4

Numbers of Practicing Gynecologists, Midwives, and Huisarts in the Netherlands, 1960–2002

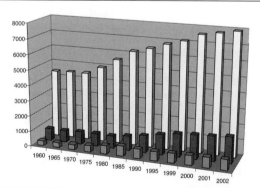

	1960	1965	1970	1975	1980	1985	1990	1995	1999	2000	2001	2002
Gynecologists	307	317	328	405	545	673	604	592	634	655	675	699
Midwives	788	778	836	850	814	945	1122	1332	1507	1578	1627	1726
Huisarts	4405	4452	4470	4937	5556	6179	6465	6814	7093	7571	7763	7939

Source: *Centraal Bureau voor de Statisktiek*; NIVEL. Numbers reflect the count on 31 December of each year.

Table 2-2
Practices of Midwives in the Netherlands, 1965–2000

Distribution of midwife-attended births

Year	Percentage of all births at home	Percentage of all births attended by midwives	Percentage of births at home attended by midwives	Percentage of births by midwives attended at home	Percentage of births by midwives attended in institutions	Percentage of births in institutions attended by midwives
1965	68.5	35.3	42.4	82.3	17.7	20.0
1970	57.3	36.7	46.5	72.6	27.4	23.7
1975	44.4	38.6	54.4	62.6	37.4	26.2
1980	35.4	39.4	58.5	52.6	47.3	29.1
1985	36.6	41.7	65.4	57.3	42.6	28.2
1990	32.1	44.8	71.2	51.1	48.8	32.4
1992	31.5	45.5	71.7	49.7	50.3	33.6
1993	30.6	46.4	73.8	48.7	51.3	34.2
1995	31.6	36.3	80.5	70.1	29.7	15.8
1996	30.3	36.1	84.4	71.0	28.9	15.0
1997	29.6	35.3	85.7	71.8	28.0	14.1
1998	29.1	36.3	89.4	71.7	28.2	14.4
1999	30.8	34.5	80.5	71.9	28.0	14.0
2000	30.3	33.9	80.9	72.3	27.6	13.4

Sources: Centraal Bureau voor de Statistiek, *1899–1989: Negentig jaren statistiek in tijdreeksen,* 's-Gravenhage, CBS Publikaties, 1989; Centraal Bureau voor de Statistiek, *Geboren naar aard verloskundige hulp en plaats van geboorte,* Voorburg, CBS, 1990, 1992; TNO, *De Thuisbevalling in Nederland. Eindrapportage: 1995–2000* (Home birth in the Netherlands. End report: 1995-2000). *TNO-Preventie en Gezondheidt,* January 2002, Leiden.

Note: Data for 1995, 1996, 1997, 1998, 1999, and 2000 are from *De Thuisbevalling in Nederland. Eindrapportage*: 1995–2000 (Home birth in the Netherlands. End report: 1995-2000). *TNO-Preventie en Gezondheid*, January 2002. Leiden. All births in the second line during these years are attributed to physicians, thus excluding births in the second line attended by midwives. The switch from data collected by the *Centraal Bureau voor de Statistiek* to data from the TNO helps to explain the sharp drop in percentage of midwife-attended births between 1993 and 1995. CBS data are population data while TNO data are from a medical registry designed for insurance purposes. CBS data were based on information collected when someone, usually the father, gave notice of the birth of a child. He was asked who assisted during the birth. When the midwife was present most of the time and the gynecologist only came in at a later stage, the father likely said that the midwife assisted. The same would happen when the child was born in hospital where midwives work under supervision of gynecologists but attend most of the births themselves. According to the CBS-data these are midwife-assisted births, but according to the TNO these are tweedelijns-bevallingen, where the gynecologist has responsibility for the birth. CBS numbers give us a picture of who actually attended the birth, while TNO data tell us who was "responsible" for the birth (even if that person did not attend the birth).

FIGURE 2-5

Cesarean Section Rates in the Netherlands and the United States, 1999–2000

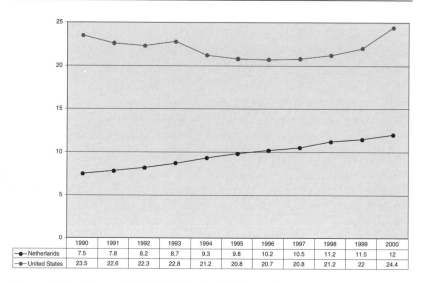

	1990	1991	1992	1993	1994	1995	1996	1997	1998	1999	2000
Netherlands	7.5	7.8	8.2	8.7	9.3	9.8	10.2	10.5	11.2	11.5	12
United States	23.5	22.6	22.3	22.8	21.2	20.8	20.7	20.8	21.2	22	24.4

Source: National Center for Health Statistics (US); *Centraal Bureau voor de Statistiek* (NL).

Another measure of how the system is working, and an oft-requested statistic about Dutch maternity care, is the rate of cesarean sections. Figure 2-5 offers a contrast between the cesarean section rates in the Netherlands and the United States. Again we find the Netherlands and the United States at opposite ends—this time on the continuum that measures obstetrical intervention at birth.

Many who learn about the Dutch system, with its continued use of home birth and its low rate of cesarean section, are curious about the infant mortality rate. In the United States, where home birth is considered dangerous and frightening, it is often assumed that high rates of birth at home must be associated with higher rates of infant death. Figure 2-6—infant mortality rates for the Netherlands, Sweden, the United States, the United Kingdom, and Canada—shows that this is not the case. In a later chapter we will look more closely at the comparative mortality rates for home and hospital birth in the Netherlands. Not surprisingly, we will discover that mortality rates for home births (with healthy mothers) are significantly lower than those found in

FIGURE 2-6

Infant Mortality Rates for Selected Countries, 1960–2000

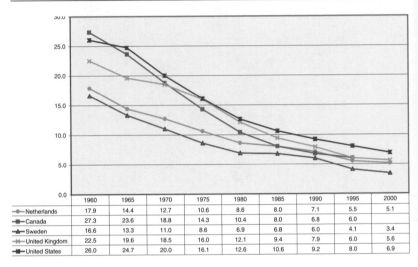

	1960	1965	1970	1975	1980	1985	1990	1995	2000
Netherlands	17.9	14.4	12.7	10.6	8.6	8.0	7.1	5.5	5.1
Canada	27.3	23.6	18.8	14.3	10.4	8.0	6.8	6.0	
Sweden	16.6	13.3	11.0	8.6	6.9	6.8	6.0	4.1	3.4
United Kingdom	22.5	19.6	18.5	16.0	12.1	9.4	7.9	6.0	5.6
United States	26.0	24.7	20.0	16.1	12.6	10.6	9.2	8.0	6.9

Source: Organization for Economic Cooperation and Development. OECD Health Data 2004, www.oecd.org

hospital births. Of course, comparisons of infant mortality rates must be done cautiously, leaving room for the fact that ministries of health in different countries count infant deaths in different ways (e.g., there is variation in the length of gestation required before a miscarriage is defined as an infant death). On the other hand, those who would justify higher rates of infant death in the United States by pointing out that countries like Sweden and the Netherlands do not have the great disparities in wealth found in the United States (after all, they argue, poor women have worse birth outcomes and there are more poor women in the United States) have a very limited definition of health care. These people somehow exclude the provision of adequate housing, education, and nutrition from their conception of the health care system.

A FINAL NOTE ON PECULIARITY

In these first chapters I have done what most do when confronted with maternity care in the Netherlands: I have highlighted the oddness of

Dutch obstetrics. But I am a social scientist, and we social scientists cannot abide oddity. We are not content to say, "This is the exception that proves the rule." We must find the pattern that lies under the peculiarity: We must discover how the exceptional case *follows* the rule. We welcome exceptions because they force us to rethink the patterns we have described, but we are not content to leave them as exceptions. In Part II we begin the work of *explaining* the Dutch difference, of putting it in its sociological place, of identifying the social and cultural features that eventuated in this unique system.

II. FORMS

HOW MIGHT we explain the peculiar characteristics of birth in the Netherlands? Where do we go to find the causes of this health care anomaly? We social scientists fancy ourselves to be explainers of social phenomena, but too often we are content to do little more than demonstrate correlations—either quantitative or qualitative—or to provide "thick description"; we are timid when it comes to explanation. Our forebears had no such fears. They marched in where we current-day angels of social science fear to tread: Durkheim boldly proclaimed the causes of suicide, even though his data were flawed; Weber had no doubts about how the forces of rationality influenced modern life; and Marx unflinchingly diagrammed the causes and effects of economic systems. Four decades ago, C. Wright Mills (1959) worried about the tendency of modern sociologists to get lost in empirical details or in flights of theoretical fancy. He called us to go beyond mere *description* to careful *explanation* of social events, to look at how our lives intersect with historical events, to distinguish private troubles from public issues, to show our fellow travelers why their lives are unfolding as they are. But explanation is not easy. Fearing to be proved wrong, we social scientists continue to shy away from it.

In Part II we move past this hesitancy and begin our search for the causes of the Dutch difference, looking at the structural features that support obstetrics in the Netherlands—its health system, professional arrangements, patterns of education, the laws governing health care, and the political environment that surrounds health care and maternity care.

3 Structuring Care

IN THE course of my research, it became my habit to ask all those I interviewed to offer an opinion on the reasons for the persistence of the Dutch way of birth. When asked his view on this question, a gynecologist, who was then serving as a member of the board of the *Nederlandse Vereniging voor Obstetrie en Gynaecologie* (NVOG: Dutch Association for Obstetrics and Gynecology), had this to say:

Because we saw it worked. You must be aware this is a small country. There is a lot of social control, also in [obstetrics]. Hospitals are easy to reach, and as I've said, most people are talking together, midwives and gynecologists. They have a rather open mind for one another. . . . We saw that there were no large emergencies, no extreme things. . . . I think there is a kind of social system, which isn't visible but which works. Why should we change? We saw that our clients liked it.

The system also appears to be very rational.

Yes, it is rational. And gynecologists—most of them—think about birth as a natural process, in which you only have to be involved if nature, to your opinion, has lost the case.

That's unusual, I think. It's certainly unusual compared to what I know of American obstetricians.

Yes, I think so. Of course, yes. People who are pregnant are not patients, they are clients. They are only patients if there is a reason for it. . . . The midwife is coming to help with your delivery. But you do it yourself. . . . Look at somebody who gets a baby! She is doing it herself! Midwives do nothing; gynecologists do nothing. A gynecologist [may put] something on the head of the baby, or take blood . . . or do a vacuum, or make an incision . . . [but] he is not really helping. He is [just] doing things.

Most of the factors mentioned by this gynecologist were echoed by other respondents: The system works, clients like it, hospitals are easily accessible, midwives and gynecologists respect each other, and (unlike obstetrical specialists elsewhere) gynecologists generally agree that birth is a natural event that rarely requires intervention. I heard other explanations as well, including: Calvinism (which creates a stoic attitude toward pain), physical characteristics of Dutch women (they tend to be large and strong and give birth easily), and the *burgerlijke* (civil, middle class) character of the Dutch (hard-working, thrifty, not given to frills or unnecessary luxuries).

In his analysis of maternity care in the Netherlands, Lammert Hingstman, a Dutch health care researcher, distills these diverse explanations into a more organized list. He believes there are four essential "pillars" of the Dutch obstetric system (Hingstman 1994, 379):

1. The special "protected" position of the midwife;
2. A generally accepted and effective screening system for high risk pregnancies;
3. A well-organized system of comprehensive home care; and
4. A sociocultural environment that regards pregnancy and childbirth as normal physiological processes.

Notice that Hingstman's list and the lists of reasons offered by others contain two types of explanations: *structural* and *cultural*. Structural explanations look to the way society is organized. Most often this means forms of *social* organization—such as health systems, insurance systems, professional regulations and the like—but structural explanations may also include the *physical* organization of society: its system of transportation and its arrangement of hospitals and clinics. Cultural explanations employ less tangible features of society—its ideas and values—to give an account of the way health care is organized. In the case of Dutch obstetrics this includes, among others, cultural ideas about the naturalness of birth, about religion, and about the proper use of medical resources.

In this chapter and the next we examine the *structural* features that give Dutch obstetrics its form. Without an extraordinary degree of organization, it would be impossible for Dutch midwives and physicians to deliver high-quality care at home and in the hospital. When we look beyond the experiences and statistics described in Chapter 2, we find a carefully designed structure that includes

- Policies that govern insurance and regulate relationships among caregivers;
- Well-organized educational programs for midwives, *kraamverzorgenden*, and specialists;

- Professional groups with a strong sense of their identity and their place in Dutch maternity care;
- Systems for monitoring the quantity and quality of care; and
- A network of roads and hospitals that allows easy access to specialist care.[1]

Birth stories from the Netherlands, including the ones I have retold here, present cozy pictures of moms, babies, dads, midwives, and physicians—pictures that can lull us into assuming that Dutch caregivers simply know how to get along and that Dutch mothers instinctively know how to give birth. But in reality, the coziness of Dutch birth is the product of a system of rules, regulations, educational programs, and arrangements between professionals, and, as we will see, the elements in this system are constantly reviewed, argued over, and negotiated.

REGULATING CARE

As noted in Chapter 2, pregnant women in the Netherlands move freely between care settings and caregivers. Lacking some sort of organization and control, these back and forth referrals would quickly become confusing, if not dangerous. If there were no rules governing the comings and goings of obstetric clients, some gynecologists might hold on to the women referred to them, reluctant to send them back to the *eerstelijn*, and, in turn, some midwives and *huisartsen* would be slow to send clients to a specialist, preferring to manage even complicated cases at home or in the polyclinic.

From the point of view of heath policy, this management of interprofessional rivalry in the Dutch system is remarkable. The system does more than simply control the competition for clients between midwives, huisartsen, and gynecologists: It also generates an unusual degree of cooperation between midwives and physicians.[2] How is this accomplished? Two features of the health/maternity care system are largely responsible:

---

1. The closing of smaller hospitals in the last few years has made access to backup care more difficult, causing some to worry about the future of home birth in the Netherlands (see Wiegers et al. 2000; Bleker 2000).

1. The insurance system, where patterns of reimbursement for health services are used to control the behavior of clients and caregivers;
2. The indications list, a set of rules (negotiated by midwives, physicians, insurance companies, and the government) that define when transfers between primary care and specialist care are to be made.

Insuring Cooperation

In all health systems, patterns of care are strongly influenced by patterns of reimbursement: Those who decide what will and will not be paid for—whether they be government bureaucrats or private insurance bureaucrats—control what happens in the clinic. When we look at the insurance regulations governing maternity care in the Netherlands, we discover a little-discussed irony. Supporters of the Dutch way of birth celebrate the fact that Dutch women are free to choose: They can get their baby at home *or* in the hospital. What these same supporters often do *not* tell you (or perhaps do not know) is that this freedom of choice is won at the cost of *limiting* the freedom of women who are expecting normal, healthy births.

In order to explain this irony and how it is related to the regulation of competition among caregivers, I must describe the rules governing maternity care in the context of the larger health insurance system of the Netherlands. The Dutch insurance system involves both the public and private sectors. Those with incomes below a specified level (set by the government, in 2003 the line was a gross salary of €31,750 per year) must be insured by the *Ziekenfonds* (Sick Fund[3]), an insurance system organized by the government, but largely administered by private insurance companies. About two-thirds of the population is covered by the Sick Fund, but contrary to the image we Americans might have of government-controlled health care, participants in the Sick Fund choose a *private* insurance company to administer their health coverage.

The Sick Fund system is subsidized by contributions made by employers, employees, and the government. Premiums are paid by a com-

---

2. For a consideration of the ethical consequences of rivalry among health care professionals see De Vries (2003).

3. *Ziekenfonds* is often mistakenly translated as "sickness fund." The more accurate translation is "sick fund," as in "fund for the sick." The plural, *Ziekenfondsen*, refers to the collection of insurance companies that offer policies within the framework of the Sick Fund.

bination of income-based contributions to the Sick Fund and fees paid to the insurer. Employees contribute 1.70 percent of their income and employers add an amount equal to 6.75 percent of the employee's income; like Social Security in the United States, this tax has a fixed upper limit on taxable salary (in 2003 it was €28,971). The insured also pays a nominal fee to the private insurer they have chosen: Those premiums range from €19.95 to €32.50 per month.[4]

All private insurance companies (*ziekenkostenverzekeraars*, or "sick costs insurers," referred to collectively as *ziekenfondsen*) must offer a "standard packet policy" (*standaardpakketpolis*) that includes coverage for basic health services for members of the Sick Fund. The government controls the content of this packet; however, those using the Sick Fund are free to purchase more services (*aanvullende verzekeringen*, supplementary insurance) from their insurance companies. Those who are privately insured—the other one-third of the population—are also free to increase the basic package of benefits and, unlike those covered by the Sick Fund, can lower the cost of their premium by adding a deductible (*eigen risico*) to their policies.

The organization of the insurance system, coupled with a law regulating health care fees—the WTG (*Wet Tarieven Gezondheidszorg*, Law for Tariffs in Health Care), passed in 1982—allows the government to control costs by specifying rules of coverage, what will (and will not) be covered. It is these rules that limit the kind of care a healthy woman can receive during pregnancy. Dutch women whose pregnancies are healthy must stay in the care of the eerstelijn: either a midwife or a huisarts. The care of a specialist in the *tweedelijn* will only be compensated when complications arise. Until recently there was an additional limit here: As a result of the government wish to promote and protect midwifery, midwives were given a *primaat*: Coverage rules required that in locations where midwives were practicing, women insured

---

4. The Dutch health insurance system also includes the AWBZ (*Algemene Wet Bijzondere Ziektekosten*, or the General Law for Extraordinary Medical Costs), which covers the cost of nursing home care, certain types of care at home, and various types of equipment. The AWBZ covers the entire population and is funded by a 10.25 percent tax on (taxable) income. In 2003 the cost for all forms of medical care in the Netherlands was €44.2 billion of which the government paid 5 percent, the Sick Fund 35 percent, the ABWZ 40 percent, and other—payments from businesses, private health insurers, and co-payments—20 percent (Ministerie van Welzijn, Volksgezondheid, en Sport 2002).

under the Sick Fund had to use their services. Thus the services of a huisarts could be used only in those places where no midwives were working. The insurance system and the primaat together created the "special 'protected' position of the midwife," mentioned above by Hingstman (1994).

Not surprisingly, there was a range of opinion about the primaat among caregivers. In general, midwives found it to be a good idea, and huisartsen found it frustrating. For midwives, the primaat was more than just a self-interested strategy. They were concerned with the quality of care offered by huisartsen. Mevrouw Zwart, the Director of the NOV from 1986 to 1999, echoed the feelings of many midwives in her explanation: "In general I think that obstetrics, like dentistry,[5] must be seen as its own specialty, where one must have sufficient experience. A huisarts has far too little experience. . . . The average midwife 'does' 100 births per year . . . [allowing her] to see clearly the problems that can arise during pregnancy."

Midwives also found frustrating the often fickle attitude of huisarts toward assisting at birth. In an interview in 1998, Mevrouw Zwart pointed out the inconstancy of huisartsen. She noted that huisartsen often say, "Let us now, when we are 30 or 40 [years old], do obstetrical work. But when we turn 50, we will say, 'I really do not want to get out of my bed in the middle of the night.' Or: 'I am not going to stay home during my vacation just to do a birth.' And then the midwife must come to the rescue."

Gynecologists had mixed feelings about the primaat. As one explained to me, "We should have very strict regulations for general practitioners to do deliveries. They can't go into practice having done 10 deliveries in a hospital ward. They have to have a lot of training . . . that's our opinion. So, there has to be a basis. Maybe one half year on a delivery ward in a large hospital. . . . But they can't . . . work in obstetrics when they've done 20 or 25 deliveries. . . . They have to be trained about the same as midwives." However, he went on to say,

If they ask us "Is it normal that they [i.e., midwives] have a primaat?" I don't think so. If somebody does his work well and can state that he does

---

5. At one point in their history, huisartsen also provided dental care.

his work everyday and does enough deliveries every year, well, why not?

Are you saying that the primaat should be removed?

Yes.

Many huisartsen I spoke with found the primaat irritating because it prevented them from providing maternity care to clients they have seen since the clients were children. In 1994, a group of huisartsen created a new association—the *Vereniging van Verloskundig Actieve Huisartsen* (VVAH, Association of Obstetrically Active Huisartsen)—to defend and promote the right of general practitioners to accompany births. The first secretary of the VVAH, Dr. T. Dorresteijn, explained the desire of huisartsen to stay involved in births: "Accompanying a birth gives you special feelings, you have a special contact with the family. . . . It's part of the whole family care. . . . It's just a very important and emotional moment in life. Why take this one out of all the other sickness? Severe sickness is an emotional moment. Dying is an emotional moment. Well, all those moments in fact the GP is connected with, and just why leave this nice thing out?"

Responding to pressure from its members, the professional association of the huisartsen, the *Landelijke Huisartsen Vereniging* (LHV, National Huisarts Association) brought suit to eliminate the primaat. The judge in that case ruled that as of 1 January 1999 the primaat would be eliminated. The government opposed the decision and filed an appeal. After prolonged negotiation between the government, midwives, and physicians, it was agreed that the primaat should be dropped in the interest of preserving home birth.[6]

In the Netherlands, control over who will and will not provide care at birth works by specification of what will and will not be reimbursed. Before the primaat was removed, a woman who really wanted her huisarts to attend her birth, even though a midwife was working in her town or city, could choose to pay for that care herself. But in fact, very few women were, or are, willing to pay these costs out of their own pockets. Privately insured women also are limited in their choice of caregiver: Patterns of reimbursement set by the Sick Funds are now deeply ingrained in the working of the system, influencing the policy

---

6. Chapter 4 offers more detail about the legal and political debates over the primaat.

packages offered to the privately insured. Thus, it is impossible to buy a health insurance policy in the Netherlands that will cover the cost of specialist care for a healthy pregnancy and birth.

Patterns of remuneration established by the health insurance system affect the clinical decisions of caregivers as well. In a conversation with a Dutch gynecologist, I noted the high number of cesarean sections in the United States and commented that U.S. obstetricians are paid far more when they do a surgical birth than when they assist at a normal, vaginal birth. She responded, "That's a good feature of our system. . . . If it's a normal delivery, or it's a vacuum delivery or a caesarian, it's all the same price [i.e., fee]. And if it takes you 2 days or it takes you 2 minutes, it's all the same price, that's the good thing. So you're not pressed by financial reasons by doing caesarians or so, that's a good thing."

Being more individualistic, we Americans are tempted to assume that even in this structure, money talks—that a woman who is willing to pay enough could get her practitioner of choice. In my interviews with gynecologists I tested this idea by asking if they would attend an uncomplicated home birth for a friend who was willing to pay cash. To most gynecologists it seemed an odd question. Their first response was puzzlement: Why would a healthy woman want a specialist in attendance at her birth? When pressed, one gynecologist reluctantly agreed that he might do it, but he would make it clear that he would be unavailable if he were not on call when the birth occurred: "If I knew you [i.e., the client] very well I would not do it. It's not wise to treat people you know well. I myself would answer 'I'm willing to, if you insist, but I think in principle you should get a midwife. If you insist, I'm willing to check or do your prenatal care, but I will never promise to be personally responsible for your individual delivery.'"

The insurance system not only affects a woman's choice of caregiver, it also affects where she chooses to give birth. It *is* true that women in the eerstelijn (the first line, or primary care system) are free to choose where they will get their babies—at home or in the hospital—but here, too, their pocketbooks are involved. A birth at home under the care of the eerstelijn is fully reimbursed. If a woman who has no medical reason to give birth in a hospital chooses a *poliklinische bevalling*, she must pay part of the cost of the delivery room. In 2003 the cost of using the delivery room was set at €404; the Sick Fund reimbursed €159.30, leaving €244.70 for the parents to pay.[7]

The basic benefits provided by the Sick Fund also cover most of the cost of the postpartum care given by a *kraamverzorgende*. The standaardpakketpolis pays for 64 hours of care given in the home, but parents must make a co-payment of €3.27 per hour of care received. A woman can choose to reduce or extend the number of hours of care received (from a minimum of 24 hours to a maximum of 80 hours); some supplementary insurance policies cover the cost of the co-payment.

By clearly defining the proper roles of midwives and physicians and by offering incentives to choose certain types of care, the insurance system offers important support for the unique Dutch way of doing birth. But the rules of the insurance system need further elaboration; the boundaries between the *eerste* (first) and *tweede* (second, i.e., specialist) lines must be clearly drawn so that women are not subjected to the whims of their caregivers when it comes to defining "healthy" and "unhealthy" pregnancies.

Indications for Cooperation

The second feature of Dutch health policy that supports Dutch maternity care—the *indicatielijst* (indications list)—offers the definitional clarity demanded by the insurance regulations. The indicatielijst, more formally known as the "Obstetric Indications List" (or, in Dutch, the VIL, the *Verloskundige Indicatielijst*), is a set of guidelines that specifies the conditions for referrals between the eerste and tweede lines. In effect, the VIL defines what "healthy" means, distinguishing between normal ("physiological") and high-risk ("pathological") pregnancies and births; these definitions are then used to identify the conditions that require midwives and general practitioners to refer their clients to specialists. Lacking the guidelines offered by this list, the preference for primary care (the eerstelijn) in Dutch obstetrics would not be possible.[8]

De Snoo, a professor of gynecology at Utrecht, first suggested the list in his 1930 text, *Leerboek voor Verloskunde* (Textbook of Obstetrics). In the late 1950s, at the request of the Sick Fund, the well-known Dutch gynecologist Gerrit-Jan Kloosterman developed

---

7. Those with private insurance can choose a coverage plan that pays all of this cost. Some insurance plans also cover the cost of a *kraampakket*, a package containing various things needed for a home birth.

8. A more complete history of the VIL is presented in Chapter 4.

the list further, and in 1973 an expanded version of the VIL appeared in *his* textbook, *De Voortplanting van de Mens: Leerboek voor Obstetrie en Gynaecologie* (Textbook of Obstetrics and Gynecology: Human Reproduction). The "Kloosterman List," as it came to be known, was endorsed by all professors of obstetrics in the Netherlands, and medical insurance companies recommended its use to physicians and midwives.

In the late 1970s and early 1980s, the *Ziekenfondsraad* (Sick Fund Council),[9] began the move toward formalizing the list by convening various commissions to review current practices and to recommend a way to better promote the coordination of maternity care services. In 1982 the Sick Fund Council organized the WBK—*Werkgroep Bijstelling Kloostermanlijst* (Work Group for the Revision of the Kloosterman List), the group that would generate the first official (i.e., government-sponsored and -endorsed) list. Among the reasons the government decided to move from an informal to a formal list was a notable increase in hospital births and large regional variations in maternity care "[creating] the impression that in some cases the medical indication [for hospital birth] was possibly requested for the wrong reasons" (Ziekenfondsraad 1987, 10).

In 1987 the WBK presented the result of its work and the official VIL was established.[10] Believing it gave too much discretion to midwives, the Dutch organization of obstetricians and gynecologists (NVOG) was not altogether pleased with the list and refused to officially endorse it. Nevertheless, it became the document that governed the policy decisions of the government and the insurance companies (see Riteco and Hingstman 1991). In the mid-1990s a new work group was formed, and

---

9. The Sick Fund Council is the governing body for health insurance in the Netherlands. Created by the 1941 law that set up the current health care system, this council makes important decisions about what sort of care will be offered, by whom, and for what fee. By statute, the membership of this council includes representatives from employers, unions, caregivers (of all sorts), hospitals, patient organizations, insurance companies, and the government. The Sick Fund Council often commissions workgroups to provide advice to the council on health policy. In 1999 the Sick Fund Council was reorganized as the *College Voor Zorgverzekeringen* (CVZ); because my research was done before this reorganization, I will continue to refer to the Sick Fund Council, here and elsewhere in the book.

10. ObGyn.net has published an English version of the Obstetric Indication List; see http://europe.obgyn.net/nederland/richtlijnen/vademecum_eng.htm

they produced a modified version of the list that has been approved by all professions delivering maternity care (see Ziekenfondsraad 1999).[11]

The VIL—Hingstman's (1994) "generally accepted and effective screening system for high risk pregnancies"—is a critical part of the unique Dutch way of birth. Having a screening system for identifying "physiological" and "pathological" pregnancies allows the Dutch to avoid the assumption, made in other industrialized countries, that all births are "potentially pathological, or high risk," and therefore must be monitored by specialists.[12] As noted above, discussions about the content of this list have not always been the most amicable, a fact we will consider in more detail in Chapter 4 when we look at the politics of maternity care in the Netherlands.

The referral structure of Dutch obstetrics, created by the insurance system and the VIL, is just one piece of the puzzle. In order for the Dutch way of birth to continue, it must also "create" caregivers who understand and follow the major tenets of the system. These caregivers are produced by the professional and educational institutions of the Netherlands.

CREATING CAREGIVERS

We have already met the major players in Dutch obstetrics: midwives, kraamverzorgenden, and gynecologists. In the following pages we examine how each profession came to be and how each is currently equipped for its role in the maternity care system. Given their central place in the Dutch system, we begin with midwives and delve most deeply into their status, both past and present.

Midwives

Midwives in other countries admire, if not envy, the autonomy of their sisters in the Netherlands. When they see the relative freedom enjoyed by Dutch midwives, they are often eager to know: How did this happen? Elsewhere in Europe, the rise of modern obstetric technology relegated midwives to the position of doctor's assistant. How did Dutch midwives escape this fate? It is clear that *current* regulations favor midwives, but how did those regulations come to be?

---

11. See Chapter 4 for more detail.
12. See Sandall et al. (2001) for a more complete description of the VIL.

Intrigued by these questions, several historians have explored the events that allowed Dutch midwives to arrive in their present position.[13] The consensus of these histories is that midwives in the Netherlands benefited from the early arrival of municipally sponsored education and regulation. Unlike their European neighbors, the Dutch believed that if midwives had the proper training and regulatory oversight they could be important figures for securing safe childbirth and promoting population growth. Rather than marginalizing midwives— a strategy used by municipal and regional authorities elsewhere in Europe—city leaders in the Netherlands sought to educate these women and put them to work in service of the townspeople.

As early as 1463, the town of Leiden appointed a *stadsvroedvrouw* (municipal midwife)—Margriete Wechels of Antwerp—who was given a small salary to see to the care of all parturient women. Her services were provided without charge to the poor; the rich were instructed to make a contribution for care received (van der Borg 1992, 44–45). Among the conditions of Mevrouw Wechels's employment, two are particularly significant: She was required to call a physician for help in complicated cases, and she was directed to train aspiring midwives. These rules promulgated in the fifteenth century foreshadow the development of midwifery in the Netherlands: The work terrain of midwives was limited to "normal" births (physician assistance was required in difficult cases), and midwifery was recognized as a distinct field of practice (student midwives should train with midwives). By the eighteenth century most towns in the Netherlands had followed the example of Leiden and had appointed *stadsvroedvrouwen.*

But not *all* Dutch midwives had appointments as stadsvroedvrouwen. During the seventeenth and eighteenth centuries, municipalities took responsibility for the regulation—and in many cases, education—of Dutch midwives in private practice. Marland (1993a, 24–25) describes the various approaches to regulation used in Amsterdam, Leiden, Rotterdam, Zwolle, Groningnen, and Utrecht; she concludes that in all cases the ends of regulation were the same: "to make the midwife answerable to the town authorities, to control her training and practice." By the end of the

---

13. What follows is only a brief summary of the history of midwives in the Netherlands. For a more complete account of the fascinating history of Dutch midwives see van Lieburg and Marland 1989; Marland (1993a, 1993c, 1995), Marland and Rafferty (1997), van der Borg (1992), Drenth (1998), Schama (1988, 481–562).

eighteenth century all "the larger and more important Dutch towns introduced statutes regulating the practices of local midwives and set up training courses and examinations to test their competence and suitability to practice" (Marland 1993a, 24).

In the nineteenth century municipal regulations and training programs were gradually replaced by national laws and state-funded education. The first national law regulating midwifery was passed in 1818. The 1818 Health Act was created to reclaim the medical system after 18 years of political subservience to France; among its rules we find formal expression of the unique Dutch approach to midwifery. First, the Act gave midwives a clear and defined sphere of practice. Midwifery was specifically included among the several *medical* professions regulated by the Act, and the competencies and duties of midwives were distinguished from those of men-midwives and obstetric doctors. Second, following the rules found in most municipalities, the Act limited the practice of midwifery to "normal" births. Midwives were to confine their practices to those births "which were natural processes or could be delivered manually, so that the midwife may never use any instruments for this purpose" (quoted in van Lieburg and Marland 1989, 299).

The Medical Act of 1865, the second major piece of health legislation in the nineteenth century, affirmed the official place of the midwife among the medical professions of the Netherlands and restated the limitations of the earlier law. In the 1865 Act, midwifery was defined as a medical profession (*medische beroep*)[14] and midwives were permitted "only to attend such deliveries, that were the work of nature, or which could be executed by hand" (quoted in van Lieburg and Marland 1989, 305).

Elsewhere in Europe, midwife regulation also began in the seventeenth and eighteenth centuries, but those laws had a slightly different character. Van der Borg explains:

> [In the Netherlands] the early use of municipal regulation of midwifery contributed to the recognition of the profession on a national level. There is evidence . . . that in other Western European countries this was less often the case . . . [in those] countries it took longer for midwives to achieve national regulation and recognition. This is especially true in

---

14. Significantly, midwifery in the Netherlands is still defined as a *medical* profession, distinguished from *paramedical* professions like physiotherapists, speech therapists, and dieticians *and* from professions like nursing and optometry.

England where there was no talk of government involvement with the occupation of midwifery until the end of the nineteenth century. In Germany and France there were isolated examples of municipal regulation of midwives [but] in these countries it was the church that played an important role in the control of midwives. (1992, 144)

Church-sponsored regulation was more concerned with assuring the good character of midwives than with their skills and education. After reviewing the early efforts to regulate midwifery in countries outside the Netherlands, Van der Borg (1992, 144) points out that the Dutch system of educating and regulating midwives gave the profession another advantage. Less regulated and less educated, "midwives in other Western European countries lacked the necessary protection from the competition of physicians and men-midwives who were becoming skilled in obstetrics."

Laws in the Netherlands provided midwives a place in the medical system and enabled them to consolidate their position as attendants in normal childbirth. Marland offers a concise summary of the distinct history of Dutch midwifery:

> The story of the Dutch midwife is not one of decline from the eighteenth century. Emphasis remained on reform, not replacement. Midwives were seen as being essential in the eighteenth century, all the better if they were *burgerlijke* [middle-class], respectable, well-trained, and a close eye kept on their activities. The functions of the midwife were curtailed in the eighteenth century—regulations forbidding her from using instruments were strengthened, her role in gynaecology and minor surgery undermined, her competence confined to normal births, falling under the supervision of doctors. *Yet her position as attendant in normal cases of childbirth was guaranteed, something not assured in other European countries.* . . . The eighteenth century laid the groundwork of a confirmation of the midwife's role in the nineteenth, with the *stadsvroedvrouwen* system forming the basis for the future organization of the midwife practice. In the nineteenth century emphasis remained on supervising the midwife's work and restricting her activities, rather than excluding her from practice. (1993b, 206, emphasis added)

In England, France, and Germany regulatory laws kept midwives on the margins of medicine. When, in the late nineteenth century, these states recognized the need to train midwives, that training occurred in maternity clinics, under the supervision of male doctors, further eroding the autonomy of the profession. Van der Borg explains:

> In the second half of the nineteenth century physicians [in other Western European countries] began to create maternity clinics. These clinics gave

men the opportunity to gain experience in obstetrics [and] as a result male obstetricians gained authority over the birth process . . . Because these maternity clinics were seen to be the necessary location for midwife training . . . midwives came under the direct authority and supervision of male obstetricians . . . Midwives became less qualified and lost their independence. (1992, 144–145)

Maternity clinics were also created in the Netherlands, but they had less influence on the practices of midwives. To understand why this was the case, and to better understand the current position of midwives, we must take a look at how Dutch midwives were educated in the nineteenth and twentieth centuries.

The Health Act of 1818 defined the midwives' sphere of competence but did little to ensure that midwives were competent. Concerned with the unreliability of training by apprenticeship, the legislature provided for the creation of "clinical schools" for the teaching of midwives. Between 1824 and 1828 six of these schools were opened, in Amsterdam, Rotterdam, Middelburg, Haarlem, Hoorn, and Alkmaar. These schools, however, were only partially successful in creating a uniformly trained midwifery workforce: In 1850, less than one-third of the 811 licensed midwives had been trained in these clinical schools (van Lieburg and Marland 1989).

A continued desire to improve the quality of midwifery care, especially in rural areas, led to the creation of state examinations in 1860 and, in 1861, the establishment of the first state school for midwives (*Rijkskweekschool voor Vroedvrouwen*) in Amsterdam. A second state school was opened in Rotterdam in 1882, and a Roman Catholic school was opened in Heerlen in 1912. These schools were an improvement on the clinical schools, both in the quality of education offered and in the number of students trained. Between 1861 and 1900 the Amsterdam school trained 1,143 students, and the Rotterdam school had 628 students between 1882 and 1900. In the early years of these schools, there was some worry about the quality of the students being recruited to the profession: Many entering students lacked a good basic education, often they had to be tutored in the basics of reading, writing, and arithmetic. But by the turn of the century, as a result of the expansion of secondary education for girls, new students were better prepared; in 1902 the midwifery schools began to use entrance exams.

The training program in these state schools lasted two years, during which time most students boarded on site. Topics included general anatomy and physiology, "special knowledge of the female parts," the care of infants and sick women, and both theoretical and practical midwifery. In 1920, a third year was added to midwifery training allowing further competence in infant and prenatal care.

Throughout the twentieth century, developments in obstetric science and improvements in midwifery education expanded the tasks permitted to midwives. In 1932, midwives were authorized to give advice and assistance to pregnant women in the second half of pregnancy, they were allowed to correct malpresentations externally, to take measures against sickness in pregnancy (under the direction of a doctor), and to give medicines (orally and by injection) in cases of weak contractions and bleeding. In 1951, the legal competency of midwives was further expanded to include the provision of prenatal care throughout the entire pregnancy, the drawing of blood, and the suturing of first- and second-degree perineal tears.

The 1960s marked a critical turning point in Dutch midwifery. During that decade a series of reforms in midwifery education were proposed: Had these proposed reforms been implemented, it is likely that the autonomous practice of midwifery in the Netherlands would have disappeared.

In the early 1960s, several important figures in Dutch obstetrics began to suggest that significant changes in midwifery education were needed. In his talk on the occasion of the 100th anniversary of the Rijkskweekschool voor Vroedvrouwen in Amsterdam, none other than Professor Kloosterman—regarded by many to be the champion of today's autonomous Dutch midwife—asserted that independent midwifery would, *and should*, eventually fade away:

> The midwife must give up part of her independence and more than in the past she must be prepared to share her responsibility and accept control and oversight of her work. She cannot and may not anticipate further expansion of her competencies. The boundary between "healthy and normal" and "not completely normal" is becoming more subtle . . . and it is possible that in the future we will no longer speak about "normal," instead we will use the word "optimal," making the terrain of the midwife . . . increasingly small. (Kloosterman 1961, 629)

Influenced by a model adopted in England, Kloosterman and others proposed a new educational program combining midwifery and nursing. Under the new plan, would-be midwives would complete a two-year nursing degree and then enroll in an 18-month course in midwifery.[15] In 1968 the government approved the new plan; in October of that year, the NRC Handelsblad (1968) announced, "Education of midwives: only nurses allowed to sit for exam."

In an interview in 1994, Dr. Jeanette Klomp, a gynecologist who worked at the midwife school in Amsterdam and was its director from 1970 to 1990, explained the events surrounding this proposed change:

In 1968 the government decreed that from August 1969 onwards only nurses would be admitted to midwifery training.

How did this happen?

In the beginning of the sixties, the end of the fifties, it was rather quiet here you know, and everyone still looked up to authorities and all that kind of thing. It was a nice, quiet period after the Second World War. And at the end of the fifties, the two midwifery organizations—we had two at that time, a Roman Catholic one and a neutral one—were quite desperate. For the number of practicing midwives was going down, the number of deliveries performed by midwives was going down, half of the young midwives disappeared after training—they went either to developing countries, or into nursing, or into quite other professions. If you look at the age distribution you'll have far more older midwives than younger ones. Under thirty years of age they were rather scarce. Because they didn't see any future in it.

The midwifery organizations did not see any solutions. So they wrote a letter, together, to the Minister of Health, or some other high authority in the Hague. They said, "We are desperate, please help us."

A few years later, the Department of Health instituted an inquiry among midwives, all practicing midwives, how their financial situation was and how they were working and how many deliveries they performed, and how they did or did not work together with GPs and other doctors, and so on.

---

15. I asked Kloosterman about his support for this planned combination of midwifery and nursing training. He replied: "Yes, that was a mistake (laughter). That was under the influence of British ideas, and also because of my cooperation with the Free University in Amsterdam. [The professor at] the Free University was very much against home confinements. I offered my outpatient service also for his students, but he refused this. He said, 'The future is for hospital confinements, and I will not educate my students in a home direction.' And I tried to compromise, and he tried to make a midwifery education in the Free University, in combination with nursing. And he asked me to give lectures for them. I did this for several years."

The results weren't very good . . . the whole situation wasn't very healthy. So then [the government] decided to have a committee to talk about it. "The position of the midwife in the Netherlands." On that committee were all the professors in obstetrics, some GPs, some other doctors and authorities from the department of Health and the *Geneeskundige Hoofdinspectie*,[16] and two midwives. Two midwives: the president of the Roman Catholic organization, and one of the neutral organization; but only the second one was active. So they were far outnumbered by doctors and other authorities.

This committee decided to get the training of midwives on a higher level. And what should that level be? That level should be first to be a nurse, to have completed a nursing training. For at that time it was felt—and that's very interesting too—that the progress of medical science was very big and very important, and that there even was progress in obstetrical science, and that now obstetrics was fitting into the whole picture of the medical science, and it was not just something apart from it, so it would be too difficult for midwives who had had three years of training to take that all in. In the future they never could practice midwifery independently, autonomously, as they had done before, so they had to fit in a medical team. How could they be fitted in medical teams? Well, to have them first trained as nurses, so they know about the medical teams and medicine, and then have them trained for midwives.

It was thought that the independent midwife would disappear. And that midwives would be working in hospitals, as they do in all other European countries, and well, help the doctor. They did not say it that way, but anyhow, that was the picture. They looked especially at England, where they were changing to the nurse-midwife.

After a few years of talks, at the end of 1965, it was definitely decided that only nurses would be admitted to midwifery training. And that they would get one-and-a-half years of training. It was not expected that the autonomous midwife would survive, but of course it would take a few years to have all people in hospital, and so on, so for the first years you still needed midwives, so they were training midwives, but it was expected that they would loose their autonomous position. It was at the beginning of 1966 that the final report of the committee appeared.

In 1966 and 1967 nothing happened, but then in 1968 the Minister of Health took the decision that he would accept the conclusion of the report and have only post-nursing training for midwives. And we had just one year to change over, you know, from the three-year training to one-and-a-half-year training.

---

16. Literally the "Head Medical Inspector," a government organization that oversees medical practice.

That was the end of 1968. We started negotiating with the Department of Health, how to change the whole program. But one thing was quite sure, that we needed more money. For you couldn't have your younger students take care of the post-partum mother, so we needed all kinds of qualified personnel, and had to intensify the training, and so on. So we asked for money, money, money. And then, in January 1969, civil servants of the department told us that there wasn't any money [laughter]. So it was decided to postpone the new training for one year and not to start with it until the end of 1970.

But in the meantime much, much, much had changed after 1966. Of course it was all a very gradual process. At that time, in 1968, 1969, there appeared to be a shortage of midwives, and the GPs were doing less and less obstetrics. So there were quite a lot of places in our country where people couldn't get any midwifery care any more. They had to go to a specialist, they had to go to hospital. And so in 1969 the Ziekenfondsen got very worried. And they wrote a letter to one of the advisory bodies of the government, the *Centrale Raad voor de Volksgezondheid*.[17]

The Centrale Raad took up the question asked by the Ziekenfondsen, and at the end of 1969 decided to study how the organization of maternity care should be in our country in the future. And that report appeared in 1972. In that 1972 report it was decided to try to keep home deliveries in Holland and that kind of thing.

According to Klomp, *money* played an important role in preserving the independent position of Dutch midwives. In the first instance, the government delayed the implementation of the new educational program because it was not prepared to pay for the expensive transition; and then, the Sick Funds complained that a decline in midwife-attended home births would drive the cost of maternity care to unacceptably high levels. But Klomp goes on to note that more than money was at work:

In 1968 and 1969 much was happening here. In society, you know, people didn't look up to authority any more; all was upside-down in the whole society, and I think in the whole Western world. Contraception was of course in the middle of the sixties very much involved. At the end of 1967 we started with abortions here in Amsterdam. Kloosterman started it. And the second feminist wave, or whatever you'd call it, just started. Women were organizing themselves to demand abortions and to demand all kinds of things. The authority of doctors was disappearing. There were all kinds of books about obstetricians and especially gyne-

17. The "Central Council for the Public Health," is an advisory body set up by the government. In 1982 this council was replaced by the *Nationale Raad voor de Volksgezondheid* (National Council for the Public Health).

cologists, how they were mistreating women. Everything was happening in that last three years or so of the sixties.

The authority of doctors was going down, and women were looking for other obstetrical help, and so they arrived at the midwife. This change came at the end of the 1960s, the beginning of the 1970s, that educated women were asking for midwifery help, and not doctors any more.

And of course, midwives are women too. Younger midwives, and other groups of midwives, in 1968, were frightened by the whole prospect of nurse-midwives. At the end of 1968, the beginning of 1969, a whole group of midwives started to talk about how to prevent the new training from happening. And they started to write letters to the Minister . . . a group of midwives of the two organizations were very active in trying to convince the Minister that he should not go on with nurse-midwifery training.

All these things together did something to convince the Minister. And in the end of 1970, in November 1970, he sent a message to parliament saying that in the future not only nurses could be trained to be midwives, but that he was renewing midwifery training, and that those who were not nurses could be trained too in future.

In her written summary of these events—contained in one of several *Klomp Cahiers* that describe critical points in the history of Dutch midwifery—Dr. Klomp (1994) unequivocally states that if the new nursing-based training had been instituted it would have been the end of independent midwives in the Netherlands. Indeed, she calls her report on these events, "The Sixties: The Midwife Nearly Disappears, Long Live the Midwife!"

After weathering this storm, midwifery education was not only reestablished as a training program for an independent profession, but gradually the leadership of important committees and institutions came into the hands of midwives themselves. Up until the early 1970s, the fate of midwives rested in the hands of committees and directorships dominated by men. Following the failed effort to blend nursing and midwifery, government commissions concerned with the work and education of midwives included a majority of midwives and women. For example, in 1987, the assistant secretary of health appointed a committee to recommend changes in the curriculum for student midwives: *Commissie Herziening Curriculum Opleiding tot Verloskundige* (Committee for the Revision of the Curriculum of Midwifery Schools). A man, Pieter Treffers—a well-known gynecologist and advocate of midwifery—chaired the committee, but all other members were midwives who were women. And by the early 1990s all three schools of midwifery were headed by midwives (Drenth 1998, 84–85).

Dutch midwives continue to be among the best-educated midwives in the world, a fact that is made more striking to many because midwifery education in the Netherlands remains *outside* the university. Those who wish to be midwives complete five years of secondary schooling and then apply to one of the four schools of midwifery, which are part of the Dutch "HBO" system-Higher Occupational Education (*Hoger Beroeps Onderwijs*).[18]

The number of students admitted to the four schools of midwifery is deliberately limited in order to guarantee every trained midwife a job (van Teijlingen 1994, 146). In the late 1990s approximately 1,000 applicants applied for the combined 120 openings for first-year students (Rooks 1997, 14); in 2000, responding to a growing shortage of midwives, the government expanded the number of openings for first-year students to 160. In 2001 the first-year class was further increased to 200; this number was upped to 240 for 2002 and scaled back to 220 in years 2003 through 2006 (Ministrie van Volksgezondheid, Welzijn, en Sport 2002).[19] The schools use a modified lottery system to select those to be admitted: Candidates are screened and those who are approved are put into a pool from which names are drawn.

In 1994 a fourth year was added to the midwifery curriculum. Midwife educators had long complained that they needed an additional year to allow better training in the conduct of scientific research and statistics. In its final report, issued in 1991, the Commissie Herziening Curriculum Opleiding tot Verloskundige

---

18. In the Netherlands, preparation for a career occurs in one of three institutions: WO (*Wetenschappelijk Onderwijs*, or Scientific Education; i.e., university education), HBO, and MBO (*Middelbaar Beroeps Onderwijs*, or Middle Occupational Education). HBO is required for midwives, accountants, managers, teachers, and so on; MBO prepares one to do police work, carpentry, plumbing, and the like. Each level requires a slightly different degree of secondary school preparation. For admission to WO, a student must have six years of preparation (in gymnasium, athenaeum, or lyceum), HBO requires five years of secondary school, and MBO students must complete four years of secondary education. A student interested in midwifery must include a specified number of science courses in her or his secondary school curriculum. In 1999 the educational system was slightly reorganized. See http://www.minocw.nl/english/index.html for details of the new system.

19. This latter increase coincided with the opening of the fourth midwifery school in Groningen. The school in Groningen is administered by the Amsterdam school.

agreed.[20] In his letter accompanying that report, Pieter Treffers made a plea for adding a fourth year:

> If the three year curriculum is maintained, we fear that insufficient time will be available for the necessary curriculum, so that parts will be insufficiently taught or ignored altogether. This will have important consequences for midwives. As an independent medical profession in the Netherlands, midwives have a key position in the obstetric care system. This system is unique and attracts attention from around the world. Essential for maintaining this system is a well-educated *eerstelijn* . . . that can prevent and possibly reduce medicalization. (Treffers 1992, 233)

The Ministry of Health, convinced of the need to maintain and enhance the professional position of midwives, eventually authorized a fourth year of education, which began in 1994.

During their four years of midwifery school, students are trained in antenatal and postnatal care; the management of normal "physiological" births (both at home and in the *polykliniek*); the identification of high-risk situations in the antepartum, intrapartum, and postpartum periods; and techniques of scientific research. In the first year the focus is on the normal physiological course of pregnancy, delivery, and postpartum period. In the second year, the curriculum shifts to obstetric pathology and related fields. In the third and fourth year students work on integrating the theoretical and practical knowledge acquired in the previous two years.

Midwifery students spend about half of their education learning in the classroom and at the "bedside" (i.e., clinical settings) and the other half apprenticing with a qualified midwife. Skills training is an important part of the curriculum, with particular emphasis on (1) diagnostic skills; (2) therapeutic skills; (3) skills needed to manage pregnancies; (4) laboratory skills; and (5) social skills.

Midwifery is the only medical profession in the Netherlands that locates its educational program in the HBO. Should the education of Dutch midwives be shifted to the university? Midwives and their supporters continue to struggle with this question. On the one hand, they recognize that the current system—the vocational school model of the

---

20. An English version of this report is available from the American Foundation for Maternal and Child Health, 439 E. 51st Street, New York, NY 10022.

HBO—protects their profession by sustaining a unique educational program that is directed by midwives, not physicians. This program imparts, if you will, "midwife knowledge" rather than "gynecologist knowledge." But, on the other hand, they are aware that university education brings with it a certain caché recognized by the public and by other professions.

I asked the director of one of the schools of midwifery if she thought midwives should be trained in the university. She responded:

> Well, I don't think so. I'm very glad with our training system and the sort of people attending this kind of school. There was a period that we had a different way of making out which one was coming to the school and which one wasn't. We tried to do some intelligence tests, but when you take the highest IQ, the most intelligent people, they very often have two left hands. They had the brains, but a midwife is not only good when she's got the brains, but she also has to do several things with her hands, and we had some problems when we had only *gymnasium* people [i.e., students trained in the highest level of secondary education]. That's generalizing, of course, but I think it's okay, the sort of people that are midwives at this moment.

She went on to add, however, that midwives strengthen their position among health care professions when they are skilled in research, prepared to do scientific studies that measure the success of their profession:

> But it would also be better when within the group of midwives there would be people doing more informal statistics . . . and *wetenschap en statistiek* [science and statistics]. Because very often they are talking about the midwives and the way they work, what they do, and the figures coming out of the care, and the ones talking about it are always other professionals and not midwives themselves. So, we [also need] scientific workers.

The issue of university education also came up in an interview with a teacher at a different school of midwifery. She too demonstrated some ambivalence about the move to university education:

> *In the Netherlands the training for midwives is not university-based. Do you wish it was?*
>
> Yes.
>
> *Why?*
>
> It gives more prestige to the profession, but it also provides more possibilities for the education. Yes, we have four years now so that's not so bad, but we want to have it university-based. I think it's because you want to make

it better every time, to improve it. Maybe, when you get a university-based education, maybe you become more independent, but maybe you're more influenced, I don't know. We don't want to be influenced, but maybe it will happen.

But why are we thinking about it? Because we know that the situation is going to change.

She went on to explain her fear that anticipated changes in the way HBO educational programs were organized would make it increasingly difficult for the four schools of midwifery to remain independent: She feared that midwifery might be demoted to the status of a paramedical profession. For her, university education was the way to preserve the autonomy of midwifery.

The tendency of modern society is to push midwives toward university education. This is happening in many other countries. In their review of the various models of midwifery education found in North America and northern Europe, Benoit et al. (2001) identify what they call "a trend toward higher education." The view is best represented by the comments of a Dutch gynecologist who is the head of obstetrics at a major university:

> I am convinced that within ten years the education of midwives will occur in a medical faculty [i.e., university]. This is our desire. But midwives do not yet share this desire. Why do I think midwife education belongs here? Our society is changing. At the university we now have separate specialists to educate us about attitude research, psychology, and ethics. Midwives can profit from this instruction as well.

He goes on to express his desire that *his* department be the location of midwifery education:

> I strongly desire for midwives to be kept up-to-date in the fascinating medical faculty here, where so much knowledge comes together, rather than have them in a separate school. Midwives are still a bit fearful of university education. . . . I am in no hurry. . . . I mention the idea every now and then, I write a piece on occasion. When I give a lecture I mention it *en passant*.

Dr. Klomp summarizes the push and pull between HBO and university education:

> I was asked by some midwives a few days ago, "Do you think we should have a university training?" Well, I'd never thought about it. . . . I think it should stay as it is: a practical training of four years. It has been, and I

hope it's staying that way, as soon as a midwife has done her final examinations, she is ready to practice extramurally, just on her own. I mean, she is a complete midwife when she finishes training.

But what I think is a very good thing, is that in the training now there is at least some time for statistics, reading articles and how to read them, the basis for ultrasound examination. They aren't ready for it all as soon as they finish training. They are midwives, well-trained midwives, who can do midwifery, but they have had a basis for other things. So the few of them that want it can go on to more scientific work, go on in ultrasound or whatever they want. And I do hope that within the next ten years or so we will have some midwives who write a thesis and get a doctorate in medicine. They are allowed to now. Our schooling system now allows them, with their midwifery training, to write a thesis and to get a doctorate at one of the universities. And then I hope we will get a few professors of midwifery, the normal physiology of pregnancy and delivery, who are midwives themselves.

In recent years there *have* been steps toward the *academisering* (making academic) of midwifery. In April 2002 the government gave its approval— and €450,000 per year support—to a masters program in midwifery, based at the Academic Medical Center in Amsterdam, in the hope of generating more scientific research on eerstelijn midwifery care (see http://www.min-vws.nl/document.html?folder=393&page=17660). In summer 2004 the midwifery school at Kerkrade moved into Maastricht, close to the Faculty of Medicine at the University of Maastricht. The school has not merged with the university, and the training will remain at the HBO level, but according to the director of the school, the new location will allow the *academiseren* of the education. The midwife school will be able to draw on the expertise of medical school faculty and share their special knowledge of verloskunde with medical students; as a result midwifery students will be better able to do research, allowing studies of eerstelijn health care to be done by those working in the eerstelijn (De Wit 2003).

The position of midwives in Dutch society also is maintained by their professional organization, the *Koninklijke Nederlandse Organisatie van Verloskundigen* (KNOV). Dutch midwives first organized in 1898, creating the *Bond van Vrouwelijke Verloskundigen* (Alliance of Female Midwives). In the early 1900s several splits, fusions, and reorganizations of the professional organization occurred, the most significant being the departure of Roman Catholic midwives for their own organization, the *R.-K. Bond van Vroedvrouwen* (The Roman Catholic Alliance of Midwives), formed in

1921. In 1926, the two major nonsectarian midwife associations joined together in the *Bond van Nederlandsche Vroedvrouwen* (Alliance of Dutch Midwives). These two organizations—"neutral" and Catholic—coexisted until 1975. In that year, they merged into one association: the *Nederlandse Organisatie van Verloskundigen* (Dutch Organization of Midwives). In June 1998, in recognition of the 100-year existence of organized midwifery, the NOV was crowned with the title *Koninklijk* (Royal) (see Croon 1998). Throughout their histories, organizations of Dutch midwives have given a sense of identity to the profession by organizing yearly meetings, publishing journals and newsletters, and representing the interests of midwives to the government, other professions, and the public.[21]

Thus we see the distinctive structural features of Dutch midwifery: It is a profession with a long history of regulation and education, with a legally defined sphere of practice, with unique and separate educational institutions, with a clear professional identity, and with a well-established professional association. We turn next to the work of kraamverzorgenden.

Kraamverzorgenden

Well-educated midwives depend on the assistance they receive from kraamverzorgenden, an occupation unique to the Netherlands. The demands on Dutch midwives are many, making it impossible for them to keep a close eye on the several women under their care who are recovering at home; kraamverzorgenden—postpartum caregivers, briefly described in Chapter 2—become the eyes and ears of the midwife, caring for women and their households while watching for any signs of illness in mother and child.

Dutch policymakers and government officials often remark that kraamverzorgenden are an important "pillar" of the maternity care system in their country.[22] In his research on postpartum care in the home, Kerssens (1991) suggests there are *two* pillars that support Dutch maternity care, the VIL (the indications list) and "good post-partum care in the home. Without good postpartum care at home we cannot ex-

---

21. For more information on the history of professional associations of midwives in the Netherlands see Drenth (1998). We will revisit the role of organized midwifery in chapter 4.

22. Recall that Hingstman (1994) lists "a well-organized system of comprehensive home care" as one of the four pillars that support Dutch obstetric care.

pect new mothers to receive their postpartum care outside of the hospital." He goes on to support his opinion by referring to a document published by the Dutch parliament: "Even the government regards postpartum care at home as an essential part of the organization of obstetric care. Without postpartum care in the home, birth at home is not thinkable" (Tweede Kamer 1988–89).

Recognizing the system of home care as an indispensable part of the Dutch way of birth, the Ministry of Health keeps a close eye on the state of the occupation delivering this care. In the late 1990s a shortage of kraamverzorgenden developed, causing concerns about the accessibility and quality of postpartum care (see LVT/NOV 1997). The minister of health responded by developing a plan to "resolve the bottlenecks in postpartum care" (Ministrie van Volksgezondheid, Welzijn, en Sport 1998). To that end, research (to better understand the causes of the problems) was begun, educational programs were revamped, and tariffs were restructured (see Borst-Eilers 2000a).

The unique occupation of postpartum caregiver has a long history in the Netherlands. Organized educational programs for kraamverzorgenden[23] began in 1899; in that year the Groene Kruis (Green Cross)—one of many "Cross Associations" in the Netherlands, organizations assembled and supported on the local level in order to provide home care, health education, centers for infants and toddlers, and the loan of medical aids—offered a course for these caregivers in Langedijk. In the early 1900s several other Cross Associations followed the example of the Groene Kruis and began to offer training to kraamverzorgenden. In 1926, the government issued a report on the education of kraamverzorgenden and established a one-and-a-half year education program; by 1940, 1,100 trained kraamverzorgenden were registered with the government. In 1943 a government committee, the Commissie inzake de Kraamhulp (Committee Concerning Postpartum Care) issued its Herzieningrapport (Revision Report); this report established kraamzorg as a recognized profession, created a uniform education for kraamverzorgenden, and laid the groundwork for a national network of

---

23. The original name for this occupation was kraamverzorgster. Although relatively few men work in this field, the name was recently changed to the gender-neutral kraamverzorgende.

kraamcentra, which would be responsible for organizing postpartum care in their region.[24]

As of 1998, there are a few different ways to become a kraamver-zorgende. The traditional route to this occupation requires a minimum of four years of secondary school followed by a three-year course of study at the MBO level. This post-secondary education includes training in general caregiving skills—clothing, bathing, and moving patients; providing information on health issues; noticing health problems; and maintaining contact with other caregivers—and specific training in care of the new mother and baby, other family members, and the tasks associated with the immediate postpartum period. In response to a shortage of these caregivers, the government created a second, short-ened training program that can be completed in 9 to 12 months by those already working in health care or 18 months for those with no experience in the health care system. Those who follow the traditional course can work in homes and in health care institutions; however, those finishing the short course are limited to working in homes (Wiegers and Beaujean 2002).

In his analysis of the role of kraamverzorgenden in Dutch mater-nity care, van Teijlingen (1990) notes that the availability of this kind of help allows women in the Netherlands to plan a home birth or a short-stay hospital birth, even if they do not have help from family, friends, or neighbors. This means that unlike Britain, where it is pos-sible to have the costs of birth at home paid by the National Health Service, home birth and short-stay births are available to *all* women, not just those in the middle class who have a network to assist them. In fact, 95 percent of women who get their babies at home or in the polyclinic use the services of a kraamverzorgende (Coffie, Wiegers, and Schellevis 2003).

Convinced that the *kraamzorg* system reduces the costs of care by free-ing up midwives and physicians, the Dutch government is eager to as-sure the quality and quantity of kraamverzorgenden. More than ten years ago van Teijlingen (1990, 365) invited health policymakers in other countries to take note, but to date none has, perhaps because there is no place for them in other systems.

---

24. See Creybas 1990 and Verbrugge 1968 for further details on the history of *kraam-zorg* in the in the Netherlands.

Gynecologists

To the casual observer, the practice of gynecology and obstetrics in the Netherlands looks identical to its practice in other European countries. When you watch a Dutch gynecologist at work in the clinic, she or he is indistinguishable from colleagues working in other highly advanced medical systems: They perform surgeries, do IVF (in vitro fertilization), and operate on unborn fetuses. And yet there is something peculiar about the practice of gynecology in the Netherlands. We have already seen that Dutch gynecologists have an unusual belief in the normality of birth and are content to consign those births to the care of midwives. This attitude helps to explain why the Dutch obstetric system continues to have the lowest rate of cesarean sections in Europe (see Figure 3-1). The training of Dutch gynecologists is also unusual. The obstetrics text that is used in all training programs in the country includes this statement:

> A form of organization in which everyone is forced to go to the hospital for delivery as in the United States, seems first to have put at the center the interests and preferences of doctors. The segregation of healthy expectant mothers at home . . . has a number of advantages: it underscores the physiological character of the event and stimulates the self-consciousness and self-reliance of the women in labor; the cozy and homey nature

FIGURE 3-1
Cesarean Section Rate (Procedures per 100 births, Selected Co

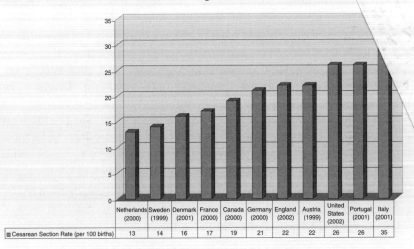

	Netherlands (2000)	Sweden (1999)	Denmark (2001)	France (2000)	Canada (2000)	Germany (2000)	England (2002)	Austria (1999)	United States (2002)	Portugal (2001)	Italy (2001)
■ Cesarean Section Rate (per 100 births)	13	14	16	17	19	21	22	22	26	26	35

Source: Declercq and Viisainen 2001.

of her environment, to which her husband also has total access, works in the same direction. (Kloosterman 1981, 390, quoted in Hiddinga 1993, 69)

You will not find a statement like this in any other obstetric text in any other country.

How can we explain these peculiarities of Dutch gynecology and obstetrics? It is wise to begin with history. In her review of the development of gynecology and obstetrics in the Netherlands, Hiddinga (1987; 1993) points out that, compared to its European neighbors, Dutch obstetric science was a late bloomer. This assessment is not original to Hiddinga. In the eighteenth and nineteenth centuries, Dutch professors of medicine expressed this same opinion. In his 1797 lecture celebrating his appointment as professor of surgery, medicine, and obstetrics at the university in Franeker, Johannes Mulder publicly wondered why "Dutch doctors seem to have contributed little to improve and expand knowledge in the fields of medicine and obstetrics." He concluded that the problem was inadequate education and insufficient legal controls on practice (Houtzager 1997, 3). A century later, in 1889, Mendes de Leon, a gynecologist in Amsterdam, offered the same opinion. He wrote, "Our fathers have shown that they were not strong leaders in [gynecology and obstetrics] (quoted in Houtzager 1997, 3).

Professorships in obstetrics did come late to the Netherlands. It is true that the University of Leiden appointed Simon Thomas as "extraordinary professor of obstetrics" in 1848, but elsewhere in the Netherlands professorships in obstetrics were combined with those in surgery up until the 1860s. In that decade, the universities of Amsterdam, Utrecht, and Groningen created separate chairs in obstetrics.

Dutch gynecologists also were slow to organize and, once established, their professional association remained quite small for decades. The *Nederlandse Gynaecologische Vereniging* (NGV, Dutch Gynecological Association) was founded in 1887; two years later NGV began publication of the *Nederlands Tijdscrift voor Verloskunde en Gynaecolgie* (NTvVG, Dutch Journal for Obstetrics and Gynecology). In 1919 the NGV had only eighteen members, by 1938 that number had grown to just eighty-eight. Hiddinga notes that at the early meetings of the NGV, typically attended by only seven or eight members, conviviality and science were mixed in equal measure. She quotes from the minutes of the NGV (in Hiddinga 1993, 64):

In accordance with the jovial character that typified our meetings, we often examined patients difficult to diagnose, and all who were present took part in the discussion. . . . Eating together, a thing that sociable doctors fortunately have always appreciated, seduced us in 1901 not to meet at all in July, but instead to have a feast for no other reason, as is mentioned in the minutes, than that summer is here.

The *Tijdschrift* also had a difficult beginning. Obstetricians from other European countries marveled that the journal could be kept going in such a small linguistic area, and, indeed, the minutes of the NGV note the following complaint from the journal's editors: "Once again it has to be stated openly here that more than once the editorial board had to deal with such a dearth of copy that it was not always possible to publish a volume in time (quoted in Hiddinga 1993, 64)." The vast majority of the references included in the articles published before 1900 came from outside the Netherlands: further evidence of the place of Dutch obstetrics in European medicine (see Hiddinga 1993, 57).

The development of obstetric science in the Netherlands also was hindered by a lack of clinical settings for the study of obstetrics and gynecology and by the absence of government support for research. The orientation toward home birth that prevailed in the Netherlands resulted in a paucity of clinical births, and hence, little opportunity for research. At the turn of the last century, the clinic at the University of Amsterdam, the largest maternity clinic in the country, was handling only around 500 births per year (Marland 1993a, 33). This fact, coupled with the lack of government support for laboratory research, led many Dutch gynecologists to seek training in Germany where the laboratories were well equipped and where clinical material was plentiful.

Today, at the beginning of the twenty-first century, Dutch obstetrics has caught up with the larger, international scientific community. Hospitals are larger and more births are occurring there—hence more "clinical material" is available—and the government is generous in its support of research. Dutch gynecologists are now regular contributors to the science of their profession, presenting and publishing papers in the "ordinary science" of obstetrics and gynecology as well as papers that review the unique situation in their country.[25]

But the modernization process occurred slowly. Up until the late 1950s there were only four university departments of obstetrics and

---

25. See Chapter 6 for more information on the science of obstetrics in the Netherlands.

gynecology, and through the 1950s and on into the 1960s a high percentage of doctoral students continued to write their dissertations in Dutch. The editors of the *Nederlands Tijdscrift voor Verloskunde en Gynaecologie* were also slow to give up on this Dutch language journal, even though—as they watched many interesting articles being offered to foreign journals—they recognized the need to join the larger professional discussion occurring outside of the Netherlands. In 1970, the editors finally reestablished the NTvVG as an English language journal, the *European Journal of Obstetrics, Gynecology and Reproductive Biology,* but the last issue of the Dutch version was accompanied by "words of sorrow and grief" (Hiddinga 1993, 71).

Modern or not, vestiges of the history of Dutch gynecology remain in current day practices. In my interviews with gynecologists and midwives, I was eager to explore these vestiges, to discover how the distinctive features of this specialty were passed on to new generations of practitioners.

Substantively, the training of gynecologists in the Netherlands is quite similar to the training gynecologists receive in other modern countries. Those who wish to enter medicine must complete six years of secondary school; they then apply directly to one of the eight universities that have medical faculties.[26] Selection for admission to medical school is accomplished with a modified lottery system: students are chosen randomly, but the odds of being chosen are increased by a good performance in secondary school. General medical education lasts six years, after which students are awarded a *basis-arts* (basic-doctor) degree. After receiving this (undergraduate) degree, a student must specialize, completing an additional three years of training—for family medicine/general practice or for a public health specialty—or four to six years of training for one of 28 clinical specialties. Training in gynecology lasts six years.

The government, in cooperation with the NVOG, controls the number of students admitted to gynecological training and the workloads they are given. The gynecologist and board member of the NVOG whose comments opened this chapter told me,

There's a real strict regulation [of the number of students accepted for training]. . . . We have a committee and they've said: "Well, every uni-

---

26. See Smal (1997) for a more complete discussion of medical education in the Netherlands.

versity hospital and its cluster, the other hospitals around it, may have 24 doctors in training."

There are eight training programs so that is . . . 192 students?

There are a little bit less, so it might be 180 now.

Does that include the people who started 6 years ago and the people who started just this year?

Yes. So there are about one sixth of that 192 a year, so it's about 36 a year or so.

That's quite a select group.

Yes, that's a select group. . . . We very strictly regulate it, and we control it. . . . Each program has to write to the board [of the NVOG] how many they have in training, and how many they will have in training on the 1st of January next year.

In an effort to balance supply and demand—walking the line between shortages and oversupply (and thus overuse) of specialist care—the government sponsors regular counts of practicing gynecologists and estimates of the need for specialists in the future (see, for example, van der Velden, Bennema-Broos, and Hingstman 2001).

The government also is making an effort to make the training of medical specialists more humane. I asked a gynecologist about the working hours of medical residents in the Netherlands:

In the United States residencies are, as you might have heard, considered to be hell. These people are made to work incredibly long hours, without sleep. Is it similar here?

It was like that, when I was in training. I have carried, for a long time, my overwork paper in my *portemonnee* [wallet], because people didn't want to believe that in one month I had one week of 122 hours work, and the next week was really very nice, it was only 67, and the next week was about 84 and then about 90. [My overwork paper] had a signature from the University that it was correct. . . . When then somebody asked me and said "Ah, well, it won't be true. 122?" And then I could show them this paper. Now . . . it's arranged by the law that assistants in training may only work for about 48 hours a week.

And that really happens?

No, it doesn't really happen, because it is not workable. You cannot say, "I think the baby is coming, but I'm sorry". . . most of them work about 55 hours a week. And they are always free of their duty the day after they work the night. So, you cannot work more than 24 hours straight. There has to be a break.

Do you think it's better?

A lot better . . . when you do your tenth delivery after 24 hours work, even if you're very experienced, it's not the best delivery . . . I can assure you . . . but there has to be *een evenwicht* [a balance]. You have to find a way to make it workable. You can't say to somebody: "Well, I go home, lady. I stop the procedure now and somebody else is coming on duty." So you have to be a little flexible.

What about the content of Dutch obstetrical education? When asked to describe the distinctive feature of gynecological training in the Netherlands, a gynecologist responded:

I don't know exactly if there is really a difference in the specific training. . . . I don't think that really there is a large difference between countries . . . every doctor, every gynecologist learns to do a delivery, learns to do a forceps, to do a cesarean, to do a laparoscopy, to take out a uterus. . . . So I don't think it is extremely different.

But this gynecologist learned his trade in the Netherlands and, not having examined obstetrical education elsewhere, he is unaware of the many subtle ways the Dutch way of birth seeps into the training of students. As we have already seen, the Dutch obstetrics/gynecology text encourages students to organize birth around the interests of the mother, not the physician. This same text also distinguishes "active" and "expectative" approaches to birth. The *active approach* assumes that all women, even those identified as "low risk" need "intensive monitoring in a hospital, often need medication and pain relief, often or always need an episiotomy, and frequently end in an artificial delivery [i.e., vacuum, forceps or cesarean]" (Kloosterman and Thiery 1977, 200). The text continues:

Others, over and against this approach (and in no other country in the Western world is this group so large and so strongly represented as in the Netherlands) begin from the standpoint that birth, for a healthy, carefully selected woman, almost never requires intervention and that attendance at such a birth can remain limited to the offering of moral support and careful monitoring with simple equipment. This is the e*xpectative approach* to birth.

The opinion of the authors about these two approaches is revealed in a later paragraph that more fully describes the expectative approach:

The departure point is that a physiologically occurring birth is optimal and cannot be improved. It is possible to intervene in certain aspects of this process (we can speed the process with drugs or instruments, we can use medication to lessen or eliminate the sensations of pain), but in the end we will always find that the obstetrical goal (a healthy child in the arms of a healthy, uninjured, happy mother) is not promoted by these interventions, but is, in fact, threatened by them.

Unlike any other obstetrics text intended for physicians who will practice in modern medical systems, this text also describes how to accompany a home birth and includes a list of the equipment needed (see Kloosterman and Thiery 1977, 216–217). Clearly, Dutch students of gynecology are given a uniquely Dutch view of birth and their role in it.

Another obvious and important difference in the training of gynecologists in the Netherlands is that their education occurs in a system that has a strong and independent profession of midwifery. Not only must gynecologists-in-training develop ways of cooperating with midwives, but by training with midwives they are exposed to an approach to birth that eschews obstetrical intervention. In their training as *basisarts*, medical students are often taught by midwives and, as residents, many student gynecologists work with midwives. My interviews yielded different responses with regard to amount and effect of this co-training. Dr. Klomp, the former director of the midwife school in Amsterdam, had this to say:

Do you think that obstetrician-gynecologists are trained differently in the Netherlands with respect to midwives? Is there something in their training that allows them to be more accepting of midwife care?

Yes, I mean, the phenomenon of midwives has always been with us. So we're used to, day and night, to receive women who are sent in to us by midwives. Even if the ideology of midwifery is not accepted by the professors, the phenomenon of midwife is always present. . . . Whether or not you like it, it's a fact.

Do gynecologists train with midwives?

No, they don't train with midwives. They're supposed to do the more simple work, I think, in the beginning of their training, but that's only in the beginning. I think the gap between midwives and doctors is getting deeper. And I'm quite convinced that obstetricians just don't know about normal deliveries.

A midwife, who teaches at the Amsterdam midwifery school, echoes these comments and makes a plea for more interaction between midwives and gynecologists in training:

> Up until now we have the luck that a lot of obstetricians and gynecologists are very aware of the importance of the Dutch system. They have confidence in midwives. But there are also a lot of gynecologists who haven't met midwives in their training, who are not familiar with this profession.
>
> *Dutch gynecologists?*
>
> Ja. So they think: "It's weird, those people are doing some things at home. Oooh, it's dangerous, they don't have a CTG [ultrasound scans]." And then, what they remember is those people going from home to the hospital; those situations where you can say: "Hmmm, could have been better." And they say: "You see, those midwives, they are doing irresponsible work." So I think it's very important that every gynecologist is doing a traineeship in a midwifery practice. So that they can see how midwives are working. How they are doing it; what their knowledge is.
>
> I think that the two professions must work together more, and must learn from each other. In some regions there is such a clash between the two professions, that the midwives are, eh, they are making fights with the gynecologists, and vice versa. They don't trust each other: "When I'm sending one of my patients I don't get her back!" There is no confidence, and I think that's important.

Research done in the Netherlands confirms that working with midwives changes the attitudes and practices of gynecologists. In their study of a sample of obstetrical units in Dutch hospitals, Pel and Heres (1995) discovered that the presence of midwives consistently lowered the use of cesarean section, episiotomy, induction, and forceps delivery. They conclude that having midwives around decreases intervention rates in two ways (116): "firstly by the midwives' continuous social support to the parturient women . . . secondly . . . midwives, by asking for justification for medical intervention, compel the obstetricians to strict adherence to [the protocols of] medicine."

Other of my interviewees noted that student gynecologists' views of birth and midwives are significantly shaped by the attitudes of their professors. A midwife, who now works in a government agency, offered the following observation:

> In obstetrics there's a difference between the south of the Netherlands, particularly Limburg, and the rest of Holland in more hospital deliveries and

more medical indications for transfers to the hospital. I have thought about why this happened. It has to do with several things, I think. It is near Belgium, it is near Germany, where there is another culture of giving birth than we know. And most gynecologists working in Limburg are trained in Nijmegen, and Nijmegen is well-known for its anti-home delivery attitude.

Are you referring to Professor Eskes?[27]

Yes, Eskes. The last few years he does not speak so loud about it, he lowered his voice a little bit about it, but it *was* true. And I think the training you have had as a gynecologist is very *bepalend* [determinative]: when you are trained in a certain way, it is a very essential part of your behavior in your profession; the ideas you have got during your study.

A professor of gynecology agrees:

[Students] have to be influenced by the people who are training them. [Students often want] to be like a clone of their professor. There are a lot of [students who] don't make their own opinion about how to work together with midwives.

So, sometimes you see a school, for example, the Free University, in that school obstetrics is: "There's a patient who is ill, who has to get a baby." And two kilometers away is the University of Amsterdam, where they say, "Somebody who is pregnant is a very healthy woman. She has proved to be healthy because she's got pregnant. And she's only ill when she's proved to be ill." Do you know what I mean?

Yes. So it is possible for you, when watching a gynecologist at work, to say without knowing the doctor's past: "This person is from the University of Amsterdam, and that person is from the Free University?"

Yes, yes. If you work together with them for three days you know . . . who their professor was, where they were trained.

I was also interested to learn how many students got their training abroad. If a large number of students leave the Netherlands for their pre- or post-doctoral training, it will undoubtedly result in the importation of a more medical approach to birth. I asked a professor of gynecology about this:

27. T.K.A.B. Eskes was well-known in the obstetric community of the Netherlands as an opponent of midwife-attended home birth. His attitude has since softened. See Chapter 6 for more details on the home birth debate among Dutch gynecologists.

Does anyone go abroad for training? You mentioned that there were a few doctors here from abroad, but do people go to England, or to the United States?

Only for small periods. For post-doctoral work, but also in training sometimes for a few months. But it's not really common. You can ask for a sabbatical year. . . . If you for your investigation you need to work [abroad] . . . the registration committee for a specialization says, "Okay, you can quit for a year and do your investigation and go on," but it's not regular.

So it is not happening enough that you would say the Dutch system will be influenced by a number of doctors getting part of their training abroad?

No, no.

Dutch gynecologists are well aware of their peculiar standing in the international community of obstetric specialists. One gynecologist, commenting on an oft-heard complaint of midwives—that she and her colleagues are too quick to intervene—said, "Our midwives will say that the Dutch gynecologists do too many cesarean sections, too many forceps, and so on. . . . Compared to the *midwives* we are American doctors [but] compared to our American colleagues, *we* are midwives, I think." Another gynecologist points out how odd it is that she prefers births to end normally:

> True, it's only exciting [for gynecologists] when there is something wrong. But still—and I think that's the difference between . . . me . . . and the big bulk of obstetricians—when I was called for a more or less complicated case, and I could end it normally. I mean, I could take some measures and see the baby born spontaneously in good condition and so on. I liked that far more than doing a cesarean. . . . It's nice to be called by a midwife and then try to judge "what can I do" and have it end normally, spontaneously.

We now have a good sense of how the professional and educational systems of the Netherlands create the caregivers needed to maintain the Dutch way of birth. Before we close our consideration of the structural supports of maternity care in the Netherlands we must briefly examine two other items: record-keeping systems and the physical infrastructure of Dutch health care.

KEEPING TRACK

The policies and professional and educational systems that support Dutch maternity care are kept in place by careful monitoring of how the system is working. We can learn much about what a society values by looking at what (it) counts and how the counting is done.

The Dutch are famous for their meticulous record keeping, and their records of births—including information about mothers and the attendant, location, and outcome of birth—are no exception. Regular records are kept by the *Centraal Bureau voor de Statistiek* (CBS), and the government and professional associations fund separate studies to monitor practices, workloads, demand for service, and supply of practitioners.

The best-known and most complete registry of information is the *Landelijk Verloskunde Registratie* (LVR, the National Perinatal Database), which collects detailed data from midwives and huisartsen[28] (in the LVR-1) and gynecologists (in the LVR-2). Begun in 1982 as a joint initiative of the midwife association (NOV), the gynecologist association (NVOG), the *Inspectie Gezondheidszorg* (IGZ, Inspectorate of Health Care), and *SIG Zorginformatie* (SIG Health care information), the LVR gathers information on over 80 percent of all births in the Netherlands. The registry includes demographic data on pregnant and birthing women and on nearly every aspect of the care given them including, among others: age, parity, ethnicity, length of pregnancy, birth weight, presentation, Apgar score, birth defect, mortality, morbidity, place of birth, attendant, referral to specialist care (and the reasons for referral), cesarean sections and other artificial deliveries, and multiple births. These numbers give a complete picture of obstetric care in the Netherlands, but, because participation is voluntary, they cannot be used as an accurate representation of nationwide trends.[29] In fact, the presentation of nationwide data is a *secondary* purpose of this registry: Its primary purpose is "to stimulate a consistent form of quality control for individual care providers and professional groups involved in obstetric care" by "stimulat[ing] peer review between colleague care providers in primary and secondary care" (SIG 1996, 99). To that end, LVR data are given to regional groups of practitioners, allowing them to

---

28. However, the participation of huisartsen in the LVR is extremely limited (see SIG 1996, 12–24, 100).

29. Participation in the LVR by both midwives and gynecologists is improving: In 1989, 76 percent of midwives and 73 percent of gynecologists were involved; by 1993 these numbers had grown to 88 percent of midwives and 87 percent of gynecologists (SIG 1996, 15).

see how their practices match up with other practices and with national totals. To date, only three summaries of the LVR have been published (SIG 1990; 1992; 1996); data from the LVR were used in a 2002 report on home birth in the Netherlands prepared by the TNO (*Nederlandse Organisatie voor Toegepast-Natuurwetenschappelijk Onderzoek*, the Netherlands Organization for Applied Scientific Research).

It is the CBS that is responsible for collecting and presenting nationwide data on birth and obstetric caregivers. Data on birth are included in the *Vademecum Gezondheidsstatistiek Nederland* (Collection of Health Statistics, Netherlands) and in a variety of special reports (see www.cbs.nl). These data come from various sources ranging from the *Gemeentelijk Basisadministratie Persoonsgegevens* (GBA, Municipally Administered Personal Data; it is obligatory for residents of the Netherlands to report births and deaths to their local government) to various regularly administered surveys of representative samples of the population including *Het Onderzoek Gezinsforming* (Research on Family Formation) and *Permanent Onderzoek Leefsituatie* (POLS, Continuing Research on Life Situation) (see CBS 1999). The *Vademecum* presents data on many aspects of birth: age of mother, parity, single and multiple births, nationality, birth weight and length, place of birth, cesarean sections, and use of contraceptives.

In 1994 an interesting change occurred in record keeping for births. One of the more important government records of birth is the CBS report, *Geborenen naar Aard Verloskundige Hulp en Plaats van Geboorte* ("Births by source of obstetric help and place of birth"). For decades this was *the* record of Dutch maternity care showing *who* was accompanying births and *where* these births were occurring. The data were gathered along with GBA (Municipally Administered Personal Data) at the municipal level. When a family member came in to report the birth—in most cases the father—the respondent was asked to fill in an additional card reporting where the birth had taken place and who had accompanied the birth. These cards were then sent to the CBS and compiled in the yearly report referred to above. In 1994, the CBS decided to "automate" (computerize) the municipal data collection system and, for reasons that could not be explained to me, the new form did not include questions about place of birth and caregiver. With the help of a researcher from the *Sociaal en Cultureel Plan Bureau* (Social and Cultural Planning Office),

Mevrouw Josette Hessing-Wagner, I inquired further into the reasons for this change. It seems in the process of automating the system, this information simply dropped out. We were told that this information

- Was not relevant to the purpose of the GBA (the GBA was intended to collect demographic data, not health data);
- Was never really part of the GBA (it was collected on a separate card);
- Had the potential to invade the privacy of citizens; and
- Was available from other sources, namely the CBS sample surveys and the LVR.

It is for these reasons that you will always find an asterisk on birth data from the Netherlands after 1993.

Another important source of information about the birth system is found in registries and records of the number of professionals in practice and in training. In cooperation with the professional associations of midwives and gynecologists the NIVEL has set up a data collection system that allows for ongoing assessment of the state of these two professions; the NIVEL uses these data to produce regular reports and—after combining these data with data on fertility rates, working habits of caregivers, new technologies, and new policies—to estimate the number of professionals needed in the future (see NIVEL 1998, 1999; Hingstman et al. 1992, 1994; Hingstman and Kenens 2002; van der Velden and Hingstman 1999; van der Velden, Bennema-Broos, and Hingstman 2001; Wiegers, van der Velden, and Hingstman 2002). The Vademecum of the CBS also reports numbers of working professionals and professionals in training (CBS 1999, 197–210).

Finally, the government and professional associations sponsor occasional research projects to answer questions about the condition of the maternity care system. Most recently, the government has sponsored research on the workloads of midwives (Jabaaij et al. 1994; Wiegers and Coffie 2002), issues affecting women's choice of caregiver and place of birth (Wiegers 1997), bottlenecks in obstetric care (Wiegers et al. 1999), an inventory of obstetrically active huisartsen (Wiegers and Hingstman 1999a), and midwives' departure and reentry into the profession (Wiegers and Hingstman 1999b).

The counting and monitoring of Dutch obstetrics reflects a general concern with the stability of the system and a specific concern with how both patients and occupational groups are faring. The government is interested in providing quality care in an efficient manner, while professional associations are interested in protecting and enhancing their position in the larger obstetric market. In any case, the counting that goes on helps to maintain the system.

ROADS AND HOSPITALS: THE PHYSICAL INFRASTRUCTURE

In looking at the variety of *social* structures that support Dutch maternity care, it is easy to overlook the obvious fact that the system needs a *physical* infrastructure to survive. Nearly all of my interviewees included the geography of the Netherlands, the quality of its roads, and the location of its hospitals among the reasons for the continued presence and success of the unique Dutch obstetrical system.

I often was told that there is no spot in the Netherlands that is more than 20 minutes from a hospital. I suspect that this is not literally true, but it is likely that very few residents of the Netherlands are more than 30 minutes from hospital care.[30] This network of hospitals is important for the maintenance of birth care in the Netherlands because it allows easy and quick transfer of home birth mothers to the care of a specialist.

There is a move in the Netherlands to consolidate specialists' practices and to close smaller hospitals, developments that cause some to fear for the future of Dutch home birth. Jouke van der Zee (2000), the director of NIVEL and a supporter of the Dutch system, observes:

> Home birth in the Netherlands is threatened by . . . the process of concentration of gynaecologists and pediatricians/neonatologists in bigger groups and more specialized hospitals which leave the common general hospital without sufficient expertise in the domain of specialized birth care. This is a real threat to home deliveries because the hospital next door might not be available in case the delivery at home meets complications.

In his inaugural address, celebrating his appointment as professor of obstetrics at the University of Maastricht, J. G. Nijhuis (2000, 17) offered the same prediction, saying that the closure of small hospitals (as a result of mergers) and the consequent increase in the distance between home and hospital makes home birth "irresponsible":

---

30. Those who live on Texel, an island in the Waddenzee must rely on the ferry to get them to the hospital in Den Helder. If a woman needs transport, the ferry will take her immediately, ignoring its schedule and even turning back to the island if it is in mid-trip.

Minister [of Health] Borst has already said that we in the Netherlands must return to a maximum of 40–60 hospitals and this will have immediate consequences. The distance to the large, consolidated hospitals shall become such that home birth in parts of our country will become irresponsible. Transport during the birth, for example, will become more complicated and take longer because of the increase in traffic congestion.

In its report on Nijhuis's address, the *Nederlands Dagblad* (2000) summarized his comments with this colorful phrase: "Mergers in the hospital world are 'choking the neck' of the Dutch system of home birth." Indeed, a year later the newspaper in Twente reported that "home birth is becoming a bit more difficult" as a result of the closing of the gynecology department at a local hospital (*Twentsche Courant* 2001).

Clearly, geographic conditions are important to the Dutch way of birth, but geography can only be a *necessary* condition for the preservation of home birth, it is hardly a *sufficient* cause. Having conducive geography, or ways of overcoming geographic problems, is not enough to prevent birth from moving to the hospital. Other small countries— for example, Belgium, the Netherlands' neighbor to the south—have eschewed birth at home. To understand the relatively slow movement of Dutch births to the hospital, we must look beyond geography.[31]

In Sum

The several structures that support the Dutch way of birth analyzed here are clearly interdependent. Insurance regulations and professional policies grew up in physical infrastructures that allowed for easy communication and transport between home and hospital, and, in turn, these rules promoted and sustained the maintenance of that infrastructure. The same is true for the relationship between the development of professional groups, the rules of practice, and the records kept.

Lying behind all these relationships, and only hinted at until now, are the political arrangements—the power to decide and to influence policy, record-keeping, and hospital networks—of Dutch health care. It is to this important structural feature of the maternity care/health care system that we now turn.

---

31. This is not to imply that countries with less hospitable geographies could not create systems of home births. Most residents of urban areas in developed nations are within easy reach of hospital care.

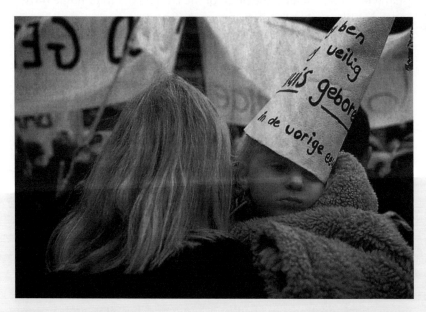

Mother and baby at a March 2000 demonstration for midwives. The child's hat says, "I was safely born at home in the last century." Reproduced by permission from ANP, the Netherlands.

4   The Politics of Care

AT THE stroke of midnight on 31 December 1999, while the rest of Europe was celebrating the dawn of the new millennium, midwives in Amsterdam were out on strike. Between 10 P.M. on the last day of the last century and 2 A.M. on the first day of the new century, midwives in the city refused to deliver babies at home or in the polyclinic. Women in Amsterdam whose babies arrived in that four-hour window of time had to travel to the midwife school at the *Slotervaart* Hospital, where temporary delivery rooms were set up and staffed by midwives who had volunteered for duty. Midwives planned this work stoppage to call attention to their heavy workloads and poor salaries.

It was a savvy strategy. Midwives knew that every news agency in the country was planning to run a story on the first baby of the new century. They anticipated that their plea to improve the working conditions of midwives would be piggybacked on these cute stories. They were right. A few news organizations *did* offer separate coverage of the strike—*Radio Nederland Wereldomroep* (RNW, Dutch Radio World Broadcast) devoted a few lines to "Short strike by midwives in Amsterdam" (RNW, 31 December 1999)—but the big newspapers tucked news of the strike into their articles about millennium babies. The *Volkskrant*, a national newspaper based in Amsterdam, mentioned the strike in its story, "Waiting for the millennium baby with candles and a wooden fetoscope [*toeter*]" (*Volkskrant*, 3 January 2000), and Rotterdam's *NRC Handelsblad* covered the strike in its humorously titled piece, "The first millennium placenta" (*NRC Handelsbad*, 3 January 2000).

The New Year's Eve strike was the first round in the midwives' organized protest against high workloads and low salaries. At noon on Sunday, 26 March 2000, a group of 40 midwives in the Hague began a similar work stoppage by symbolically turning in their midwife bags and other tools of the trade. From noon until midnight midwives refused to attend births at home or in the polyclinic; as in Amsterdam, extra delivery rooms were prepared in a local hospital, and three midwives stood ready to accompany the births of women who otherwise would have delivered at home.

March 2000 was a month of protests for midwives, all timed to coincide with a parliamentary debate about the "crisis in midwife care," scheduled for the 30th of the month. In the weeks leading up to the debate, midwives held public demonstrations in cities throughout the Netherlands, including Breda, Gouda, Leiden, and the Hague. On the day of the debate, 2,000 midwives and their supporters converged on the *Binnenhof*, home of the Dutch parliament, and loudly protested against their working conditions. The demonstration had something of a party atmosphere. Protestors waved banners:

> *Verloskundigen uitgeperst*
> *meer poen*
> *anders is het niet te doen*

(Midwives squeezed, more "dough," otherwise nothing can be done)

> *Verloskundigen verlossen u van uw baby's,*
> *maar wie verlost hen van de werkdruk?*

(Midwives deliver your babies, but who will deliver them from the [high] workload?)

Midwives passed out balloons declaring, *Help De Verloskundigen!* (Help the Midwives!), *Wij Willen Meer Vroedvrouwen* (We Want More Midwives). Dutch singer Angela Groothuis entertained the crowd and activist Astrid Seriese loudly called the names of *haar vroedvrouwen* (her midwives) asking the assembly to do the same. Clients, politicians, *huisartsen*, and specialists took to the podium to defend midwives and support their claim for better working conditions.

Why all this commotion? As we have seen, midwives in the Netherlands are the envy of midwives around the world: They are well-educated, they are free to practice in a variety of settings—home, polyclinic, and hospital—and they have a great deal of autonomy and independence. In the Netherlands, midwifery is a *medical*—not a *paramedical*—profession: Midwives need no supervision from a specialist physician. Given their strong position in Dutch health care, why did midwives feel the need to mount a nationwide demonstration?

Over the last decade Dutch midwives began to recognize that they were overworked and underpaid. They remained proud of their unique position in the world, but they noticed that they were working very hard and were not earning a salary commensurate with their status and responsibility. Up until 1994 midwives were expected to accompany 165 births per year: The government established an expected yearly salary for midwives and that amount was then divided by 165, called the "standard workload" or *normpraktijk*,[1] to arrive at the remuneration given for each birth (complete with pre- and postnatal care). Midwives working elsewhere in the world were flabbergasted when told of this expectation—165 births per year? Complete with prenatal and postnatal care? With (on average) approximately half of those occurring in women's homes? Even a clinic-based midwife, who has the advantage of attending several women at the same time in the same place, would find it difficult to supervise that many births in one year. And for this daunting amount of work, midwives were paid Dfl 65,000 per year (approximately €30,000[2], far less than salary given to other medical professionals).

In the course of the parliamentary debate on that last Thursday in March, Els Borst, the minister of health, tacitly admitted that she had long recognized the plight of midwives. She said, "Midwives have been very late to sound the alarm bell . . . in the last years they have kept themselves busy with the quality of their profession and not with their income position" (quoted in Berkelmans 2000, 336). To be fair, the ministry had taken some steps to deal with high workloads and burnout among midwives. In 1992, responding to a request of the NOV (Dutch Organization of Midwives), the ministry financed a study of work and workloads among independent midwives. The subsequent report, published in 1994, confirmed that midwives were being overworked; the authors noted that midwives who wished to work only 40 hours per week must limit themselves to 117 births per year (see Jabaaij et al. 1994; Bakker et al. 1996). As a result of this research, the minister reduced the yearly workload to 150 births (still a daunting number) and increased the number of students accepted to the three schools of midwifery from 90 to 120.

---

1. See Scheerder 1997 for a complete discussion of the way health professionals in the Netherlands are paid.

2. In 1994, the guilder (Dfl) was the unit of currency. For the sake of consistency, I will convert guilders to euros, using the 2.2 conversion rate fixed when the euro was introduced on 1 January 2002.

In the days before the demonstration and debate, Borst announced that she would further reduce the midwives' workload, to 120 births per year, and open up an additional 40 places for first-year midwifery students. Even so, the minister came under heavy criticism for waiting so long to take action and for giving insufficient attention to the salaries of midwives. The chairperson of the parliamentary committee holding the hearing (*Vaste Commissee voor Volksgezondheid, Welzijn, en Sport*, Permanent Committee for Public Health, Welfare, and Sport) accused Borst of waiting until "five minutes before midnight" to "pull a solution out of the magician's hat." Several members of the committee pressured the minister to lower the normpraktijk to 90 births per year and to increase the remuneration for each birth so that midwives' salaries were brought up to Dfl 120,000 (€54,600).

In spite of this and other scattered voices of disapproval, midwives seemed quite pleased with the result of the work stoppages and demonstrations they organized on their own behalf. The vice-chair of the KNOV commented,

> The actions, and especially the demonstration in the Hague, have had a positive effect on our profession and on our image with the public. . . . We collected 50,000 signatures, sent an "action bus" on a tour through the country. . . . The strikes in the Hague and in Leiden received the full attention of the media. The strikes resulted in the KNOV receiving an invitation from minister Borst to have a discussion before the debates in parliament. The demonstration in the Hague was the absolute high point: 2000 people were in attendance. (Van Crimpen 2000, 437)

In her letter to the Parliament's Permanent Committee for Public Health, Welfare, and Sport, explaining the changes, Minister Borst (2000b, 1) noted, "Pregnant women who wish to give birth at home must be able to make this choice. This clear directive for midwife care is my intrinsic policy goal. Bottlenecks that threaten this goal must be eliminated."

The new regulations took effect on 1 July 2000. The normpraktijk was reduced to 120; the tariffs were increased, pushing the norm salary from Dfl 65,000 (€30,000) to nearly Dfl 100,000 (€45,500); *District Verloskundige Platforms* (DVPs; Regional Midwife Support Offices) were created—offices that will help midwives reduce the number of hours spent in activities not related to client care, such as negotiations with insurers and hospitals; and in September 2000, 160 new students (as opposed to 120 the previous year) began their studies in midwifery. Because of continued concern about the shortage of midwives, the Ministry of Health, Welfare, and Sport further expanded midwifery education in September 2001, authorizing a fourth school in the Northern part of the country—in Groningen—thereby expanding the number of places for first-year students to 200, with further increases in the following years (240 in 2002 and 220 for years 2003 through 2006). These strikes, protests, and government acquiescences to midwife demands show undiminished support for a profession that, elsewhere in the world, struggles for official recognition—not to mention financial assistance. The success of Dutch midwives in the *Binnenhof* shows them to have political power not commonly found in an occupation that is dominated by women and lacks the prestige of a university education. The structures we reviewed in Chapter 3—the insurance system, the *primaat*, the VIL, the educational system, and the arrangements between professions—are sustained by the unique political system of the Netherlands. To understand this important *structural* support for Dutch midwifery, we must look to the way power is distributed in the Netherlands, both on the national level and within the health care and maternity care professions.

POLITICS IN THE NETHERLANDS[3]

Students of the professions in the United States, well-versed in the way powerful professional groups use their influence to create policies that promote and protect their interests, are surprised by the many government decisions that favor midwives over physicians. How is it that a prestigious group of physicians lacks the power to shape government decisions in a way that favors their interests? In the United States those who wish to see midwifery and the opportunity for home birth expanded have been repeatedly defeated by powerful medical lobbies (De Vries 1996).

---

3. This is a very brief description of a large topic. For further information see Shetter 1997, Andeweg and Irwin 1993, and Rochon 1999. The Web site for the Dutch embassy offers an official description of the political system in the Netherlands, see http://www.netherlands-embassy.org/fn_country.html.

As we have already seen, the training of Dutch gynecologists makes them less inclined than their American counterparts to expand their scope of practice at the expense of midwives; but *if* the NVOG decided to embark on a campaign to solidify and extend the power of gynecologists over midwives, they would find it extremely difficult. In the United States, wealth and prestige are easily wielded to garner favorable legislation. Lax campaign financing laws allow monied organizations to gain legislative favors in exchange for the hefty contributions politicians need to be (re)elected. By way of contrast, the political organization of the Netherlands, with its parliamentary government and electoral system, make it very difficult to buy influence.

The Dutch parliament consists of two houses: the First Chamber (*Eerste Kamer*) has 75 members who are elected by provincial councils and whose duties include discussion and review of legislation; the Second Chamber (*Tweede Kamer*), where the true political power of the country lies, has 150 members who are chosen by direct elections held every four years.

In all national and regional elections, the Dutch use a system of proportional representation, where seats are allocated to political parties in accordance with the percentage of votes received; for example, if a party wins 10 percent of the vote, it will occupy 10 percent of the seats in the representative assembly. A Dutch ballot presents the voter with a list of candidates arranged by party; the voter chooses one person and votes are then tallied, first by *party* and second by *person*. In parliamentary elections, the quota that is used to determine how many seats are allocated to each party is devised by dividing the total number of valid votes by 150 (the number of seats). The party fills those seats with its highest vote-getters and with party members high on the list of candidates.

It can take as little as 0.66 percent of the overall vote to obtain a seat, a fact that allows a large number of political parties and movements to flourish. Ten parties currently sit in the Tweede Kamer (see Table 4-1). There are three large political parties in the Netherlands: the PvdA (Labour Party), CDA (Christian Democratic Alliance), and VVD (People's Party for Freedom and Democracy). The PvdA was founded in 1946 and has its roots in the trade union movement. Its aim is to be a social democratic party with supporters in all social classes. The CDA was formed in 1980 as a merger of three confessional parties: the Catholic People's Party, the Anti-Revolutionary Party, and the Christian

Historical Union. These parties had been cooperating for some years in response to secularization in Dutch society, and, for the most part, the CDA bases its policies on religious principles. The VVD, founded in 1948, represents the conservative[4] tradition in Dutch politics. The smaller parties represented in Parliament are the left-leaning liberal Democrats '66 (D66); the Green Left Alliance (a merger of communists, pacifists, and greens); the small left-wing Socialist Party; the fundamentalist Protestant SGP, the Protestant Union (a merger of two conservative parties: the GPV, Reformed Political Alliance, and the RPF, Reformed Political Federation); and the Pim Fortuyn List (the remnants of the party established by the charismatic Pim Fortuyn, who was assassinated in May 2002).

The funds needed to keep these political parties running are collected by means of membership dues. Some parties receive business donations, which they must declare, but individual members of parliament may *not* accept such donations.

After the elections to the Tweede Kamer have been held, the existing government resigns and various party leaders in the parliament, who think they can form a coalition government that will control a majority in parliament, begin a process of negotiation. A person called a *formateur* is

TABLE 4-1

Seats and Parties in the Tweede Kamer

Seats in the House of Representatives

Political Parties	1994	1998	2002	2003
Christian Democratic Alliance (CDA)	34	29	43	44
Dutch Labour Party (PvdA)	37	45	23	42
People's Party for Freedom and Democracy (VVD)	31	38	24	28
Socialist Party (SP)	2	5	9	9
Pim Fortuyn List (LPF)	—	—	26	8
Green Left Alliance (PPR, PSP, and CPN)	5	11	10	8
Democrats '66 (D66)	24	14	7	6
Protestant Union (GPV and RPF)	—	—	4	3
Calvinist Political Party (SGP)	2	3	2	2
Liveable Netherlands	—	—	2	0
Total	150	150	150	150

Source: http://www.netherlands-embassy.org/ (accessed 24 April 2003).

---

4. What we in the United States see as *conservative*, the Dutch refer to as the *liberal* tradition, referring to an economic liberalism that calls for a minimal role for the state.

appointed by the Queen to consult with each party regarding possible coalition partners. It usually takes several weeks before the formateur—the architect of the new coalition—successfully organizes a new government. The current government of the Netherlands, headed by Prime Minister Jan Balkenende, is a coalition of the CDA, the VVD, and the D66.

Several features of this system make it difficult for lobbyists, whether they are representatives of professional groups or other interests, to control policy decisions. The large number of active and successful political parties in the Netherlands requires negotiations and alliances between groups in the formation of government, assuring representation of a variety of interests and complicating the work of lobbying groups. In a winner-take-all system, lobbyists can go directly to the party in charge; in the Netherlands, those who wish to influence policy have to find a way to appeal to parties from the left, the center, *and* the right. The Dutch system also makes it difficult to "buy" politicians: Votes are counted first by party, not by persons, and donations to individual candidates are not allowed. Reelection to office does not depend on getting large sums of money, rather it is based on effectiveness of representing the interests of constituents.

Mirroring the structure of politics, government agencies are carefully organized to give representation to all interested parties. The Sick Fund Council is a good example of this democratic representation. For more than 35 years—until its reorganization as the *College voor Zorgverzekeringen* (CVZ, the Board for Care Insurance) in 1999[5]—the Sick Fund Council made the important decisions about what sort of care was to be offered, by whom, and for what fee. By statute, the 35 members of this council included representatives from employers, unions, caregivers (of all sorts), hospitals, patient organizations, insurance companies, and the government. Each representative had an equal voice, and negotiation and compromise were used to reach decisions. Thus, *if* Dutch gynecologists had wished to move all births to the hospital they would have been forced to argue, on equal footing, with those who desired to protect the choice to give birth at home, including Dutch midwives, consumer groups, insurance companies, and government officials.[6]

---

5. See chapter 3, note 9.

6. The former minister of health summarizes this situation (Borst-Eilers 1997, 18): "Embedded in a long history of consensual processes of consultation and policy debate, health policies are shaped by the interaction between government and organized interest groups."

Some have characterized the Dutch way of sharing power as a *democracy of interests,* a system that guarantees a voice to all who have a stake in a particular issue or policy. This style of government, characterized by negotiation and accommodation, has played an important role in preserving home birth and the autonomy of midwives.

In his study of the "politics of accommodation" in the Netherlands, Lijphart (1968; 1975) classifies the type of democracy practiced there as *consociational.* According to Lijphart, consociational democracy emerges in nations with a *segmented society* and a *cooperative elite.* Those who are unfamiliar with the social and political history of the Netherlands might find it odd to hear this country described as segmented. Looking in from the outside, Dutch society seems homogenous. But up until the 1960s, the Dutch population was clearly and cleanly divided into groups described by the Dutch as "pillars" (*zuilen*). The roots of *pillarization* (*verzuiling*) go back to the Reformation, but the pillarized system blossomed fully in the late nineteenth century with the rise of socialist and liberal pillars. Gladdish explains:

> Originating in the 1880s when confessional movements sought to mobilise their followers into self-conscious communities, [pillarization] became in the 1920s the dominant and most conspicuous feature of social organisation. Trade unions, educational bodies, welfare schemes, cultural associations and the media, all became orchestrated on the basis of would-be hermetic pillars topped by political parties. (1991, 28)

Hooker adds,

> At the height of *verzuiling,* almost all social activities were voluntarily segregated on the basis of philosophical views. For instance, there were separate Catholic, Protestant, Liberal, and Socialist sports clubs, newspapers, schools, insurance companies, labor unions, agricultural associations, and political parties. The *zuilen* did not start to break down until the 1960s. (1999, 46)

During the period when Dutch society was fully pillarized, the government was forced to find a way to incorporate the interests of each pillar in its decision making; as a result a series of informal "rules of the political game" (Lijphart 1968, 122–138) emerged, rules that encouraged negotiation and accommodation. In the 1960s and 1970s the pillars began to disappear, but the rules of politics remained. The Dutch inclination toward a politics of accommodation is most clearly seen in the widespread use of "external advisory commissions" (EACs) in policymaking. EACs are created by the government to offer advice on new initiatives or revisions of existing regulations; EAC members include representatives of interest groups as well as civil servants and academics considered to be experts in the policy area under consideration.

Rochon points out, "As the number of confessional organizations in [Dutch] society has declined . . . the role of confessional organizations in EACs has shrunk in favor of EACs composed of representatives from various professional associations" (1999, 165). Because EACs give professional organizations and other interest groups direct access to the policymaking process, the incentive to use money to enhance access is eliminated. This results in more balanced deliberations between competing professions. Rochon explains,

> Formalization of the role of EACs in the policy development process—that is, making them part of the corporatist system . . . has the side benefit of making it unnecessary for interest-group representatives to pour money into politics in order to gain access to the policy making process. The relatively low cost of Dutch electoral campaigns is due to many factors . . . but the availability of institutionalized access to the policy process . . . contributes to the small role of money in politics by eliminating much interest-group incentive to make contributions. (1999, 166)

The midwives and physicians I spoke with were well aware of how the "democracy of interests" in the Netherlands influenced the way maternity care was delivered. Politically astute Dutch midwives, those who had seen how laws governing maternity care professions were made elsewhere, recognized the protection they are afforded by the way power is distributed in their society. One of the more outspoken midwives in the Netherlands told me,

> Physicians [in the United States] have such political power . . . and such cultural power too, I would say. . . . With that power they can . . . convince people that all births should be hospitalized, "this is dangerous, you know, home birth is only for people who are partly crazy and . . ." And that's convincing, because of their political and cultural power.

> In the Netherlands, gynecologists . . . have cultural power, I think. They're widely respected, but they cannot . . . go to the Ziekenfondsraad and convince this group that all births should be in a hospital.

> *Why do you think Dutch gynecologists lack that power?*

I think because of the way decisions are made about health care here . . . the Netherlands is called the "democracy of interests". . . . With all our *raads*, these councils, there's this scrupulous attention to making sure that the unions are represented, the *werkgevers* (employers) are represented, the insurance companies, private, public, the *hulpverleners* (caregivers), so everybody, every interest is represented. . . . There's 1,000 midwives and 6,000 *huisartsen*. There is a huisarts-interest and a midwife-interest, and they can meet together and talk, and one cannot win over the other automatically. In the United States . . . the obstetricians have money to give the politicians. . . . That's a democracy of money and prestige, in America.

Do you think it is more democratic in the Netherlands?

In that sense, yes. Midwives have a seat on the Ziekenfondsraad, and the gynecologists *niet* [not]. The LSV has a seat, the *Landelijke Specialisten Vereniging* (National Specialists Association), but they represent pediatricians and internists and cardiologists and . . . so they have one seat for all of those, and the midwives have their own seat. So it just won't happen that they could come in some day, the LSV, and say: "All births should be moved to the hospitals." Because that's just one voice. And then you have the insurance companies and they're saying "How much does this cost?" And then you have a midwife who is saying "I don't think so" and you have the *werkgevers* (employers) and the unions saying "The costs might be [too high]." It just cannot happen.

For their part, physicians recognize that their power is *limited* by the Dutch concern to allow all interested parties a voice in policymaking. A representative of the *Landelijke Huisartsen Vereniging* (LHV, National Huisartsen Association) explained,

[It] is the "democracy of interests," the former Secretary of Health Care has said once, when he was confronted with the system here. All the interests are lobbying together. . . . There is always an immense circling around of interests, but none is given the advantage.

So huisartsen have no stronger voice than midwives.

Ja . . . people are seeing the necessity of the advantages of the midwife being cheaper, being at home [and] we [i.e., huisartsen] haven't got the access to politics, to the policies as you [in America] have as chairman of the Ways and Means Committee.

We're a society of very slow change. We experiment and we try to see good habits being translated into legislation. Which is also a *remmende* (braking) factor, it slows down developments. The lawmaking process in the health care system is very slow. It's very difficult with all these special interest groups . . . they're all lobbying in the Hague and circling around, but not like usual . . . when there is a change, it is normally backed by all parties, and all groups.

Which takes a long time.

Ja.

POLITICS IN MEDICAL AND MATERNITY CARE

The larger political environment of the Netherlands sets the tone for political negotiations elsewhere in Dutch society.[7] Policy decisions regarding labor, housing, education, transportation, and other public issues involve all stakeholders in a process of negotiation, accommodation, and compromise. This does not suggest that all parties are always satisfied with the outcome or that negotiations are always calm and civil. In the case of maternity care policy, we have already hinted at two lingering conflicts:[8] (1) a disagreement between midwives and huisartsen over the primaat and (2) gynecologists' refusal to approve the VIL. Because maternity care in the Netherlands is so well organized, we are tempted to conclude that midwives, huisartsen, and gynecologists get along well, cooperating in a friendly manner, each respecting the roles assigned to the other by government policy. But these two long-standing arguments between professions remind us this is not the case. Even though both of these conflicts have now been resolved, a closer look at their history and the process that resulted in resolution allows us to see how the politics of the professions shape Dutch obstetrics.

The Primaat

It is no surprise to discover that the two *eerstelijn* providers of maternity care in the Netherlands have long struggled with each other. It is also not surprising that much of this struggle has revolved around the primaat—a regulation that advantaged midwives by requiring women to seek midwife care if it was available in their neighborhood. While it was in place, huisartsen believed that they and their clients were disadvantaged by the regulation and they often felt that midwives used

---

7. See Giaimo (2002) for a broader consideration of how political structures affect medical systems and medical reform.

8. See Chapter 3.

the primaat capriciously and abusively. In my interview with Dr. T. Dorresteijn, the first secretary of the VVAH (Association of Obstetrically Active Huisarts), he described one such case for me:

> Some years ago there came two midwives in Dokkum,[9] but the huisart-sen there kept all the [maternity] patients for their own. So they were accused [by the midwives] and they were taken to the court. The two midwives were supported by the NOV. They accused the huisartsen of *oneerlijke concurrentie*. Unrighteous. [Literally, "dishonest competition."] Well, the midwives were in *het gelijk gesteld* [their action against the huisartsen was upheld]. They got their rights.

> Then the whole matter was transferred to the *Europese Hof* (European Court) in Strasbourg. And there the huisartsen got their rights. And later on they have agreed to come to this *samenwerkingsverband* (agreement for collaboration). The patients . . . can choose the midwife or the huisarts. When the huisartsen do the deliveries they are, eh . . . the money is collected from the sick fund by the midwives and 70 percent of it goes to the huisarts, and 30 percent they [i.e., the midwives] can keep as compensation.

> *Even though the midwives might do nothing? If they don't see the woman for prenatal or postnatal care? They still keep 30 percent?*

> Yes.

Needless to say, Dorresteijn found this compromise *oneerlijk* (dishonest).

These feelings on the part of huisartsen have a long history. In 1963, a huisarts touched off a broad discussion of the primaat when *Medisch Contact*, a weekly journal for Dutch physicians, published his complaint about the use of the primaat by a midwife who moved to his town. He and his partner had a well-organized practice, including prenatal, obstetric, and infant care, in a rural area:

> One day a young woman came to one of our villages [and] hung up her shingle, *"Verloskundige"* (midwife), and proclaimed that our practice, and the practices of two neighboring colleagues, were her "work area." We protested. What medical interest is the young woman serv-

9. It is significant that this episode took place in the Frisian town of Dokkum. Dokkum was the home of the much-celebrated early eighteenth century Dutch midwife, Catharina Schrader. Schrader kept a detailed record of her practice and her life— *Memoryboek van de Vrouwens*—which has been edited and published in Dutch (van Lieburg 1984) and English (Marland 1987), giving us a well-documented glimpse of obstetric practice in her era.

ing? On what grounds was this part of our income taken over? It is depressing to come home from an exciting birth and to think that you have done it all for nothing. But the interest of the young woman from the city is, in our village, completely protected. (Huisarts 1963, 95)

I questioned Mevrouw Zwart, who was then the executive director of the KNOV, about the more recent case—the one involving the two midwives in Dokkum. Her response highlights the midwife/huisarts difference of opinion about the primaat: Huisartsen often said the primaat was created to save money, but midwives asserted that the primaat was designed to promote quality of care by allowing the most experienced birth attendants—midwives—to provide care at birth:

> *Dr. Dorrestijn told me a story about some huisartsen practicing in Dokkum. Two verloskundigen in a nearby village decided to extend their area, causing these doctors to lose their Ziekenfonds reimbursement for accompanying birth. Do you think this is reasonable?*

> I know the case he is talking about. . . . If you take a huisarts who does only eight or six births per year, I must ask myself about the quality of that care. If, during your office hours, you see one woman who is six months pregnant, and then you must wait another half-year until you see another woman at that same stage of pregnancy, that is naturally completely different from the practice of a midwife where a number of women at the same stage of pregnancy arrive for prenatal care every day. Everyday midwives are busy with prenatal care. I think you must look at this fact if you want to figure out what is reasonable in this situation.

I heard, in my many discussions about the primaat with midwives and huisartsen, a standard set of responses about why one caregiver was to be preferred over the other. Huisartsen stressed the value of continuity of care, and midwives emphasized the importance of the expertise that comes from experience.

These comments from a representative of the *Landelijke Huisartsen Vereniging* (LHV) summarize the case made by many huisartsen, that it is important for a woman and her caregiver to have a long-standing relationship:

> [When a woman goes to a huisarts] it is someone she has known for a long time . . . she has been his patient for a long time, and then she knows: "I trust this [doctor]." When she goes to a midwife she doesn't know her. She never has seen the person . . . [all she knows is] "when you're becoming pregnant you have to go to a certain address where a lady is who says she is a midwife, and she can deliver your baby" and that's the most

dramatic experience, in my words. It's new to her. She is not assured. I hope her help is good, but . . . when you're going to your doctor, you've known him already for years, and you know how he reacts, you know his voice, his face and his treatment. You've heard of course in your neighborhood how he, how he worked with the other deliveries. What are the experiences [of] women in the neighborhood. So the atmosphere or expectation about the abilities of the huisarts I think are quite different from the expectations of what to get from the midwife. And those are all factors that contribute I think to the assurance that when the doctor is in charge you can feel safe. These are the small things, but they build together the position of the delivery at home system in the Netherlands, I think.

This last comment, about building the system of home birth in the Netherlands, reflects another argument that was often made by huisartsen, that huisarts care at birth is more inclined toward home and, thus, more economical. In the same interview the LHV representative explains why huisartsen are better equipped to keep women from unnecessary trips to the hospital and the specialist:

There is a special link between the huisarts and the patient . . . when the patient wants to go to a doctor, free of charge, he has to go to the doctor who he has registered with. And the Sick Fund is paying to give that help. So you have to go always to the same doctor. Who has known you, who knows your problem, he knows your father, maybe your mother, your sisters, your environment, your employer maybe. So he knows you and he has known you for years. So that's, I think, one of the reasons why you have to move through so many channels before you can go to the hospital . . . or to a specialist. Because you have to argue your case before your GP, before you may move. He allows you, in a way, to move to the hospital. The doctor, the huisarts, has learned that part of his job is to keep the people out of the hospital—that's the way we see them, eh, that's the general feeling that you have to keep people as long as possible out of the hospital, the "second line." And that means arguing with patients. The patient may get angry, and you have to learn to cope with it, and maybe they become aggressive, because they want to have a prescription now and they want to have a specialist now. But you have to learn to cope with that problem, to teach your patients not to want too much at the same time, and take it at ease and come back tomorrow and we'll see what the situation is then. And that is also part of this system.

The research of Dr. M. Springer, professor of general medicine in Leiden, was often used to support these observations. Springer (1991, 1987) examined the obstetric practices of a number of huisarts and discovered that compared to midwives, huisartsen are *more* likely to accompany births at home and *less* likely to refer a woman to specialist care. The easy conclusion of this research is that maternity care by the huisarts is *cheaper* than care given by midwives, undermining the value of the primaat as a cost-saving measure.

Midwives insisted that the primaat was not primarily about saving money, it was about ensuring the quality of care. As Zwart noted, huisartsen are too busy with their practices to gain the experience needed to accompany birth: Six or eight births a year are too few to maintain the expertise needed to be a competent birth attendant. An Amsterdam midwife concurred:

> *Do you think it's important that the midwives keep the* primaat?

> Ja. Because you know, most of the *huis*-doctors don't know anything about pregnancy. . . . I prefer that *huisartsen* concentrate more on what their profession might be. Because, eh, here in Amsterdam, when somebody calls a huisarts, it can take days before this huisarts will come to see the patient. And I think they should do their own work, more correctly. And then they got enough to do.

Dr. O. Bleker, professor of obstetrics at the University of Amsterdam, agreed:

> A huisarts must have a specific minimal number [of births] per year. And otherwise he should be so wise as to stop it. . . . Practical obstetrics, of the eerstelijn, is midwifery. Beyond any doubt. . . . Some GPs obviously are very well able to do normal pregnancy and delivery adequately [but] a minimum per year is indicated then, for instance 15 or 20. That's more than most of them are doing . . . in practice now."

What about Springer's data on huisarts-accompanied births? Is it true that care by the huisarts is cheaper than midwife care? Zwart, from the KNOV, had this to say:

> *What do you think of Professor Springer's research? He is making the point that a government interested in saving money would notice that huisartsen are a better bargain.*

> The doctors that do obstetrics are, in general, working in rural areas. Thus, if you wish to compare, you must compare midwives working in rural areas with *huisartsen* working in rural areas.

> *He didn't do this?*

> No. So you cannot say, "Better care is given by *huisarts* that do obstetrics." I do not believe it. . . . He said that increasingly few *huisartsen* are doing obstetrics, but those that do are doing almost all births at home. That is true only because obstetrically active huisartsen are more often working in rural

areas where people are still accustomed to birthing at home. Thus, you must also compare areas.[10]

Frustrated by the continuing disagreement, and spurred on by the VVAH, in March of 1994 the LHV began a legal procedure against the *staat* (the Dutch government) to have the primaat removed.[11] A lawyer employed by the LHV explains:

I've heard that the LHV is working to remove that primaat.

For us it's, eh . . . The *Ziekenfondswet* (Sick Fund Law) was established in the war, by the Germans. But the thinking had been going on for years, of course. And one of the things the Germans, or under the German occupation I should say, established was the primaat of the verloskundige, the midwife. And probably in those years they [i.e., the midwives] were the lesser factor and also the *zwakke partij* (weak party), the underdog, in that discussion. And the general practitioners had big practices, so they didn't mind too much when a midwife came in their area. But the numbers of midwives were always small, and the birth rate was high. And each doctor, each huisarts, had his deliveries. Quite a lot. But in due time the population growth diminished . . . and the number of midwives grew. . . . those factors are combining into a struggle in the rural areas where a midwife establishes herself, because the primaat has a consequence that the Sick Funds ends the agreement with the doctor for his deliveries. That's a consequence.

When a midwife establishes herself in your vicinity, the sick fund ends the agreement on the deliveries, *de verloskunde praktijk* (obstetrics practice), and the patients have to move, have to go to the midwife when they want to have their delivery in *natura*. That's their insurance package. And of course the huisarts opposes to this, but when the law is the law, the Sick Fund has to do what the law says, and as a consequence he loses 60 percent of his [maternity care] population; as far as this *obstetrie* (obstetrics) is concerned there remains 40 percent.[12] But his experience, as the Germans say his *Fingerspitzengefühl* he has to see quite a lot of patients so he can remain [keep] his marksmanship, because a childbirth is quite an experience. And when he starts to lose his grip, his knowledge on this field, because he doesn't do it any more with 60 percent but 40 percent, he thinks . . . "We can't

---

10. De Miranda (1996) and the *Werkgroep Verloskunde 2000* (1996) made this same argument in their evaluations of Springer's research.

11. The LHV brought their case against the state (i.e., the Dutch government), not against the midwives or their organization, because it is the state that promulgated and enforces the primaat.

12. Recall that the primaat applies only to women insured under the Ziekenfonds, actually about 64 percent of the population.

do it any more for the 40," and the midwife takes the other 40 percent privately insured patients. And that's still going on, a steadily growing erosion of the tasks of the huisarts doing deliveries at home.

And it has gone on such a—unnoticed almost—on such a scale that almost, I believe, only 20 percent of the Dutch huisartsen does do verloskunde (obstetrics) still. And the ladies are creeping in, and they are saying that it is a natural job, and so on, and so on, and so on. And that is the main reason. The law, also. There is nothing left but the law, and that's the reason why the LHV has decided about half a year ago to take it to court. That will take about two years, to see what's happening, what our supreme court will say about it.

You're taking this case to the supreme court?

No, no, not yet, but it is a Hague court, and then it's to an appeal court, and then I think we're coming to the high court. Not directly, no, no. But the importance of the matter is such that in all probability it will end there [in the high court].

Is the Ziekenfondsraad *involved in this legal action? Do they have an opinion?*

The Ziekenfondsraad is first of all the *toezichthouder* (an oversight organization); it has to control and check the applying of the law by the sick funds. That is the prime task of the Ziekenfondsraad. To observe and watch and criticize the sick funds for their task. And as the Ziekenfondsen are only applying the law, the Ziekenfondsraad also has no opinion.

Really?

Maybe the individuals, but officially not. They are a bit pro the midwife. Because of the underdog position. . . . We are always cheering the loser, the smaller party.[13]

Before the legal action was taken, did the LHV consult with the (K)NOV?

Quite a number of times, but they are *onvermurwbaar* (unyielding). Thanks to the primaat in the law, they are gaining. And it would be unwise, I think, of them when you find out that you're winning in the end

---

13. This estimation appears to have been correct. A staff member of the Sick Fund Council admitted to me, "In Holland, for centuries midwives have been doing the work perfectly. And they know everything about that part of the work, and it has grown into the current system, and so we say 'Well, let them do it. The GP has a lot of other work to do.' But I can imagine that some GPs like to do it very much. That is possible. But it's some kind of employment policy, you know. When all those GPs do the births, the midwife is gone." When I asked why the LHV was pursuing this case he replied, "I think it is [for] purely financial [reasons]."

to give up your greatest . . . *troef* (trump card). . . . They are prepared to do all kinds of things, opening up practices of midwives . . . [helping] GPs [gain] experience and so on and so on. And talk and talk and talk, but nothing like a joint venture to the parliament, to the government, to abolish the primaat. In about 10 years I think there is hardly any huisarts anymore who will be doing obstetrics. That's a black scenario, I know, but some people say it's going to be like that.

On 27 December 1995, the court in the Hague found in favor of the LHV, declaring that as of 1 January 1999 the primaat would no longer be in effect: Women insured by the Sick Funds would be free to choose between a midwife and a huisarts. A spokesperson for the LHV responded to the decision (*NRC Weekeditie* 1996, 3): "All efforts to work with midwives to find a solution failed. It is very important that patients now will have a free choice." But, as the lawyer at the LHV predicted, this decision was not the end of the story. The government was not pleased with the decision and appealed to a higher court.[14]

Midwives have a slightly different perspective on the proceedings. Mevrouw Zwart of the KNOV offered this view of the events leading up to and surrounding the court decision:

> The huisartsen said that the [Dutch] state had never intended this law [i.e., the primaat] to exist. But the law has been in place since 1966. Before this time there was no law, but a *ziekenfondsenbesluit* (Sick Funds policy). And the origin of that policy lies in the Second World War. 1941. Thus the LHV claimed, "This is a rule of an occupying government."

> But that is not true, because when the Germans established this rule they looked at the policies under consideration in the Netherlands and it was those policies they put into place. Thus the primaat was a Dutch idea. And after the war, all policies put in place during the occupation were reviewed to see which should be maintained. In 1946/1947 the Dutch government said: "We will keep this policy [the primaat] and other policies we will allow to expire." And that decision lasted until 1966 when the primaat became a definite law.

> *So the LHV claimed that the primaat should be thrown out because it was established under the occupation.*

---

14. The appeal delayed the lifting of the primaat, but after lengthy negotiations, it was decided that in the interest of preserving home birth—which required more trained attendants, that is, both midwives and huisarts—the primaat should be lifted.

Ja. I recently read a very interesting article that said, "If the LHV argues this point it could very well become a boomerang, because the way huisartsen practice today is the result of the very same policy."[15]

What happened at the hearing?

I was there. And when the judge asked: Why was this rule established?" the lawyer for the huisartsen said: "It was only about money. Economic motives. And its continued existence hinders competition."

The judge then asked the government attorney the same question, and she had no other answer. She said: "Yes, economic motives."

Economic motives for the state?

Ja. It was cheaper to pay the midwife than the huisarts. But that was just a very small part of the argument. The most important part was: the quality of the midwife is better than the huisarts. And that argument was never made. So I jumped up and asked if I could say something. And the judge said . . ."Refused." So I sat down.

We had given the government attorney all the articles and arguments relevant to our position. . . . But she was not ready with the information. I think she was too weak—one must go to America for a real, quality lawyer [laughter].

When the case was over, it was declared that the midwife in the Netherlands is in such a good position that the primaat is no longer needed. We agreed with the first conclusion and were happy, but we were not happy that the primaat was abolished.

After the decision, we urged Minister [of Health] Borst to take the case to a higher court. And we said, if you take this case to a higher court, allow us to be a party to the proceeding, allow us to explain our interests to the judge. She hesitated, but in the end she agreed to send it to a higher court. And now the LHV no longer wishes to speak to us. And we are now waiting to see the outcome of this case.

Is this the highest court?

Yes, if the LHV loses, it is not possible for them to take this to another judge in the Netherlands. Perhaps they can take it to the European Court.

---

15. The Dutch are sensitive about this topic—the roots of the current health system in the German occupation. It is true that in 1938 the German government passed a similar law for the promotion of midwives; it was argued that healthy Aryan women could easily have their babies at home under the care of a midwife and that this would free physicians to care for wounded soldiers.

Where is the negotiation? The accommodation? The compromise? In the case of the primaat we see the interests of two professions coming into conflict, and we see very little give and take. The huisartsen accuse the midwives of being "unyielding." The midwives believe the huisartsen are exaggerating their case and claim the doctors are unwilling to speak to them.

As we have noted, compromise takes time, health policy changes slowly. In 1991, the Sick Fund Council published a report on the future of obstetric care in the Netherlands in which the professional organizations of huisartsen and midwives declared they were prepared to compete and went so far as to offer strategies that would further the interests of their profession (Ziekenfondsraad 1991, 59–70; appendix 5). In the mid-1990s, the period in which I conducted most of my interviews, the value of the primaat was being argued in court. But, true to form for Dutch politics, by the autumn of 2000, while awaiting the results of the appeal on the primaat, midwives and huisartsen had softened their positions and moved toward compromise: In an October 2000 report, the Minister of Health stated that she had every expectation that she would be recommending the ending of the primaat pending an agreement between the LHV, the VVAH, and the KNOV (Borst-Eilers, 2000c). How did this happen?

As early as the summer of 1994, I could see midwives becoming less defensive about holding on to the primaat. The director of one of the midwife schools had this to say:

Since 1941 the midwives have had the primaat. Do you think that is what has preserved autonomous midwifery here?

Ja, I think it's important. Because of the primaat we have been able to keep our group of clients. The primaat also has prevented the medicalization of birth. I think the primaat was very important at that moment.

What do you think now about the LHV and the effort to remove the primaat?

I think that at this moment I'm not so afraid for the primaat . . . What I'm afraid of is that there are too few midwives. That's why I think we need more workers. So if the primaat is going out, you need a lot of workers who do a very good job, and then the clients are coming automatically to the profession. So I'm not afraid for the primaat, I'm more afraid for the quality of the work of the midwives. Because I think not all midwives work in a way that the clients are coming to the midwife. Because what midwives are doing now, they have too big practices, and they work with four or five midwives. And I think that's too big, because then you don't have, what we say, the midwife knows her clients and has her *vertrouwen*, how do you say . . .

Faith? Trust?

Ja, so the client has vertrouwen in de vroedvrouw. But if you work with five midwives, you see them one or two times in pregnancy, so you don't know the women. So then they can go to the doctor, to the huisarts, because he is always the same. And so I'm more afraid for the kind of work we are doing now than for the primaat. And I think midwives don't realize that enough.

For this midwife, then, the future of Dutch midwifery did not lie in keeping the primaat, but in the way care is organized and the number of midwives in practice. Another midwife echoes her opinion:

I hope that the primaat has just lasted long enough to stabilize the system, and to create a strong midwifery profession in Holland. . . . I mean, if it hadn't lasted for twenty or more years, then probably the profession would have gone. Then I think we would not have made it, as a profession. Now, we have a very strong position, I think, in the birth market in Holland.

In the mid-to-late 1990s health care administrators also began to wonder about the advisability of keeping the primaat. From their point of view it seemed the primaat had outlived its usefulness. This excerpt from a July 1995 interview with a staff member of *Zorgverzekeraars Nederland* (Health Care Insurers Netherlands), an organization that includes and represents all the companies that provide health care insurance in the Netherlands, gives us a glimpse of the insurers' standpoint:

I find the primaat . . . strange. I find it out of date and old-fashioned. . . . Look, the privately insured can choose to go to the huisarts or to the midwife, and if you have always had a good relationship with your huisarts, and he offers obstetric care, you can go to your huisarts. And if you know a good midwife then you can choose to go to her. Now, *"vrijheid, blijheid"* (freedom, happiness). But a person insured under the Sick Funds cannot go to her huisarts; she must always go to the midwife. . . . That is no longer from this time, that is old-fashioned. . . . I find that ridiculous. . . . This cannot continue.

The (K)NOV and the LHV should come to an agreement . . . [but] the (K)NOV is very concerned about the loss of work, that many huisartsen will begin with obstetrics. I do not believe it. Because who is sitting there, ready to jump? I think nine out of ten huisartsen will say, "Go ahead and do that. It is working well and I will send all of my patients, including the privately insured, to the midwife.

In the midst of these gradually changing opinions about the primaat, the government stepped in and played an instrumental role in helping the midwives and huisartsen solve their disagreement. In September 1999 the Minister of Health organized an EAC—the *Stuurgroep Modernisering van Verloskunde* (SMV, Steering Committee for the Modernizing of Obstetrics)—asking them to develop policy for obstetric caregiving in the twenty-first century, policy that would strengthen the eerstelijn and stimulate more home births. In keeping with the Dutch idea of getting broad representation of all stakeholders, the committee included, among others, representatives of the KNOV, the VVAH, the LHV, the NVOG, the *Nederlandse Vereniging voor Kindergeneeskunde* (NVK, Dutch Association for Pediatrics), *Zorgverzekeraars Nederland* (ZN, Care Insurers Netherlands), *Landelijke Vereniging Thuiszorg* (LVT, National Association for Home Care), and the Ministry of Health.

Drawing on several reports about the state of affairs in Dutch obstetric care—especially the "Inventory of Obstetrically Active Huisartsen" (Wiegers and Hingstman 1999a), a report that showed a decline in the number of huisartsen doing obstetrics, and "Bottlenecks in Caregiving by Midwives" (Wiegers et al. 1999), a descriptive study of a variety of problems in the provision of midwife care—the SMV recommended a number of policies favorable to midwives but also made it clear that the future of eerstelijn obstetric care and home birth required lifting the primaat and bringing more huisarts into obstetric practice:

> Given the fact that the proposals of this steering committee to an important degree are based on the principle of cooperation it is advised that the primaat of midwives in the Ziekenfondswet be abolished, on the condition that the organizations involved come to good agreements on their relationship and collaboration. (SMV 2000, 34)

Recognizing the concerns of midwives about the quality of huisarts care, the SMV recommended a new, optional course of study in obstetrics for huisarts-in-training and a certification process for obstetrically active huisarts that would require a minimum number of births per year and continuing education. (SMV 2000, 11–14).

As a result of the work of the SMV, it appeared that the decision in the pending appeal about the primaat had become moot. In September 2000, Wiegers summarized the situation:

> I really think that the primaat will not last much longer and that the decision of the higher court is waiting on the final report of the Stuurgroep

Modernisering Verloskunde. . . . In practice, the primaat no longer works to limit competition between huisartsen and midwives. At this moment, they have too much need of each other simply to meet the demand for obstetric care. The primaat now is a "*sta-in-de-weg*" (obstacle) because—by prohibiting payment for patients insured by the Ziekenfonds—it works against the huisartsen who wish to help with the growing demand for care. [So] the primaat is still in force, but it will not last long.

In the resolution of this disagreement about the primaat we see the slow working of the Dutch process of compromise and negotiation. We also see that midwives are not disadvantaged in the presentation and defense of their interests. The lengthy debate over the VIL gives us another view of the same dynamic.

The VIL

The "Obstetric Indications List" (VIL), briefly described in Chapter 3, is a set of guidelines that specifies the conditions for referrals between the *eerste* and *tweede* lines, a list that distinguishes normal ("physiological") and high-risk ("pathological") pregnancies and births. Because the VIL defines the relationship between midwives and gynecologists, it is not surprising that it has been the site of protracted debate and disagreement. Although gynecologists promulgated the list, subsequent revisions of the list by government-appointed committees were not to their liking. Among other objections, gynecologists were concerned that the revisions gave too much power to midwives and huisarts. A closer look at the history of the disagreements over the VIL gives us further insight into the unique politics of the professions in the Netherlands.

There are several histories of the VIL, but all are in Dutch, making them inaccessible to non-Dutch-speaking scholars (see Schellekens 1987; Riteco and Hingstman 1991; Hiddinga 1998; Drenth 1998). A brief review of these histories is necessary to set the stage for an analysis of the recent debates over the VIL.

The idea of an indications list began in 1930 with the publication of the first edition of *Leerboek voor Verloskunde* (Textbook for Obstetrics) by De Snoo. In this text De Snoo, a gynecologist, pointed out that careful prenatal care could prevent certain pathologies of pregnancy and birth. In particular, he identified toxemia in pregnancy, abnormal positioning of the fetus, and narrowing of the pelvis as medical indications for a hospital birth. Before the publication of De Snoo's text, there was only one indication for a hospital birth and that was a *social*, not medical, condition: inadequate living space.

Over the subsequent years the Sick Funds were presented with additional medical indications for a hospital birth. In order to help clarify what was becoming a confusing situation, the Sick Funds went to Professor Kloosterman for advice. In 1958, at a meeting of medical advisors to the Sick Funds, Kloosterman offered his reflections on a list of indications for the intervention of a specialist in pregnancy, birth, and the postpartum period. His comments helped bring some order to a situation where many lists of medical indications were circulating, but the Sick Funds, realizing they needed a more formal list—one that was commonly accepted—went to the government for help.

Among other things, the Sick Funds were concerned that uncertainty over the conditions that warranted transfer to the hospital was contributing to an increase in the number of hospital births. Responding to this concern, the government convened several committees in the late 1960s and 1970s to examine the state of obstetric care in the Netherlands (see *Centrale Raad voor de Volksgezondheid* 1972; 1977; Sikkel 1979). In general, the reports of these various commissions affirmed the preference for birth at home and emphasized the need for good cooperation between midwives, huisartsen, and gynecologists. Although none of these reports created a government-endorsed list, they did point to the lists found in obstetrics texts as models for decision-making. As a result of these discussions and reports, the "Kloosterman list"—an expanded list that appeared in Kloosterman's (1973) textbook, *De Voorplanting van de Mens: Leerboek voor Obstetrie en Gynaecologie* (Textbook of Obstetrics and Gynecology: Human Reproduction) and was supported by all professors of obstetrics in the Netherlands—came to be the informal law of the land.

In 1983, prompted by a proposal from the NVOG, the Sick Fund Council undertook a revision of the Kloosterman list. To carry out this revision the Council organized the WBK—*Werkgroep Bijstelling Kloostermanlijst* (Work Group for the Revision of the Kloosterman List). As was true of the SMV, this EAC included representatives from midwives ([K]NOV), huisartsen (LHV), gynecologists (NVOG), pediatricians (NVK, *Nederlandse Vereniging voor Kindergeneeskunde*, Dutch Association for Pediatrics), postpartum caregivers (*Nationale Kruisvereniging*, National Cross Association), health insurers (VNZ, *Vereniging van Nederlandse Ziekenfondsen*, Association of Dutch Sick

Funds; and the KLOZ, *Kontaktorgaan Landelijke Organisatie van Ziekenkostenverzekeraars*, Contact Group for the National Organization of Health Insurers), the Health Inspector (GHI, *Geneeskundige Hoofdinspectie*), and the Sick Fund Council. The group also included an independent expert in the person of Dr. van Alten, a gynecologist.

The government had several reasons for acceding to the request of the NVOG. Not only was there confusion about the official status of the list, but the government was also concerned about the improper use of services. A sharp increase in the number of women under the care of a gynecologist for pregnancy and birth and large regional variations in maternity care made it appear that medical indications were being used improperly (Ziekenfondsraad 1987, 10).

The WBK began its work in May 1983. At the outset they affirmed the basic assumptions of the Dutch obstetric model:

> Considering that pregnancy, birth and the postpartum are, in principle physiological processes and that, in a situation where no complications are expected, birth can take place at home, the WBK has formulated the following basic assumptions:
>
> - The pregnant woman can, in principle, be accompanied by an eerstelijns obstetric caregiver unless an indication exists or develops which calls for a tweedelijns caregiver.
>
> - The pregnant woman can, in principle, give birth at home (or in the hospital, in the case of a "relocated home birth") unless an indication exists or develops which calls for birth in the hospital. (Ziekenfondsraad 1987, 12)

In determining the obstetric policy for each indication the committee took into consideration the following:

1. The source and severity of the complication that increases risk;
2. The possibilities of preventing the complication;
3. The possibilities of timely detection of the complication;
4. The possibilities for intervening in the complication.

Using these four aspects, the committee developed decision criteria that allowed them to "translate obstetric risks into obstetric policy" (Ziekenfondsraad 1987, 15). These criteria were used to create a list of 124 indications with a referral policy for each. The possibilities for referral fall into four categories:

- **Eerstelijns obstetric care (A):** The woman remains under the care of the eerstelijns caregiver and the birth can take place at home (or in the polyclinic).
- **Tweedelijns obstetric care (C):** The woman is referred to the care of a tweedelijns caregiver and the birth takes place in the hospital.
- **Risks requiring consultation (B):** The determination of a need for a referral requires consultation with a gynecologist. The gynecologist gives advice after seeing the woman. With this advice and a thorough consultation, the eerstelijns caregiver determines the need for referral and bears responsibility for the referral decision.
- **Medium situation (B→D):** In a number of situations the obstetric risk for mother and child require that the birth take place in a hospital, but allow for accompaniment by an eerstelijns caregiver

The 124 indications are divided into four categories: (1) diseases that can negatively influence pregnancy and birth or be negatively influenced by pregnancy and birth; (2) indications based on obstetric history; (3) indications that develop during the prenatal period; and (4) indications that develop during birth. Each indication has a specific referral policy associated with it. A few examples: an umbilical cord prolapse during birth is classified as "C": a case requiring specialist care; loss of amniotic fluid during pregnancy is a "B": a case requiring consultation; previous abortion is regarded as an "A": a case to be cared for by a midwife or a huisarts.

In June 1986 the WBK sent a preliminary version of its report to the directorates of the (K)NOV, the NVOG, the LHV, the NHG, and the NVK, asking for their reaction.[16] Because it was a *preliminary* report, the WBK asked that this first draft of the list be kept confidential: It was to be shared only with a few experts who could offer advice on its content. The boards of directors of the midwives, huisartsen, and pediatricians ([K]NOV, LHV, NHG, NVK) supported the report and offered some useful amendments. The NVOG, however, was not as sanguine. For a variety of reasons, the association of gynecologists found the new list unacceptable and asked for the continuation of the discussion of its content. In the course of its exchange with the NVOG, the WBK learned, much to its disappointment, that the gynecologists had ignored its di-

---

16. This review of the fate of the VIL is based on Schellekens 1987, 621–623.

rective to keep the report confidential. Dr. Schellekens, the medical adviser of the Ziekenfondsraad, comments, "It appeared that the gynecologists leaked the report and distributed it nationally. The WBK regrets this action because it caused gynecologists to come to premature judgments about a report that would later be revised" (1987, 622).

The WBK and the directorate of the NVOG met in October 1986 and had an "intensive exchange" of ideas about the content of the report. In December of that year, as a result of that meeting and the comments received from the other organizations, the WBK sent a revised list to the NVOG. The changes did not satisfy the gynecologists; in January 1987 they informed the WBK that they were once again rejecting the report.

One of the strongest objections of the NVOG centered on the role of eerstelijn caregivers in the determining the need for referral. The gynecologists were particularly worried about the "B" situation because they did not trust midwives and huisartsen to make decisions about the proper level of care. In their response to the WBK, the directorate of the NVOG also made the (somewhat curious) argument that women should be allowed to freely choose a caregiver and the place of birth. In summary, the NVOG declared itself to be "extremely concerned" about the effect the implementation of the proposed rules would have on the quality of obstetric care.

After "thorough deliberation" on the response of the NVOG, the WBK dismissed their objections. They found the first at odds with longstanding obstetric policy: "The eerstelijns obstetric caregiver is specifically educated to be responsible for carrying out the referral policy; the selection system of obstetric care in the Netherlands is based on this fact." The second argument of the NVOG—that women should have free choice—was seen as in direct conflict with the organization of health care in the Netherlands, where the eerstelijn acts as a gatekeeper. The third concern, about the quality of care, was seen as a simple difference of opinion; after all, the WBK saw the new list as a step toward *better* and *more responsible* obstetric policy.

Recognizing the strong negative reaction of the gynecologists and the potential bias of the committee in their defense of its work, the WBK asked a number of professors of obstetrics, who were not involved with the revision of the list, for their reaction to the list and to the objections of the NVOG. The professors gave clear and strong support to the position of the WBK. With this support and with the support of the other professional organizations, the committee submitted the list to the Sick Fund Council with no further changes.

The Sick Fund Council did not immediately approve the report; they too considered the objections of the NVOG. The members reviewed the role of the eerstelijn in determining the course of care and, with the exception of the member from the LSV (the National Specialist Association), agreed that it was a typical function of the eerstelijn to decide, in consultation with the specialist, when a referral is necessary. In April 1987 the Sick Fund Council sent the new VIL to all midwives, huisartsen, gynecologists, and Sick Funds, defining the list, not as mandatory, but as "very important" (*zwaarwegend*, literally "heavy weighing") advice.

The official appearance of the list set off a flurry of letter writing between the Sick Fund Council and the professional organizations involved in obstetrics, as well as a number of articles in the professional literature (Schellekens 1987; Huisjes 1987; T. Eskes 1987; Lems et al. 1987; van der Lugt et al. 1991; Riteco and Hingstman 1992a; 1992b). In these letters and articles, the NVOG persisted in its rejection of the new VIL. At one point in the exchange of letters between the Sick Fund Council and the directorate of the NVOG, the secretary of the council, Dr. van der Kooij (1990), felt compelled to remind the gynecologists that "the *Verloskundige Indicatielijst* is not intended to be a consensus of all caregivers. The list is the very important advice of the Ziekenfondsraad, which includes a member from the LSV (National Specialist Association)."

Why did the NVOG object to this new version of the list? After all, it was the gynecologists who first saw the need for, and who created, a list of medical indications. In an appendix to a letter sent to the chair of the Sick Fund in October 1991—intended "to enter into a discussion of the obstetric situation in the Netherlands"—the chair of the NVOG, Dr. M.D. Kloosterman (the son of G.J. Kloosterman), and its "first secretary," Dr. H.A.M. Vervest, summarized the criticisms of the list by the NVOG. The criticisms fall into four categories:

1. Criticism of the reasons for the creation of the WBK: An increase in medical indications for specialist care and regional variations in the use of specialists are *also* caused by improvements in medical

technology, changing societal opinions, and new ideas about the most appropriate caregivers at birth. The WBK gave no consideration to these.

2. Criticism of the working-methods of the committee: The committee had only *one* representative from tweedelijns obstetric caregivers, and this person was not appointed by the NVOG. The other members of the 15-person committee were all representatives of the eerstelijn. The final decision of the committee, made by a majority, reflects insufficient involvement by the NVOG.[17]

3. Criticism of the terminology used and the decision criteria: There are several problems here, including:
   • Improper use of the term physiological pregnancy and no use of scientific criteria to define low, some, and high risk;
   • Continual confusion about the ideas "referral policy" and "obstetric policy";
   • Improper recognition of the expertise of the gynecologist;
   • Creation of the list based on consensus, not proper decision-making criteria; and
   • The NVOG completely disagrees with the opinion that the eerstelijn may decide, and remain responsible for, obstetric procedures in the case of medium and high-risk situations. The midwife may ask for the advice of a gynecologist, but does not have to follow that advice. In the medium-risk situation this means that the midwife does the birth, which, in our opinion, has increased risk, and the gynecologist is expected to stand by in the case of complications.

4. Criticism of the scientific foundations of the obstetric policy for many of the named indications.

---

17. In an interview, a midwife explained that the NVOG felt inadequately represented on the WBK because the gynecologist asked to serve on the committee was "midwife friendly:" "It's quite a history about this medical indication list, because the board of the Sick Fund initiated talking about the old Kloosterman list, and the NVOG was involved, but there was not enough feedback during the process of creating the list, the NVOG says. I know the gynecologist, who was on this committee . . . Bennebroek Gravenhorst from Leiden, and he is a very nice . . . person, and he is convinced about the qualities of the midwives, so they blame him. There was a time when he said, 'I'm stepping out of the NVOG, they make the work so hard for me,' but he stayed in it. Treffers [former professor of obstetrics at the University of Amsterdam] said so as well. There were public fights between Treffers and the NVOG about the list and all those things . . . oh, a bad history."

The gynecologists also had specific objections to the referral policies associated with some of the medical indications. In a commentary issued in January 1987, the NVOG presented detailed objections to 35 of the 124 medical indications. For example, the WBK classified the presence of an IUD (intrauterine device for contraception) during pregnancy in category "A," a situation suitably handled in the eerstelijn (Ziekenfondsraad 1987, 15); the gynecologists believe this indication falls into the "B" category, requiring consultation, because of the "increased chance of bleeding, spontaneous abortion, premature rupture of membranes, and premature contractions" (NVOG 1987).

It became clear that the strong objections of the gynecologists to the new VIL were hampering the working relationships between gynecologists and caregivers in the eerstelijn. In an effort to work their way around this problem, the government commissioned a study of the implementation of the new list. In 1990 researchers at the NIVEL[18] sent surveys to all practicing midwives (1,068) and gynecologists (611), and to a sample of huisartsen (1,708),[19] soliciting their opinions about the new VIL and its creation, and asking about their use of the list. The response rates were good (midwives, 60.5 percent; gynecologists, 67.1 percent; huisartsen, 53 percent) and analysis of nonrespondents indicated only slight differences with those who did respond (Riteco and Hingstman 1991).

The research showed that midwives and gynecologists were in accord about the basic assumptions of the Dutch system but differed sharply in their opinions and use of the revised VIL. Figure 4-1 shows that midwives and gynecologists agree with the two basic assumptions used by the WBK as the basis of their work: Barring complications, a pregnant women can give birth (1) under the care of midwife or a huisarts, (2) at home.

But when asked about the revisions that resulted from those assumptions, midwives and gynecologists parted company. Unlike midwives, gynecologists were not convinced that the old list needed revising (Figure 4-2), and they were not pleased with composition of the group that was given the responsibility for those revisions (Figure 4-3).

---

18. See Chapter 2, note 1.

19. There were *two* samples of huisartsen: a random sample of 596 and a stratified sample (based on the distribution of huisartsen who were attending births) of 1,112.

FIGURE 4-1

Do you accept the 2 assumptions of the WBK? (in percent)

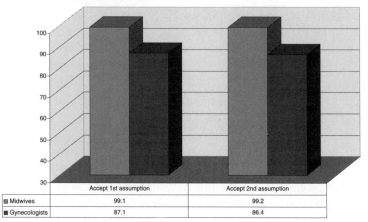

	Accept 1st assumption	Accept 2nd assumption
▨ Midwives	99.1	99.2
■ Gynecologists	87.1	86.4

Source: Riteco and Hingsman 1991, 56.

Note: Midwives, 1st assumption, N = 640; midwives, 2nd assumption, N = 636; gynecologists, 1st assumption, N = 387; gynecologists, 2nd assumption, N = 383.

FIGURE 4-2

The old VIL was in need of revision (in percent)

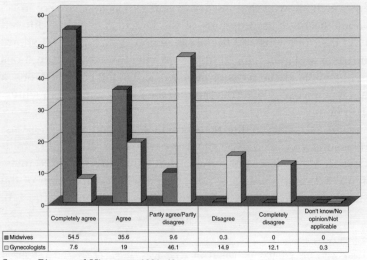

	Completely agree	Agree	Partly agree/Partly disagree	Disagree	Completely disagree	Don't know/No opinion/Not applicable
▨ Midwives	54.5	35.6	9.6	0.3	0	0
□ Gynecologists	7.6	19	46.1	14.9	12.1	0.3

Source: Riteco and Hingsman 1991, 43.

Note: Midwives, N = 640; gynecologists, N = 395.

FIGURE 4-3

Are you in accord with the composition of the WBK (in percent)

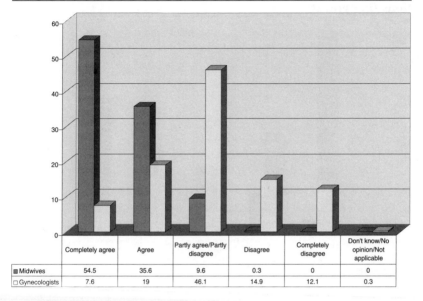

	Completely agree	Agree	Partly agree/Partly disagree	Disagree	Completely disagree	Don't know/No opinion/Not applicable
■ Midwives	54.5	35.6	9.6	0.3	0	0
□ Gynecologists	7.6	19	46.1	14.9	12.1	0.3

Source: Riteco and Hingsman 1991, 45.

Note: Midwives, N = 630; gynecologists, N = 382.

Reflecting the position of the directorate of the NVOG, practicing gynecologists indicated their uneasiness with allowing an eerstelijns caregiver to decide on when a woman should be referred to specialist care (Figure 4-4). Opinions about the list were reflected in action: Midwives were far more likely to report using the list than were gynecologists (Figure 4-5).

In the interviews I did in 1994 and 1995, I found the opinions of midwives and gynecologists had changed little, if at all, from those recorded by Riteco and Hingstman. The following comments are typical. In discussing her opposition to the new list, this gynecologist called attention to problems with allocating responsibility for cases in the "gray zone":

> The problem is the "gray zone." Low risk is no problem, high risk is no problem. But it's just in between. And I think that the main problem is that the midwives ask the gynecologist's advice and then when the advice is there they just ignore it. That's the main problem that the

FIGURE 4-4

The eerstelijns can determine the referral policy in "B" situations (in percent)

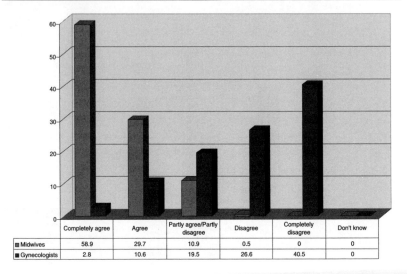

	Completely agree	Agree	Partly agree/Partly disagree	Disagree	Completely disagree	Don't know
▨ Midwives	58.9	29.7	10.9	0.5	0	0
▣ Gynecologists	2.8	10.6	19.5	26.6	40.5	0

Source: Riteco and Hingsman 1991, 60.

Note: Midwives, N = 632; gynecologists, N = 395.

gynecologists have with that list. If they ask you for advice, I think well, it should be followed. You can discuss about it, but it's more common that the advice is followed. That was the discussion in the gray zone. They [the midwives] don't want to take over responsibility and then they want to go on with the patient. So if something goes wrong it's our [the gynecologists'] responsibility.

They want you to see the patient and know everything and then they want you to say "okay go ahead. I'll be there if you need me." You are responsible. If I'm responsible, I want to be responsible. I want to treat the patient myself. Or very close by.

How do you think the Ziekenfondsraad will solve this problem? The midwives seem to be quite happy with the list from '87.

Of course. We have the responsibilities and they can go on. It's all a question of money. I don't know what the solution is. I think the gray zone will be described more clearly. But you can always ignore the list. By just having a discussion. But the midwives . . . they don't like you to tell them that maybe it's better to take over. They want to make the decision. But they don't want the responsibility. And it's also a question of money I

FIGURE 4-5

To what degree do you use the new VIL? (in percent)

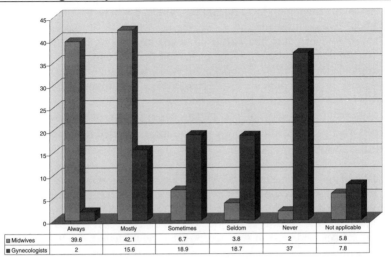

	Always	Mostly	Sometimes	Seldom	Never	Not applicable
Midwives	39.6	42.1	6.7	3.8	2	5.8
Gynecologists	2	15.6	18.9	18.7	37	7.8

Source: Riteco and Hingstman 1991, 78.

Note: Midwives, N = 639; gynecologists, N = 397.

think, and it's a question of prestige, a matter of status, they want to have the same position as the doctor, I think.

In her last sentence, this gynecologist *does* suggest a new wrinkle, an issue left unexplored by Riteco and Hingstman: money. Hers was not the only comment I heard on the effect of the revised list on the financial fortunes of the professions. Several of my interviewees observed that the new VIL would affect the flow of patients between midwives and gynecologists. When asked what she thought of the revised VIL, a midwife replied:

I think it is a good document. Good to work with. The sad thing is that the specialists still refuse to recognize the list.

Why have the gynecologists refused to recognize the revised list?

When you handle the list as a guideline for obstetrics, when you do it in the way it is meant, it can mean that in a certain practice of gynecologists there [will be] less clients than before you used the list, and that is money! That's always the thing. . . . But they say "it's not money, it's the principle" and things like that, but that's not true.

What will happen to the list?

I hope that in contacts with the Sick Fund Council, the (K)NOV, the huis-artsen organization, the LHV, and the NVOG it will be possible to agree about two or three indications on the list which are in discussion the most. And of which the parties involved say "oh well, we better can change that indication." Maybe then, after that discussion, it is more acceptable for the NVOG. I hope, but it is like walking on a rope, and balancing. It is very difficult, the discussion about this matter.

A former professor of obstetrics, a supporter of the work of the WBK, also believed that money played an important role in shaping attitudes about the revised list:

[When the list] came out in '87, an enormous turmoil started, because the effect of the list would be that less would be done by specialists and more would be done by primary caregivers . . . the list was not accepted by the board and the majority of the members of the NVOG. It was accepted by the Ziekenfondsraad, it was accepted by the midwives, by the general practitioners . . . but it was not accepted by the obstetricians and they protested against it. And until now there is no agreement and almost no talks about the subject, because the subject is so difficult to manage.

So no one wants to open up the subject again?

Well, I think the midwives would be prepared to talk about it, but they would be prepared to talk about revision of the new list, while the obstetricians won't talk about revision of that list . . . they'll only talk about revision of the *old* list, they don't accept the new list at all. And I think the main reason why the emotions are so high on the new list is financial.

In addition to being uncomfortable with the way the revised list allocated responsibility and remuneration, gynecologists were concerned about the lack of evidence for some of the policies of the WBK. Here is a gynecologist's comment on the need for more evidence:

In 1988 . . . our society said, no, no deal, we stick to the old system. And still, in 1994, we stick to the system. And it's always my advice to stick to the system. The reason is very simple. I want the facts and figures from the simple system. And if they are perfect then you can allow more risk factors to be given to midwives. But if you don't have the facts from that period you're absolutely doing crazy things.

But in fact the midwives are using the new system. If it is not supported by evidence why are they doing that?

It's very easy, because they attract more women. They are doing crazy things.

Another gynecologist, a member of the NVOG's board of directors, protested that the list was too limiting. He was concerned that the list could not anticipate the many factors that influence the relationships between caregivers and between caregivers and their clients.

Our general opinion is that our midwives are well-trained, intelligent women and men [and] they can give a good selection. And that in most parts of Holland there is a good relation between midwives and gynecologists, so [when they have] doubts about the selection they can talk about medium risk [cases] and decide. Together with the specialist. There are some spots in Holland where it is not well arranged; when a midwife has a bad relation with the gynecologist, and she asks the opinion of the gynecologist, the gynecologist always takes the patient into his practice and then does the delivery. But I think in most places there is a rather good working together.

But the NVOG has not officially approved the new Kloosterman List?

Absolutely not. We haven't approved. And that's coming back to what I said: it's no science. There are people who are at medium risk. You can't make three lists. It might be even possible that somebody who has no medical indication, like we say, but is already four years by a gynecologist, is pregnant after three abortions and a lot of fuss. Still she has a very good pregnancy, no problem at all. But she still stays by her gynecologist, because she has a relation there, she feels well there. Why bring her to a midwife? She will arrange it like that—that she comes back to the gynecologist. So, we don't think that there has to be a real specific list. Of course you can make a list, but this list doesn't have to be law, yes? And in that part of Holland where there is no good relation between the two groups, it's used as a law. And then it's really difficult. If you don't talk with one another, the list doesn't work. And if you talk with one another, the list doesn't have to work.

And you can have somebody who has a really strict medical indication, but which says, "Please, let me try again with the midwife. I'll come to the hospital; she'll be responsible, and as soon as something changes she will call the gynecologist. But please . . . I've had such a bad experience, I'm afraid of the hospital." Well, most gynecologists will say: "Try it with your midwife, and we'll come when there's something wrong. Of course you have your own responsibility then. If you have lost two liters of blood the first time and you want that, okay. You want it. We are not responsible for it, if we are called in and you have lost a lot of blood again." But it's what I said. And this doesn't work. Because it's no science, because you have to talk it over, because the patient is involved.

Gynecologists and the government were clearly at an impasse. Eight years after the VIL was issued, the specialists still refused to accept its recommendations. It is remarkable that this conflict did not create serious problems in the delivery of maternity care; the rejection of the list by gynecologists *could* have disrupted patterns of referral and communication between the eerstelijn and the tweedelijn. In fact, during this period most clients never even noticed that caregivers were engaged in a serious disagreement about policy; in the absence of an agreed upon list, midwives and gynecologists relied on their long history of working together to guide their referral decisions. Problems were also headed off by the fact that the government classified the revised list, not as a legal mandate, but as "serious advice," allowing room for disagreement and negotiation.

How was the impasse over the VIL broken? As with the primaat, the government brought all interested parties together and allowed them to work together to find a solution. After reviewing the NIVEL report, and the many problems with the implementation of the new list it identified, the medical adviser of the Sick Fund Council organized a series of deliberations between the (K)NOV, the NVOG, and the LHV/NHG. These informal deliberations continued for nearly four years until November 1994, when the Council decided to create a more formal commission, an EAC called the *WerkOverleg Verloskunde* (WOV, Obstetric Work Consultation). The WOV included representatives of the three professional groups, an advisor from the *Inspectie Gezondheidszorg*, and staff from the Sick Fund Council. Their task was the "stimulation and development of cooperation between obstetric caregivers and the identification of areas that need special attention . . . an important [one being] the Verloskundige Indicatielijst" (Ziekenfondsraad 1999, 2, 10).

In December 1998, the WOV produced the *Vademecum Verloskunde* (Ziekenfondsraad 1999)—a document approved by the directorates of the KNOV, the NVOG, and the LHV—which contained a revised Indications List, guidelines for the use of echograms, a list of qualifications for caregivers, and advice for promoting cooperation between members of the professions providing maternity care.[20] The document opens with a mission statement:

> Characteristic of this *Vademecum* is an effort to promote quality, efficiency, and cooperation. Quality and efficiency are achieved by making balanced agreements, which are based on the highest degree of scientific evidence and on decisions reached by consensus between the obstetrically involved professional organizations. The advice of this *Vademecum* can only be implemented on the basis of cooperation. Therefore, this *Vademecum* is also intended to stimulate close cooperation between the obstetric professions.

With the publication of the *Vademecum*, the problems of the WBK list were resolved; all three professional groups approved the new list:

> The governing boards of the Royal Dutch Organisation of Midwives (KNOV), the National Association of General Practitioners (LHV) (with the approval of the Dutch General Practitioners' Fellowship (NHG)) and the Dutch Association for Obstetrics and Gynaecology (NVOG) declare the ratification of this report during the General Meeting of the members of their professional organisations.

> The governing boards of the three professional associations strongly advise their members to use the recommendations in this report in practice and when collaborating with other caregivers providing obstetrical care. (Ziekenfondsraad 1999, 4)

On its face, the list approved in 1998 is not that different from the one that was strongly contested by the NVOG. The indications for referral now fall into *six* categories rather than four: (1) preexisting conditions, not gynecological; (2) preexisting conditions, gynecological; (3) obstetrical history; (4) conditions that develop during pregnancy; (5) conditions that develop during birth; and (6) conditions that develop during the postpartum. The four possibilities for referral remain the same, except that the "medium situation" (Situation "D") of the old list is now called *Verplaatste Eerstelijns Verloskundige Zorg* (Relocated Eerstelijns Obstetric Care). And the foundational assumptions of the list continue to favor the eerstelijn: The medicalization of birth is decried, the value of home birth is affirmed, the expertise of

---

20. An English translation of the *Vademecum* (abridged) is available at each of the following web sites: http://www.jiscmail.ac.uk/files/MIDWIFERY-RESEARCH/ official_dutch_obstetric_guidelines and http://europe.obgyn.net/nederland/default. asp?page=/nederland/ richtlijnen/vademecum_eng.

eerstelijns caregivers is recognized, and the eerstelijn is seen as having the expertise and authority to make referrals.

There are, of course, a few small differences between the new list and the one prepared by the WBK, and it is these small differences—in procedure and content—that explain why the directorates of all three groups accepted the *Vademecum*. After the difficulties of the WBK report, the Sick Fund Council realized that if consensus among the obstetric professions was to be achieved, a new process for revising the list was required. A member of the council pointed out that if the list was to generate "optimal commitment" from the professional groups, the representatives must be "authoritative" members of their professions (Bultman 1999, 58). This time around, representatives of the professions were chosen by their organizations and remained in continuous communication with their respective boards. The council also stepped away from the process, acting only as facilitator and allowing the *Vademecum* to be a product of the professional organizations themselves, not of a government agency.

In terms of content, the new list goes to great lengths to clear up the confusion and disagreement over cases requiring consultation between the eerstelijn and the tweedelijn (Situation "B"). The *Vademecum* states that if, after consultation, no transfer occurs, the responsibility for the case stays with eerstelijn. Furthermore, the *Vademecum* offers 11 detailed guidelines for Situation B (the *overlegsituatie*), explaining the responsibilities of both the eerstelijn and the tweedelijn.

The *Vademecum* also acknowledges that there might be situations that fall outside the list, situations where the wishes of the client should be considered. In a section titled, "The Wish of the Woman," the *Vademecum* explains that although midwives and huisartsen are not qualified to accompany a patient with a "high risk" pregnancy, gynecologists *are* capable of accompanying low-risk pregnancy and birth. Echoing the comments of the gynecologist from the NVOG quoted earlier, the report goes on to suggest that a "special relationship" between a woman and a gynecologist (as a result of extended treatments for infertility, for example) might call for making an exception to the list and allowing a woman to stay with her gynecologist even though no complications are expected. A few paragraphs later, however, the report maintains that the desire for an efficient division of labor in obstetric care requires that requests of this sort should be honored only in "highly exceptional cases" (Ziekenfondsraad 1999, 15–16).

Unlike the WBK, the *Vademecum* builds in a certain amount of tentativeness. The reader continually is reminded that an indications list must be constantly revised in light of changes in society and science. In several places it is noted that no list can be absolute, that deviations are possible, and that the list should be seen as just one part of a larger cooperative working relationship among professionals. Like the WBK, the *Vademecum* was issued, not as a legal mandate, but as serious (zwaarwegend) advice.

Negotiating the Primaat and the VIL

What do we learn from the details of these political battles between midwives and physicians? In many ways, the arguments over the primaat and the VIL look like the classic battles between professions: Each occupational group is seeking to protect its turf, arguing that their special expertise gives them jurisdiction over obstetric policy (see Abbott 1988). Indeed, the facts of these cases remind us that there is not something magical about obstetric caregivers in the Netherlands. As elsewhere on the planet, doctors and midwives have sharp disagreements, they see the world in different ways, and these differences will be manifest in the way each professional group wants to organize obstetric care.

Unlike other modern nations, however, the Dutch have a system in place that prevents doctors from translating their professional opinions into law. In the deliberations and negotiations described here, we see the government balancing the scales between midwives and physicians. By way of contrast, gynecologists in the United States have been able to use their power, both political and cultural, to fashion rules and regulations in *accord* with their opinions. Thus, the widely shared belief of American gynecologists that birth is fraught with danger—making home birth the equivalent of child abuse—has shaped laws about midwifery and, more importantly, is used to justify insurance company rules about the type of obstetric care that will be covered. This is not the case in the Netherlands. As a Dutch gynecologist assured me, "as long as the government pushes [midwives] they will survive, of course."

POLITICS IN PRACTICE

The position of the midwife is enhanced by the way political power is arranged and distributed in the Netherlands, but legislative assemblies and government councils and commissions are not the only sources of political power for Dutch midwifery. Quite apart from the formal regulations and government directives, the micropolitics of day-to-day practice afford ways of wielding power to midwives in the Netherlands and elsewhere.

Midwives working outside the Netherlands, with a less-favored position in the rules governing health professions, must often resort to strategies of subversion to gain power in the workplace. For example, nurse-midwives in the United States have found ways to keep women walking during labor, to do perineal massages, to provide food and drink to laboring women, in spite of hospital regulations that prohibit these practices (see De Vries and Barroso 1997). Dutch midwives—legitimate and respected members of the eerstelijn of the health care system—have little need for the subversive tactics used by midwives in the United States, but they have become quite skilled in translating the formal power given them by government regulations into a more informal means of control over gynecologists.

The formal arrangements of the VIL suggest that gynecologists are the ultimate advice-givers: Even though midwives and gynecologists negotiate as colleagues, the last word, formally, belongs to the specialist. But midwives are well aware of how to use their power of referral—remember that the Dutch health care system mandates that specialist care be given only on referral from the eerstelijn (i.e., a midwife or a huisarts)—to gain control over the behavior of gynecologists. If a midwife believes a gynecologist is treating patients poorly or is actively discouraging women who have been sent for consultations from getting their babies at home, she can simply cease sending women to this specialist. Eventually, the gynecologist shunned will notice and will call to ask what might be done to once again receive referrals. This strategy works best in areas where several hospitals are competing for clients, but even midwives in rural areas report traveling extra distances (with their clients who choose a polyclinic birth) to avoid undesirable practices in local hospitals. A midwife explains:

How would you characterize your relationship with gynecologists?

Good . . . because we have more hospitals here. It means that you can bargain with them. You can more or less do what you want to do as long as you give care. But you can make your own decisions.

What does that mean: "to bargain with them?"

Like, for instance, if there is somebody who has a third-degree tear . . . a few years ago, in the one hospital the women could be sutured and then they could be sent home. And in another hospital they'd have to stay for a whole week. Which is very old-fashioned, but nobody ever challenged that. So then I had somebody with a third-degree tear, and I called the hospital where she had to stay for a week, and I said to them, "She wants to come to your hospital, but . . . if she goes [to a competing hospital], she can be sutured and then she can be sent home. Could you do the same thing in your hospital?" At first they said "No," and when I asked them again they said "We haven't talked," and then the third time they said "Yes, alright." That's how you can bargain with obstetricians.

If we cannot get something from one hospital, we'll go to another hospital and we'll negotiate. And then we'll let the first hospital know that we negotiated with the other hospital, so would they also let us have the same.

And if not, you won't be coming there.

Ja. Strong, eh?

Another midwife, in a different city, describes the same strategy:

I work with three hospitals, and one of those hospitals was boycotted for years and years. We refused to go there. We told the patients: "No, we are not going to . . ." Because we did not like the way the gynecologists practiced. Because, for example, you had a delivery, you sent the woman there, let's say with a few centimeters dilation, and then you'd come there, after a few hours, and the baby could have been born with a vacuum. They just interfered . . . we refused to work there.

A few weeks ago there was a new gynecologist starting to work there; a woman who comes from the AMC (Amsterdam Medical Center) and had worked in Alkmaar. And they had a reception, to introduce her, and at that reception they really were on their knees . . . "If we, please, would we come back?" And they wanted to change everything, and things would never be done this way again, and they . . . and they would do everything we wanted, and . . .

And we were sitting there, a lot of midwives were there, and we put a lot of questions . . . "Will you stop that? And won't you do that? And is it possible to do this? And . . ."

So the boycott worked?

Ja.

STRUCTURING PREFERENCES AND PREFERENCING STRUCTURES

Chapters 3 and 4 reviewed the structural arrangements that allow the Dutch way of birth to continue. Many social scientists would end their analysis here: These are the features of Dutch society that explain their peculiar way of getting babies born. But to stop here leaves us with only half an explanation. These features of Dutch society—its politics, its educational system, its organization of health care and the healing professions—explain the autonomy of midwives and the persistence of home birth, but they also generate new questions: Why have the Dutch created these structures, why did they choose to favor midwifery in a way that none of their neighboring countries did?

In an interview with a gynecologist who had just been elected president of the NVOG, I asked if midwives and gynecologists were equal partners. She responded,

> [Midwives and gynecologists are] not equal. I'm not equal to a cardiologist. I have my own field and in my own field I can take my responsibilities. . . . And [midwives], for physiology it's no problem. But if there is pathology, they are not a medical doctor. They have another education than we have. So in that kind of view, they are not equal. They have another education. They go to midwife school for 4 years. We have a training of 14 years.

> *Would you say that their expertise is in physiological childbirth? Are they more expert in that than gynecologists?*

> Yes. They are used to physiology. We are not. We are used to high-risk patients. So a gynecologist will always look with that knowledge to a pregnant woman, I think.

Even with an awareness of all these structural factors that support midwifery and home birth, it is surprising to hear these words coming from the mouth of a gynecologist, the president of her professional association. This physician makes a case for the superiority of her education, and yet she concedes that midwives are experts in "physiological" (i.e., normal) birth. This is a highly unusual attitude for a gynecologist in a Western country. As a midwife from New Zealand put it in a presentation to Dutch midwives, "We would kill to have your kind of gynecologists [in our country]" (quoted in ten Berge 2001, 611). If we are to understand this attitude on the part of gynecologists in the Netherlands, if we are to gain a thorough understanding of why the

Dutch created a system that favors midwives and home birth, we must look *beyond* the structural features of maternity care—we must look to the cultural climate in which this system exists. In so doing we will begin to understand that health care reform cannot succeed without paying attention to the cultural foundation of medical structures.

III. FORMING

WHY IS midwife-attended home birth a practice that some sectors of Dutch society, including the government, feel is worth preserving? Why have no other European countries shown a preference for birth at home? We have seen that the distinctive organization of the Dutch political system played an important role in maternity care policymaking, but how do we account for the Dutch approach to politics? Why do the Dutch favor negotiation and compromise? These important questions compel us to extend our analysis, to consider the fundamental role culture plays in the organization of medical systems.

There is a temptation to attribute the uniqueness of maternity care in the Netherlands to an accident of history, to one or two events that brought about the anomaly that is Dutch obstetrics. But one forceful personality or one historically contingent policy decision could not sustain Dutch maternity care in the face of the modernization of obstetrics. Something broader, and—unfortunately for the social analyst—less tangible is at work here. To answer our questions about the structure of Dutch maternity care we must ask: Are there peculiarities in the culture of the Netherlands that explain its continued use of home birth? Social scientists get nervous when the discussion turns to "national culture." In our increasingly multicultural world, anthropologists and sociologists are loath to affirm a concept that somehow implies a singular, hegemonic national identity. But in our haste to distance ourselves from earlier, less thoughtful analyses of cultural traits, we must not lose sight of the fact that social structures emanate from cultural ideas. In explaining the cultural sources of Dutch maternity care policy, we learn important lessons about the forces that create health systems and hold them in place.

5   *Doe Maar Gewoon* (Just Act Normally): Dutch Culture/Dutch Birth

I have bin the longer aboutt the discription of this place etts., because there are soe many particularities wherein it differs (and in som excells) allsoe beeing my selff somwhatt affectionated and enclined to the Manner off the Countrie.
—Peter Mundy, 1640, apologizing for his detailed description of his visit to the Netherlands (Mundy 1925 [1640], 81)

I AM not the first to be fascinated by the distinctive culture of the Dutch or to think about how their cultural ideas influence the way they organize their society. For centuries, travelers, foreign diplomats, journalists, business people, and social scientists—some well-trained, some not—have commented on the peculiar habits, ideas, and behaviors of the Dutch.

Among the more well-known of these observers is the American writer, Henry James. Like many other nineteenth century travelers who visited the Netherlands, James was impressed by the cleanliness of the streets and sidewalks,[1] observing that the canal walks were "periodically raked by the broom and the scrubbing brush and religiously manured with soapsuds." Watching a Dutch housemaid—"redolent of soapsuds" and armed with a "queer little engine of polished copper" squirting water over "the majestic front of a genteel mansion"—James reflected on the Dutch preoccupation with eliminating dirt:

> [Her] performance suggests a dozen questions, and you can only answer them with a laugh. Does she imagine that the house has a speck or two which it is of consequence to remove, or is the squirt applied merely for the purposes of light refreshment-of endearment, as it were? Where

---

1. Mary and Percy Shelley (1989 [1817], 77) described Rotterdam as "remarkably clean . . . the Dutch even wash the outside of their houses." Dreiser, in his 1913 travelogue of Europe, refers to Haarlem as a "spotless town" and speaks of the "kindly, cleanly realism . . . of simple Hollanders" (495).

could the speck or two possibly have come from unless produced by spontaneous generation: there are no specks in the road . . . nor on the trees whose trunks are to all appearance carefully sponged every morning. The speck exists evidently only as a sort of mathematical point, capable of extension in the good woman's Batavian brain, and the operation with the copper kettle is, as the metaphysicians would say, purely subjective. It is a necessity, not as regards the house, but as regards her own temperament. (James 1972 [1875], 380–390)

Simon Schama, a more recent traveler to the Netherlands, opens his widely praised social history of the Dutch Golden Age (1988) with a portion of this quote from Henry James. Like James, Schama is intent on exploring the mysteries of the Dutch temperament, on describing and analyzing the distinctive features of the Dutch character: the "Batavian brain." He uses travelogues, diaries, books of moral instruction, and other products of everyday life to examine the reasons for the distinctive school of art that emerged in the Netherlands during the Golden Age. In his book, Schama demonstrates important links between the culture of the Dutch and the form of their art:

> Dutch painters worked with the same pigments as their Italian and Flemish counterparts, but somehow the end result was distinctly different. And it is how the end result came about that concerns me. For there was something special about the Dutch situation—its fortune and its predicament—that . . . set it apart from other states and nations in baroque Europe. (7–8)

But are these varied efforts to describe, as Schama (6) puts it, the "community of the nation" anything more than oversimplifications, suited to entertain and intrigue the readers of travelogues? Can we use descriptions of the customs, habits, values, and thought-ways of a society for serious social analysis?

In defense of his efforts to describe the *conscience collectif* of the Netherlands, Schama tells the story of the "drowning cell," a uniquely Dutch form of punishment/rehabilitation used on prisoners who refused to work. According to reports of tourists who visited the Netherlands in the seventeenth century, the Dutch would place incorrigibly idle prisoners in a small room that gradually filled with water: The only way for the prisoner to avoid a watery death was to abandon idleness and set to work emptying the cell of water by means of a hand pump. After review of a variety of historical records, Schama admits some doubt that the drowning cell actually existed, but he goes on to say,

Suppose [the drowning cell] was only a popular and perennially repeated myth, would that obviate its historical importance? . . . As a punitive myth—and still more as an exercise in regulated terror—the drowning cell drew its psychological force from the watery depths of Dutch culture . . . the frightening experience inflicted, *in extremis*, . . . an intensive rehearsal of the primal Dutch experience: the struggle to survive rising waters. . . . Shaken down to the elemental essentials, it must have been argued, even the most vicious and abandoned person would respond with the effort and perseverance that would, at last, proclaim him a member of the Dutch community. (24)

In descriptions of the drowning cell, whether real or imagined, Schama finds expression of peculiar Dutch ideas about water, industry, idleness, and punishment. By listening to the stories of the drowning cell, we can better understand the values of the Dutch and we see the connection between social practices and intangible ideas.

As an art historian, Schama is particularly concerned with artistic representations of Dutch life;[2] he is eager to explain the unique features of Dutch art in the Golden Age. As a sociologist of medicine, I am concerned to discover how Dutch midwives and physicians, who worked with the same developments in the obstetric arts as their European counterparts, came to develop a maternity care system that was distinctly different. And, in order to answer that question, I must look in some of the same places explored by Schama and his predecessors.

We must tread carefully here. To suggest that there may be something we can identify as "Dutch culture" and that it may have some effect on the way maternity care is organized and delivered is to open an anthropological can of worms that was tightly sealed four or five decades ago. In spite of renewed interest in the idea of "national culture," also referred to as *national character* (see, for example, Wilterdink 1994; Chamberlayne et al. 1999; Hofstede 2001), anthropologists remain embarrassed by the fact that the notion had some currency in their discipline in the 1930s and 1940s. Their embarrassment is understandable: Studies from that era often used a poorly developed concept of national culture and, more importantly, the very idea of national culture awakens painful associations with its misapplications in World War II. Today we recognize that to

---

2. Schama (1988, 9) claims that the use of visual evidence allows him to see the collective conscience of the Dutch in its proper habitat and in action, "rather than prone and eviscerated on the sociologist's dissecting table."

posit a static national culture, rooted in soil and blood, is to ignore the fact that culture is emergent, negotiable, and varied.

Skepticism about the use of the concept of national character is further justified by explanations of social organization that rely on overly simple notions of culture. Kloosterman offers an amusing report of a naïve cultural explanation of Dutch home birth given by a few members of the British parliament who were visiting an academic hospital in Amsterdam:

> To my great surprise, they suggested that the fact that so many Dutch women had their babies spontaneously, without any anesthesia, was related to our Calvinism. The Calvinist view is to give birth to children in sorrow. The Dutch would keep anesthesia from women in labor because of the Old Testament. That idea never occurred to me before. It is an interesting viewpoint, but it is not mine. It is obvious that we try to make childbirth as pleasant and painless as possible. (Quoted in van Daalen and van Goor 1993, 194)

Misuse of a concept, however, is not sufficient reason to abandon it. We can acknowledge that notions of national culture have an undeniable tendency to oversimplify the complex and competing systems of meaning in a society *without* discarding them or ignoring their contribution to human interaction. In his analysis of the stereotyping of Dutch society, van Ginkel (1997) casts a wary eye on the characterizations of the Dutch made by tourists and armchair social scientists, and yet he insists that observable and important differences between national cultures exist:

> Often firmly held opinions [about the character of the Dutch] are confirmed by a very thin selection of data. Nevertheless, [the Dutch] feel or experience, in a general sense, separation from people of other nationalities and cultures. . . . It is this subjectivity, it is these we-feelings, that color our self image and our images of others. . . . It is not for nothing that we in the Netherlands so often speak of "we" and "ours." There may be talk of a globalizing process, such that national boundaries are erased, but still we are confronted with cultural differences, for example, concerning time consciousness, manners, norms, eating habits, codes of communication, political arrangements, and so forth.[3] (39)

---

3. See also Dreiser (1913). Describing his travel from Germany into Holland, he says (490), " I was in Holland now . . . I felt . . . I was in an entirely different world. Gone was that fever of blood which is Germany. Gone the heavy, involute, enduring Teutonic architecture. The upstanding German—*kaiserlich*, self-opinionated, drastic, aggressive— was no longer about me. The men who were unlocking trunks and bags here exemplified a softer, milder, less-military type. This mystery of national temperaments—was I never to get done with it?"

Van Ginkel's assertion is supported by a remarkable convergence found in the numerous descriptions of Dutch culture offered over the last five centuries. Consider for a moment the best-known modern account of Dutch culture, an account offered by Ruth Benedict, an American anthropologist who did her research in 1944 under the auspices of the United States Office of War Information (OWI).[4] In her work, Benedict described the Dutch as moralistic, individualistic, freedom-loving, tolerant, self-assured, proud, ironic, modest, clean, prudent, thrifty, conservative, domestic, oriented toward the nuclear family, earnest, and melancholy (see van Ginkel 1992, 1997). Most, if not all, of these traits are included in accounts of the Dutch dating from the sixteenth, seventeenth, eighteenth, and nineteenth centuries *and are also found* in that most recent form of the travelogue—guidebooks for business people working in a foreign culture (see Van der Horst 1996; *NRC Handelsblad* 2001b). These modern-day guidebooks echo the observations of travelers who visited the Netherlands between 1500 and 1900; in both, the Dutch are characterized as energetic (*werkkracht*), clean (*zindelijk*), lovers of freedom (*vrijheidzin*), tolerant (*tolerant*), virtuous (*deugzaam*), friendly (*vriendelijk*), good-humored (*humorvol*), not presumptuous (*niet hovaardig*), skilled in trade (*vaardig in de handel*), resolute (*kordaat*), sober (*nuchter*), thrifty (*spaarzaam, zuinig*) materialistic (*materialistisch*), miserly (*gierig*), phlegmatic (*flegmatisch*), cold (*koel*), and narrow-minded (*bekrompheid*).[5] An explorative study of images of national character conducted in the early 1990s by the European University Institute (Florence, Italy) generated an almost identical list of Dutch characteristics, leading one of the researchers to conclude that "national images . . . are fairly well-known . . . and they are not new. All of them can be found in literature dating back to the seventeenth, eighteenth, or nineteenth century" (Wilterdink 1994, 48).

Of course it can be argued that this convergence of opinion about the characteristics of the Dutch is the simple result of stereotyping—

---

4. The OWI was charged with assembling information about America's enemies and about residents of the occupied countries of Europe and Asia. Because of the war, Benedict had to do her research at a distance. She interviewed Dutch citizens living in the United States and collected information from historical works, travel journals, news stories, and the like. Her work was intended to help American troops in their interaction with the liberated Dutch.

5. See van Ginkel (1997, 15–27) and Schama (1988, 53–54).

visitors, and more recently, social scientists, simply find what they expected to find. Interestingly, the Dutch themselves agree with these observations. A recent ten-part television series broadcast in the Netherlands asked the question: *Bestaat Nederland Wel?* (Does the Netherlands exist?). The creator of the program, Herman Belien wondered if it was still possible to speak of a unique Dutch culture in a globalized, multicultural world. In answering his question, he discovered, as he put it, "remarkable constants in our [i.e., Dutch] history," including "tolerance, pragmatism, and an inclination toward business" (quoted in Giesen 1999, 23).

What do these features of Dutch character have to do with the organization of the maternity care system in the Netherlands? Because social scientists have rejected the idea of national character and, consequently, emphasized the local and contingent nature of culture, sociologists of medicine have used the concept of culture in a very limited way: When culture is mentioned by medical sociologists, it is almost always used as an explanation of the difficulties in the interaction between clients and caregivers. I assert that culture has a *broader* and more important impact on health systems. An exploration of the connection between Dutch culture and maternity care policy in the Netherlands shows that the way health care is organized and delivered is inextricably linked with cultural ideas.[6]

If one looks carefully at the international literature on health policy and health practices, it is possible to see glimpses of culture's influence on the organization of health care, even in cases where this influence goes unnoticed by the authors. Consider an article on regional variation in the treatment of heart attacks in the United States by Pilote and her colleagues (1995). Their research uncovered great disparities in how doctors in different regions of the country respond to heart attacks, disparities the researchers found difficult to explain (571, emphasis added):

> This study demonstrated marked regional variation in the management of acute myocardial infarction in the United States. The variation was found in the use of both medications and procedures. The discordance

---

6. In a similar vein, Chamberlayne et al. (1999) describe how cultural ideas influence the organization and delivery of welfare services in Europe, and Hofstede (2001) describes how culture affects the way organizations work.

between the approach to management in New England and that in the other regions was a surprising finding; New England had a lower rate of use of procedures and a more evidence-based use of medications. Regional variation in the use of cardiac procedures was *not* explained by differences in patient profiles or in the incidence of complications related to myocardial infarction. However, we found a strong relation between the availability of angiography in a region and the number of procedures performed there. This association was less strong in New England than in the other regions, suggesting that there are other important explanations for the different way of managing acute myocardial infarction in New England.

Their findings beg for a cultural explanation, but the authors mention only physician attitudes and a variety of structural factors; they push no further. They never consider the way regional cultures—found among patient groups and in the medical community—might influence attitudes and structures.

More to the point is Kirejczyk's (2000) study of the way the science that undergirds health care is influenced by culture. After comparing the significantly different policies of the Netherlands and the United Kingdom with regard to the use of human embryos in research he concludes:

> The diversity of solutions [to the ethical problems presented by research on embryos] in the relatively culturally homogenous Europe suggests that different national cultures . . . play a significant role in the creation of policies that regulate scientific developments.

Several cultural ideas have important consequences for the Dutch view of the appropriate way of accomplishing birth and hence, for the way the Dutch organize maternity care. In the following pages, I consider various cultural traits that have a direct connection to the system of birth care in the Netherlands. In particular, I look at Dutch ideas about:

- Home, family, and the roles of women;
- Pain, the body, and the use of health services and medicines;
- Thriftiness and rationality;
- Heroes; and
- Solidarity.

Each of these cultural elements could be the subject of a book-length study. My intent here is to be suggestive, to encourage social scientists to give more serious consideration to the link between cultural ideas and the organization and delivery of medical care, and to persuade policymakers to incorporate cultural analysis into plans for the reform of health systems.

HOME, FAMILY, AND THE ROLES OF WOMEN

The most logical place to begin our analysis of the influence of culture on maternity care policy is with Dutch ideas about domestic life. Birth in the Netherlands is conceived as a family event that should occur in a comfortable and cozy setting. In my discussions with Dutch women about their choice of where to give birth, I heard—over and over—that home was the preferred place of birth because it was more *gezellig.* *Gezelligheid* is often translated as *coziness,* but in fact there is no single English word that captures the full meaning of the term. Cozy comes close, but gezellig also implies warmth, affection, contentment, enjoyment, happiness, sociability, snugness, and security. Many Dutch women find it more gezellig to get a baby in their own bed, surrounded by family and friends. As one woman put it, she "had no desire to exclude her children from being part of the event. . . . The baby was born at 6:45 in the morning, and just fifteen minutes later my other three children were standing around the bed, admiring their little brother. And that is something I would never give up" (quoted in De Haan and van Impe 1983, 91). For the Dutch, birth at home is regarded as gezellig in a way birth in the hospital can never be. To understand why this is true, we need to look more closely at Dutch ideas about home, about the family, and about the roles of women.

Home

Domestic confinements fit well with Dutch conceptions about home. According to Rybcinski (1986), the Dutch are responsible for our current notions of "home" as a place of retreat for the nuclear family. The Dutch were the first to develop single-family residences—small, tidy, well-lit homes—ideally suited for a married couple and their children. According to Rybcinski, "Privacy and domesticity, the two great discoveries of the Bourgeois Age, appeared, naturally enough, in the bourgeois Netherlands." He attributes this to the culture and geography of the lowlands. On the cultural side, he notes that the Dutch of the seventeenth

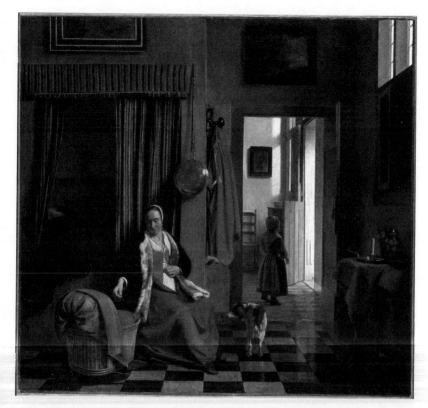

Pieter de Hooch, The Mother, c. 1659–60. Gemäldegalerie, Berlin, Germany

century were characterized by "unruffled moderation, an admiration for hard work, and a financial prudence bordering on parsimony. Thrift evolved naturally in a society of merchants and traders who, moreover, lived in a country which required a constant communal investment in canals, dikes, sluices, and windmills to keep the North Sea at bay" (54).

This interaction between culture and geography was manifest in the design of Dutch homes:

> Simplicity and thrift were apparent in the way the Dutch built their houses, which lacked the architectural pretension of townhouses in London and Paris, and which were built of brick and wood instead of stone. These materials were used for their light weight, since the boggy soil of the Low Countries frequently required pile foundations, the cost

of which could be reduced if the foundations carried less weight. . . . The expense of building on canals and pilings dictated that street frontages be reduced as much as possible; as a result, the building plots in Dutch towns were extremely narrow, sometimes only one room wide. (55)

The most efficient way to build these narrow houses was in rows, where adjoining houses shared the walls that carried the weight of the building. With this method of construction, the front and rear walls had no structural function, giving builders—eager to further reduce the weight of the walls—the opportunity to replace bricks with windows. These large windows not only reduced weight but also brought light deep into the interior of the home.

The paintings of Vermeer, de Hooch, and de Witte give us a glimpse of the clean, bright interiors of Dutch homes of the seventeenth century. These small homes were the center of life for the nuclear family, known in Dutch as the *gezin*. The idea of the home as a place of retreat for the gezin was further nurtured by the fact that household size in the Netherlands was smaller than elsewhere in Europe. Households in the Netherlands were small because, among other things, Dutch society discouraged the hiring of servants, imposing a special tax on those who paid for domestic help: "As a result, most homes in the Netherlands housed a single couple and their children . . . the family centered itself on the child and family life centered itself on the home, [a way of life that] occurred [in the Netherlands] about a hundred years earlier than elsewhere [in Europe]" (59–60). Rybcinksi goes on to point out that the Dutch disinclination to use servants helped to bring about what he calls the "feminization of the home." Women in all social classes, from the highest to the lowest, were responsible for household chores; it was women who maintained domestic order. Dutch men now had to accede to the demands of their wives to not smoke inside, to take off their shoes, and to stay out of certain rooms of the house:

> The imposition of a special code of behavior within the house was considered odd by foreign visitors . . . stories of the strictness, if not tyranny, of the Dutch mistress abounded [pointing] to a change in domestic arrangements. Not only was the house becoming more intimate, it was also, in the process, acquiring a special atmosphere. It was becoming a feminine place, or at least a place under feminine control. . . . It resulted in cleanliness, and in enforced rules, but it also introduced something to the house which had not existed before: domesticity. (74–75)

The importance of the nuclear family, coupled with the domestic role of women and the tidiness and brightness of Dutch homes made home—increasingly a sphere under feminine control—the logical place for birth. And as this brief summary makes clear, Dutch ideas about families and women are deeply intertwined with the physical and cultural structure of their homes.

The Dutch Family and the Roles of Women

Several observers of Dutch culture describe the Dutch as *huiselijk*; we might say *homey* or, as Benedict noted, "oriented toward the nuclear family." But is the Dutch family distinctive? Can study of the Dutch family help us understand the continued preference for birth at home? We know that family members have a direct influence on a woman's choice of where and with whom to get a baby. Wiegers (1997) research on the birth choices of Dutch women has shown that "the choice to give birth at home or in hospital is based primarily on social factors, with the confidence of family and friends in home birth . . . listed [among] the strongest determinants of choice" (70), but the influence of the Dutch family over birth practices extends beyond this direct effect.

Dutch homes are unique, not just because of the way they are built, but because of the life that goes on inside them. Historians, economists, and demographers who have studied the Dutch family have identified several unique features of households in the Netherlands, features that distinguish them from families in neighboring countries.

It is widely agreed that the Dutch were the first among modern nations to experience the "nuclearization" of the family. According to van Daalen (1993; 1988) the Dutch family nuclearized in the late seventeenth and early eighteenth centuries, earlier than the other nations of continental Europe. This fact might explain why Dutch is the only Germanic language that has a distinct word for the nuclear family: *gezin*. Other Germanic languages use a more generic word for family that must be qualified to denote the group that includes only mother, father, and children: in German, *kernfamilie* or *kleinfamilie*; in Norwegian, *kjernefamilie*; and in Swedish, *kärnfamilj*.

Historians also tell us that the quality of family life in the Netherlands differed from that of its neighbors. The bourgeois model of the family—a model that prized motherhood and expected all women to become wives and mothers and to care for children, do the cooking and the laundry, and keep a clean home—was found in the upper classes of Europe as early as the late 1500s, but it did not become the dominant household form for all social classes in Europe until the eighteenth and nineteenth centuries. In the Netherlands, however, the bourgeois model had already become the prevailing family form in all classes in the sixteenth and seventeenth centuries (Pott-Buter 1993, 48).

Although the bourgeois family model is often associated with the repression of women, Dutch women enjoyed remarkable freedoms. Unlike their sisters in other European countries, Dutch women could make "commercial contracts and [notarize] documents and had the formal qualifications needed for active commercial business dealings" (Pott-Buter 1993, 66). Schama reports that travelers in the Netherlands were "disconcerted" by "the apparent freedom that apparently respectable Dutch women enjoyed in comparison with their contemporaries elsewhere":

> Public kissing, candid speech, unaccompanied promenades all struck foreigners, and especially the French, as shockingly improper, even though they were repeatedly assured of the impregnable chastity of the married woman. . . . Outside the house women assumed an informality that seemed much too audacious for their own good. At the end of the sixteenth century, Fynes Moryson had been aghast at Frisian women embracing and defecating in public, assuming regular control over the family budget, skating at night until the city gates were locked, and most astonishing of all, feasting through the night in taverns ten or twenty miles from home. (Schama 1988, 402–403)

In seeking to explain this paradox of freedom and restriction, historians look to the character of the marriage relationship. Economically speaking, Dutch women—as the wives of farmers, fishers, and traders, the primary occupations in the Netherlands—assumed a great deal of responsibility for managing the family and its resources, giving them unique privileges, but always in the context of the family. Dutch Calvinism, with its emphasis on affection as the core of marriage, also contributed to the unique position of Dutch women in the family.[7] According to Schama,

> At the core of the [Dutch] marriage bond was affection, tenderhearted sentiment, love. . . . Calvinist teaching, at least in Holland, did not at all

---

7. It is noteworthy that in his description of Amsterdam, Dreiser (1913, 497) includes an account of lunch with "Madame J., the wife of an eminent Dutch jurist," in which he comments on her "ideal marriage."

subordinate love to obedience but rather exalted it as the indispensable quality for a godly union. . . . Most modern historians of the family have assumed an evolution from "patriarchal" to "companionate" styles of marriage, and have busied themselves with tracking experience along a line drawn between that point of departure and its destination. By these lights, the seventeenth century Dutch seem to have been indeed pioneers on the frontier of friendly, loving marriages. (1988, 421, 424)

Pott-Buter summarizes the distinct position of women in the Netherlands:

> In short, the relatively favorable economic features of Dutch society in the seventeenth century, such as an important trade sector and high productivity in other sectors, combined with Calvinism, may have coincided with a rather different position for women, compared with that of women in other countries. The dominance of the family household, in which married women especially played a central role and in which they were valued as partners or business partners and prized as mothers, came to shape preferred behavior much earlier in the Netherlands than in other countries. (1993, 54)

The situation of women in Dutch families—where they enjoyed a degree of freedom within the gezin, and where there was a strong identification of femininity with home and the gezin (see Pott-Buter, 1993)—resulted in distinctive patterns of fertility and labor force participation. If you ask a demographer to identify the distinguishing features of Dutch women in the twentieth century, you will be told about their extraordinarily high rates of fertility and low rates of participation in paid labor, each of which suggests that Dutch women were more domestically oriented than their sisters elsewhere in Europe.

Fertility rates for Dutch women, as compared to those of women in other Western European nations, remained remarkably high throughout the first two-thirds of the twentieth century:

> After 1910, Dutch Total Fertility Rates [average number of children born per woman per calendar year] were higher than those in [Belgium, Denmark, France, Germany, Sweden, and the United Kingdom]. . . . Since the 1970s Dutch fertility rates have been between those of the other countries. (Pott-Buter 1993, 181–182)

Figure 5-1 shows the fertility rates for women in nine European countries between 1950 and 2000; note that Dutch women have the highest rates of fertility in the period 1950 through 1970. In the 1970s, Dutch rates fell to coincide with rates in the rest of Europe.

FIGURE 5-1

Fertility Rates, 1950–2000, for Selected European Countries

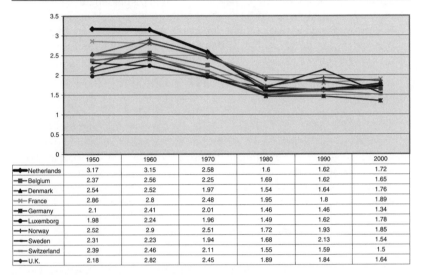

	1950	1960	1970	1980	1990	2000
Netherlands	3.17	3.15	2.58	1.6	1.62	1.72
Belgium	2.37	2.56	2.25	1.69	1.62	1.65
Denmark	2.54	2.52	1.97	1.54	1.64	1.76
France	2.86	2.8	2.48	1.95	1.8	1.89
Germany	2.1	2.41	2.01	1.46	1.46	1.34
Luxemborg	1.98	2.24	1.96	1.49	1.62	1.78
Norway	2.52	2.9	2.51	1.72	1.93	1.85
Sweden	2.31	2.23	1.94	1.68	2.13	1.54
Switzerland	2.39	2.46	2.11	1.55	1.59	1.5
U.K.	2.18	2.82	2.45	1.89	1.84	1.64

Source: Data for 1950–1980, Keyfitz and Flieger 1990; 1990 and 2000 data from OECD.
Note: Number of births divided by the number of women aged 15–49.

The involvement of Dutch women in paid labor is also unique. Until very recently, Dutch women have been conspicuous for their lack of participation in paid labor. Figure 5-2 illustrates this fact: Compared to these six other European countries, Dutch women had the lowest rates of participation in paid labor from 1900 through 1990.[8] The low rate of participation by women in the work force is a source of consternation in the Netherlands, because it results in what Dutch officials see as unfair placement of their country in some international measures of development.

> As recently as 1995 the Netherlands was startled by its low standing in the *Gender-related development index* (GDI) of the United Nations. On the *Human development index* (HDI), a general measure of well-being in a country, the Netherlands ranks fourth in the world . . . [but] on the GDI the Netherlands is ranked twentieth. This low position is caused by the relatively large difference in earned income between men and women

---

8. The relatively low number of women professors in the Netherlands is another reflection of the Dutch attitude toward women. In a 1998 study of 19 European nations, the Netherlands had the lowest percentage of women full professors (5.0) and associate professors (7.0) (European Communities 2000, 10).

FIGURE 5-2

Labor Force Participation of Women Aged 25–49 Years, 1900–2000, for Selected European Countries (in percent)

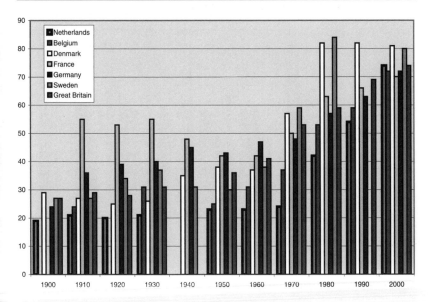

Source: Pott-Buter 1993; Centraal Bureau voor de Statistiek.

in our country, a difference that is caused, in turn, by the relatively low work-participation of women together with a high number of Dutch women who do part-time work. (Social and Cultural Planning Office of the Netherlands: 2000b, 49)

In their explanation of the low place of the Netherlands in the GDI, the Social and Cultural Planning Office highlights another distinctive feature of the involvement of Dutch women in paid labor: a very high rate of part-time work. Compared to their European sisters, many more Dutch women engage in paid labor on a part-time basis, giving something of a false picture of the degree of involvement of Dutch women in the labor market. Figure 5-3 compares the Netherlands with six other European countries on the percentage of women doing part-time work, the average workweek for all working women (in hours), and on labor force participation of women expressed in full-time equivalents. Commenting on the high rate of part-time work by Dutch women, the Social and Cultural Planning Office notes:

FIGURE 5-3

Proportion of Female Workers That Work Part-Time, Average Work
Week for Women, and Labor Force Participation for Women in Full-
Time Equivalents for Selected European Countries

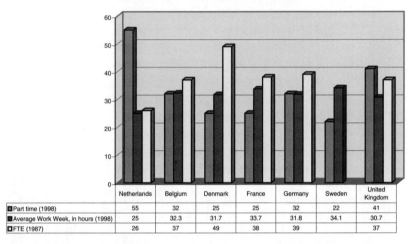

	Netherlands	Belgium	Denmark	France	Germany	Sweden	United Kingdom
▣ Part time (1998)	55	32	25	25	32	22	41
▪ Average Work Week, in hours (1998)	25	32.3	31.7	33.7	31.8	34.1	30.7
▢ FTE (1987)	26	37	49	38	39		37

Source: Part-time data and average work week, Social and Cultural Planning Office
2000a, 213–215; FTE data, Pott-Buter 1993, 205. The FTE figure for the United Kingdom
is limited to Great Britain.

The extremely high percentage of part-time work in the Netherlands can be
probably accounted for by the special position of (married) women in the
Dutch labour market. For the longest time, Dutch women's participation in
the labour force was amongst the lowest in Europe. This partly explains
why in the recent past the Netherlands did not have many childcare centers. . . . In turn, when increasing numbers of married women entered the
labour market in the early 1980s, this shortage of childcare facilities was the
reason women tended to work part-time. In countries with childcare facilities, like Denmark or Sweden, women took full-time jobs more frequently,
while in Southern Europe (except for Portugal) most married women
stayed out of the labour market. A factor that may have played a role here
is that the labour conditions, legal position, and social security benefits of
part-timers are well arranged for in the Netherlands, in contrast to many
other countries. (2000a, 214)

The importance of the gezin is also reflected in the working patterns of
men. The average workweek for men in the Netherlands is the shortest in
the European Union; this holds true for men in part-time *and* full-time jobs
(Social and Cultural Planning Office of the Netherlands 2000a, 215). It is
not clear what Dutch men are doing in their time away from work, but

there is evidence that at least some are at home with their children. Although more women than men take parental leave (28 percent and 12 percent, respectively), according to a 1998 study (Bruning and Plantenga), the share of Dutch men who exercise their right to parental leave is among the highest in Europe. Furthermore, the number of days of parental leave taken by women and men in the Netherlands does not differ by much (men average 45 full-time days and women 50, see Grootscholte, Bouwmeester, and de Klaver 2000).

These facts about Dutch families and Dutch women are connected to the position of midwives and the preference for home birth. Pott-Buter notes:

> Now, in 1990, there are still some reminders of the long period in which motherhood and fertility were of the utmost importance: the national health system provision for pregnancies, deliveries and medical child care is one. The majority of babies used to be born at home; in 1975 the figure was reduced to about 50 per cent and by 1991 this percentage had fallen to 35, internationally still a high percentage. The father is and always has been usually present at the delivery. (1993, p. 187)

But what is the mechanism of this connection? In his ruminations about the effect of Dutch ideas about the family on the Dutch way of birth, Kloosterman had this to say:

> Perhaps it is part of the explanation of [maternity care in] Holland: the backbone of our population were fishermen, seamen and farmers. And all these folks need independent women . . . seamen very often come home twice a year and for the rest of the time he is at sea. A farmer also needs a woman who works with him as much as he himself. They share the burden of life. That is perhaps the reason why they accept that a woman is independent also during delivery.

Kloosterman's explanation that women's strong and independent place in the family resulted in their jurisdiction over birth, supervised by midwives at home, is interesting, but perhaps too simple. Van Daalen (1988), a Dutch sociologist, offers a more nuanced analysis. She believes that the early nuclearization of the family hindered the hospitalization of birth. In other European countries the nuclearization of the family occurred simultaneously with industrialization and was marked by the increasing use of professional help for events once attended by family members: birth, sickness, and death. Having nuclearized earlier, the Dutch family resisted the institutionalization of birth and death:

Institutional birth [which was becoming popular in the early nineteenth century] did not fit well in Dutch society . . . in 1826, the Rotterdam city council declared the "national character" to be in opposition to the establishment of maternity clinics.

Dutch family life was organized in a way we call "modern," far before the emergence of professional groups and institutions that, in the last 100 years, have become closely involved with the cares and concerns of the modern family and that . . . have undermined the autonomy of these families. Could it be that the Dutch have developed a family culture that offers more possibilities to resist such professional interference? (Van Daalen 1988, 432)

Van Daalen (1988, 433–434) claims that this same tradition of resisting professional interference in the affairs of the family explains the slow movement of married women into the paid labor force, their limited use of professional childcare, and the less than generous policies for maternity leave in the Netherlands.[9]

Writing in the late 1960s, Dutch sociologist Goudsblom commented on the distinctively important role of the family in shaping the character of Dutch society. Goudsblom asked himself whether the Dutch family still possesses any "typically Dutch" features; his answer neatly summarizes Dutch ideas about the family and home:

This is a precarious question; the simplest answer would be to repeat that *the* Dutch family does not exist. This, however, seems too easy a way out. After all, there is a common stereotype that the family in the Netherlands plays a more prominent role in social life than in neighboring countries. This stereotype, moreover, can be supported by some official figures: for example, there are fewer cafés in the Netherlands and people go less often to the cinema. Such figures reinforce the generally shared assumption that the Dutch seek comfort first of all in the family, that they cherish the private rather than the public sphere. . . . Within the narrowly confined domestic circle [women cultivate] the virtues of primness and neatness and the pleasures of homely coziness or *gezelligheid*. (1967, 136–137)

The central place of the home, in both its physical and social manifestations, and the important place of women in the gezin are seen in the postpartum rituals of the Dutch. Unlike their European neighbors, the Dutch use ritual to frame the postpartum, or *kraam* period. Not only do the Dutch have an organized system of postpartum care, but rela-

---

9. Especially when compared to the Scandinavian countries, see the Social and Cultural Planning Office of the Netherlands, 2000a, Chapter 7.

tives and friends celebrate the kraam period by decorating the house (often with a stork in the front yard), eating *beschuit* with *muisjes* (zwieback with pink and blue colored bits of licorice candy), and by well-organized kraam parties and visits.

These ideas about domestic life provide the cultural and historical backdrop for health policies that encourage birth at home, managed by midwives. It is this preference for home that led to the creation of policies that favored and supported birth at home.

PAIN, THE BODY, AND THE USE OF HEALTH SERVICES AND MEDICINES

Dutch ideas about the body, about pain (its value and the degree to which it can, and should, be borne), and about the need for medicine and medical consults have a rather straightforward influence on the way birth care is organized. A Dutch midwife explains the connection between attitudes toward pain and the maternity care system:

> I think the important thing in Dutch obstetrics has been the attitude towards pain. In Holland the pain at giving birth is still considered completely normal, and it is considered abnormal if you need pain relief.
>
> *But how does that work? Why doesn't this attitude exist across the border, in Germany, or France, or Belgium?*
>
> It's very strange. I also think the key of midwifery in the United States is . . . if women don't change their attitude towards pain, they will never get it back. And because in Holland they think it's absolutely normal to have pain and that you can stand it, and that you need it, otherwise you don't have a good experience, that's why we haven't lost it. An important reason. Because if you need pain relief, a birth immediately gets medicalized. Without pain relief it stays in the hands of midwives. And I think why Dutch women don't need relief . . . I think that's really a combination of culture and the no-nonsense attitude.
>
> *Nuchterheid?* (temperateness, soberness)
>
> Yes. This no-nonsense . . . "Don't develop self pity, you've got to do this job." And I think if this should change, it's a big threat to midwifery. If pain relief will come in birth practice, it will be the end of midwifery as well. I really think so. And I think that in any country where this attitude towards pain doesn't change, they will never get midwifery back. Never.
>
> *So you're saying that in the United States midwifery could never seriously regain a place unless women think differently about pain.*

Yes. I really would stand up for that statement. I'm going to Chicago in September. And one of my workshops, my speeches, will be about attitudes towards pain, and the enormous impact it has on the system. And, not only on the system, but also on the feelings of women.

If you don't have the pain in birth, you just totally take out the soul of the whole event. But more basically, more no-nonsense-wise, if you have pain, the pain itself is valuable. If you have pain, first it gives you reason to put yourself in a safe place. If you would suddenly have the urge to push while you were shopping, it would be hazardous for your child. So the pain is a sign: "Hey, let's call the midwife, let's go home, let's clean a little." So it's a way to survive, the pain is a survival thing.

And another thing is that if you have pains during the event of birth, the endorphin is coming through your blood, which gives you this enormous nice feeling, which you always have in your blood when you are running a marathon, and then all of a sudden the baby is born and the endorphins go on. And I think that's the big function of pain, that it gives you this enormous endorphin level, which nourishes your mother-instinct. . . . It is simply a big injection of instinctive love.

I think that the reason why Dutch midwifery is so important is that it gives a very strong, basic family life; it gives a very strong instinctive connection to your children, so you are more tolerant when your child is horrible. It gives you more connection, bonding, and you can give more offerings[10] . . . you suffer more, endure more. And therefore I think this pain-culture in Holland, . . . it gives women so much more joy in birth and mothering, especially when your children are small.

I cannot imagine this [feminist position] that you have a right not to want pain and that you then think you are emancipated. [If] . . . you don't want that pain, you don't take responsibility of what your body natural-wise does, you let your body completely be exploited by the medical establishment, the male medical establishment. . . . And to think that you cannot stand [pain], to even think that it doesn't have any use, you completely disrespect your body.

Dutch ideas about pain and the value of medication, implicit in the comments of this midwife, are reflected in their relatively low use of pain and other medications compared to other nations in the European Union (see van Andel and Brinkman 1997, 153; Kooiker and van der Wijst 2003). Figure 5-4 provides evidence of these distinctive Dutch ideas. Compared to their European neighbors, the Dutch go to the doctor less often and use fewer prescribed and over-the-counter medications.

---

10. This midwife is likely confusing the English *offer* with the Dutch *offeren*, which means, "to sacrifice."

FIGURE 5-4

Contact with Doctor and Use of Medication and/or Vitamins in the Last Two Weeks, 1996 (in percent)

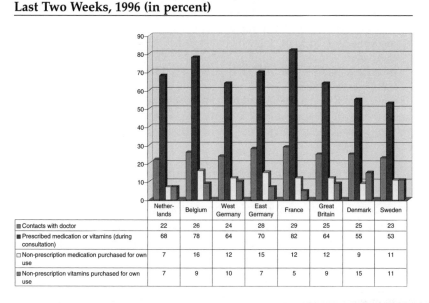

	Nether-lands	Belgium	West Germany	East Germany	France	Great Britain	Denmark	Sweden
▨ Contacts with doctor	22	26	24	28	29	25	25	23
■ Prescribed medication or vitamins (during consultation)	68	78	64	70	82	64	55	53
□ Non-prescription medication purchased for own use	7	16	12	15	12	12	9	11
▨ Non-prescription vitamins purchased for own use	7	9	10	7	5	9	15	11

Source: Social and Cultural Planning Office 2000a, 282.

In seeking to explain the Dutch approach to the use of medical services and medications, the Social and Cultural Planning Office of the Netherlands falls back on a cultural explanation:

Differences in medical consumption appear to be determined largely by culture. One important aspect is the way in which people from different cultures deal with pain and discomfort. This has also been seen in the United States among immigrants from different cultural backgrounds. Americans with Irish, Polish or Anglo-Saxon roots are more likely to soldier on and hide their pain than Americans with Italian or Latino roots, who tend to express their discomfort. They are therefore also much more likely to visit their doctor and request medication.

Characteristics of the health care system naturally also have an impact on consumption, but offer no full explanation. One example is use of medication. In France and Belgium people have to pay a contribution towards many medicines, whereas this is rarely the case in the Netherlands. However, consumption of medication is much higher in France and Belgium.

[In an earlier report, the *Social and Cultural Surveys 1999,* we] pointed out that the cultural dividing line between Northern and Southern Europe can be ascribed to the influence of the Protestant Reformation, which had little impact in the southern countries belonging to the Roman Empire. Protestantism brought a culture of austerity, rationalisation and scientific analysis. This led to the view that medication should be used only when there is no alternative and if it has proven effective. These barriers are much less evident in southern countries. The more scientific approach to medicine is reflected in the way in which randomised clinical trials spread from Great Britain and the United States via Scandinavia and the Netherlands. Evidence-based medicine is highly developed in the Netherlands, at least on paper. This is much less so in the southern countries. (2000a, 282–284)

Professor Klomp has a novel explanation for why the use of anesthesia at birth never caught on in the Netherlands. In the course of an interview I asked her what she thought about the oft-mentioned notion that Calvinism led Dutch women to avoid pain relief in labor. She said she did not think that was true and went on to offer a more historical/sociological theory:

I don't think [the Calvinist heritage of the Netherlands has encouraged the avoidance of anaesthesia]. I have my own theory . . . that is that Queen Victoria accepted medical pain relief with her seventh or eighth child already. And of course, as soon as your queen accepts it, the aristocracy wants to have it, and then the upper-middle class. . . . Well, the children, the daughters of Queen Victoria married into all European monarchies. Prussia, Germany, Scandinavia, but not Holland. We never had close ties with Queen Victoria and all her children. So there was never any need here. Our queens didn't accept any anaesthesia with their births, so there was never any reason for our upper-middle classes and so on to ask for anaesthesia. I think Queen Victoria's acceptance of general anaesthesia with one of her last deliveries has been very important for the other European countries, except Holland.

In seeking to more fully understand the Dutch approach to pain and the appropriate use of medicine, we must look to another feature of Dutch culture, *zuinigheid,* or thriftiness. This aspect of culture leads to a careful weighing of the pros and cons of the use of anesthesia at birth and inclines the Dutch to preserve home birth as a less expensive option in maternity care.

ZUINIGHEID (THRIFTINESS) AND SENSIBLE SOCIAL POLICY

The Dutch are often characterized as being careful in matters of money, a trait with connotations both positive (thriftiness) and negative (cheapness). Duke De Baena, a Spanish diplomat who spent several years in the Netherlands, offers a typical and somewhat pejorative description of this trait:

> There is no question but that in their mode of living the Dutch have an acute sense of thrift. . . . I must admit that from time to time when living in Holland, I have been irritated, and showed my irritation (with no result I fear) by the enormous importance the Dutch attach to something as insignificant as deciding whether a *dubbletje* (a ten cent piece) or a *kwartje* (a twenty-five cent piece) is the correct tip to leave in a certain place. . . . I honestly feel that every Dutchman receives a certain education which trains his character and finally leads him to behave as if he were a chartered accountant. (De Baena 1975 [1966], 25)

Some 35 years after De Baena published his observations, the Social and Cultural Planning Office of the Netherlands documented the continued, now slightly qualified, presence of zuinigheid among the Dutch:

> Although the Dutch are not extravagant in their leisure pursuits, to refer to the Netherlands as a Calvinist island in a hedonist Europe would be going too far. The Scandinavians would be more deserving of this title. For instance, the Dutch regard free time as just as important as work, whereas in almost all the other countries studied, people felt that work was considerably more important. The Dutch also account for a very high proportion of foreign tourism. The Netherlands has a large number of domestic (mostly commercial) and foreign television stations, probably because it has an extensive cable network. We have just as many television sets per 1,000 inhabitants as in other European countries, but we watch them less. No country has fewer cinemas per capita. . . . According to one survey, the Dutch read more books than people in other countries, but this is not reflected in spending on books, which is fairly low. In terms of participation in "higher" forms of culture, such as visits to museums and classical concerts, the Netherlands is by no means exceptional. Some Calvinist austerity might still be reflected in the amount of money the Dutch spend on their holidays. We spend an average of 30% less than other Europeans when we are on holiday abroad. Only the Irish and Spanish spend less. We also spend less in cafes and restaurants, although more than the Scandinavians. (2000a, 62–63)

A reporter for the online newspaper, the *InterNetKrant*[11] gives a pithy summary of these findings (14 September 2000):

> The Dutch are much more thrifty than the average European. We often go on vacation, but it must not cost too much. When we visit the café we spend little and we prefer to rent a video rather than going to the cinema. The Social and Cultural Report, delivered to Premier Kok yesterday, shows that the old cliché of the thrifty Hollander is still true, even though our average gross income of 50,000 guilders a year makes us one of the richest countries in Europe.

The thriftiness that marks the habits of Dutch individuals is also visible in Dutch social policy. Policymaking in the Netherlands is a very rational process involving careful, controlled studies of policy alternatives. The progressive social policies for which the Dutch are famous are rooted in an institutionalized willingness to experiment with unusual policies, testing their efficacy and efficiency—a willingness that allows the government to avoid moralistic stances on controversial issues. This frame of mind shapes Dutch policy on soft drugs, on prostitution, on euthanasia, *and* on the location of births. The government has funded many studies to examine the safety, cost, and desirability of home births and has made policy decisions based on those studies (see, for example, M. Eskes 1989; Wiegers 1997). The most recent of these studies openly acknowledges that the research was initiated because of a concern that "the steadily decreasing number of home births . . . threatened to diminish the home birth rate to a level where home birth would no longer be a viable option [and that] the increasing number of hospital births would lead to unnecessary medicalisation of pregnancy and childbirth"(Wiegers 1997, 1).

Caregivers are aware of the way zuinigheid influences maternity policy. A representative of the LHV (*Landelijke Huisartsen Vereniging*) told me,

> I think when you want to introduce in the States a system like this, you have to create general practitioners and midwives the way we do, in the area itself, and to make the law that they [i.e., patients] can get their help free only by the person who the States think is the most appropriate to do so. Because of course here the midwife is the cheapest. A midwife is cheaper than a doctor, than a huisarts.

---

11. See http://www.ics.ele.tue.nl/ink/

You mean cheaper in their costs to the Ziekenfonds.

To the cost of the *Ziekenfonds*. And of course when they're delivered at home it's cheaper than in the hospital. Of course. So when you're . . . looking for a system which looks for the most, for the cheapest way, you have to select always the cheapest provider, and make him given the *primaat*.

HEROES

Those who take a package tour of Europe will notice, if they are paying attention, that cities in the Netherlands are strikingly different from other European cities. I am not speaking of the ubiquitous canals, although these do give a distinct Dutch flavor to city life. There is another unique feature of the urban landscape in the Netherlands. When you walk the streets of London, Paris, or Madrid you are surrounded by large monuments celebrating the heroes of the country; in the Netherlands these monuments are noticeably absent. Stroll through Amsterdam and you will *not* see monumental sculptures, although you may bump into one of the two most famous sculptures in the city: *Het Lievertje,* a 30-inch-tall statue of an anonymous child, or the much-photographed three-foot-high statue of Anne Frank. Beaver (1987) notes: "Until the late 19th century there was no equestrian statue in the [Netherlands]; they are still most untypical. Heroic monumentality is simply un-Dutch."

This eschewing of the heroic permeates Dutch life, where children are reminded, *"Doe maar gewoon, dat is gek genoeg"* ("Just behave normally, that is crazy enough"), and *"Kom niet boven de maai veld"* ("Don't stick out above the mown field," implying that if you do, you might get your head cut off!).

In his review of the Dutch experience of, and approach to, war in the sixteenth and seventeenth centuries, Schama concludes:

Even though professional soldiers . . . played a crucial role in the defense of the Republic in the seventeenth century, they went conspicuously without honor in the patriotic culture of the time. . . . For both practical and principled reasons . . . war had come to be regarded in the Dutch Republic with a mixture of aversion and dismay. . . . [T]he marked unwillingness of the Dutch to allow the martial ethos status or dignity in its culture . . . separated it from the absolute monarchies,

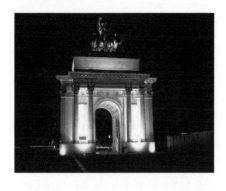

Wellington Arch, London

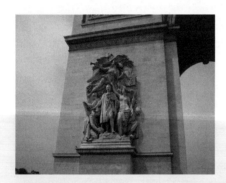

Detail from the Arc de
Triomphe, Paris

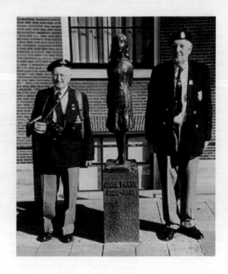

Statue of Anne Frank, Amsterdam

where whims of knightly valor and godlike indestructibility could be entertained at court. (1988, 240, 253)

The Dutch saw their dominance during the Golden Age as a result of their commercial, rather than their military, prowess. Rival nations found this annoying:

> The Dutch understanding of their own commercial power was that it op-
> erated independently of, and in spite of, military interruptions. And in
> this respect, there was some truth to the disdainful assertion of their en-
> emies that policy was made according to the prudential criteria of an en-
> larged merchant corporation rather than those becoming a great state.
> (Schama 1988, 253)

More recently, the Dutch have been forced to rethink their am-
bivalent approach to the military. In the summer of 1995 Dutch
troops were part of the United Nations force that was sent to the
Balkans to help keep the peace. Dutch soldiers assigned to protect
the Muslim citizens of Sebrenica were involved in a tragic series of
events. Out-manned and lacking a strong military tradition, the
Dutch force was overwhelmed by Serbian soldiers, who were allowed to round up men and boys and ship them off to be executed.
The inability of the Dutch force to protect these civilians caused
much soul-searching in the Netherlands, questioning whether they
were a people capable of heroic acts of war. A report concerning the
use of Dutch troops in peace missions issued five years after the incident in Sebrenica concluded that decisions to involve the Dutch
military in keeping the peace were often made with insufficient care.
Echoing the observations made about the Dutch military in the seventeenth century, the report noted:

> The political considerations that form the groundwork for the decision
> to allow Dutch troops to be involved in the so-called UN peace missions
> are more often based on maintaining prestige for "Corporate
> Netherlands" (*BV Nederland*) than on a careful weighing of the situation
> and the risks that might be run by the troops. (Quoted in *InterNetKrant*,
> 4 September 2000)

Gynecology in the Netherlands reflects this Dutch tendency to
downplay the heroic. In marked contrast to obstetricians in the
United States—who are *inclined* to heroically intervene, rescuing a laboring woman from protracted pain and life-threatening complications with surgery (episiotomies, forceps, and cesarean sections) or

medications—gynecologists in the Netherlands shun the role of hero. During interviews several Dutch gynecologists went out of their way to mention that they do not take a heroic approach to birth. The following is typical:

Why is the Dutch maternity system so different?

I think maybe it has a lot to do with the history of our country. We always have been a very individual, self-assured, emancipated people; a little bit mistrusting anyone, including doctors. I always say hospitals are dangerous . . . And maybe it has to do with the character of the people, that the doctors think with a little bit of relativity about their own duties and possibilities. We are not so much heroes, we do our best. That's the difference.

Is this attitude something Dutch gynecologists learn as part of their training?

No . . . I don't think the training is much different . . . in fact . . . it's so easy to play that role of the hero during a delivery. But [the mother] goes home with that lousy husband of hers, and not with the hero gynecologist. . . . When you respect your patients, even in delivery, or just in delivery, or utmost in delivery, you must play a very respectable, [but] tiny role. Do things, but do it not aloud. Do things, but . . . You understand? Not playing the hero . . . It's very easy to play the hero. When you are young and become a specialist of course you like to play the hero, but . . . no one is helped by it. . . . It diminishes her own role, of doing a lot of the performance, of the labor, of the work, you tiny[12] the role of the husband. . . . It's nonsense.

Ja, it gives you a lot of presents. I must admit that. But good doctors don't get a lot of presents. Very authoritative doctors, dictators, get a lot of presents. They get their special public and a lot of presents. But that's nonsense.

[When you play the hero] you don't let [your patients] grow. [You should] just play your role in a very simple way. . . . You're there, like a tiger sleeping in the sun, I sometimes say. With just one eye open to do the correct thing in the right time. Just a moment, and then you sleep again.

This refusal to stand out, to be heroic, to "come above the mown field" is linked to a final cluster of values that have helped shape Dutch maternity care policy, values that revolve around the notion of solidarity, the responsibility of all for each other.

---

12. Belittle, diminish.

SOLIDARITY

When comparing the health insurance systems of the Netherlands and the United States, most policy analysts note that the Dutch system reflects a higher degree of "solidarity" among the citizenry. We are told that the idea of a guaranteed basic package of benefits, of controls on the price/cost of services, and of limited access to certain services works in the Netherlands in a way that is impossible in the more individualistic, market-driven United States. But what is the nature of this Dutch solidarity? How is it maintained in the advanced capitalist economy of the Netherlands? What sustains the Dutch culture of negotiation, where the interests of all are considered in policy decisions? Answering these questions will allow us to understand how the structures that support midwife-attended birth at home persisted in the Netherlands and disappeared elsewhere.

The foundations of Dutch solidarity are found in unique features of Dutch social life, including (1) the polder model and its roots in *verzuiling,* (2) the peculiar Dutch notion of the *vergadering* (meeting), and (3) the Dutch insistence that everything should be *bespreekbaar* (speakable).

The Polder Model and Verzuiling

In the late 1990s, the Dutch were widely praised for a model of economic cooperation that was dubbed the "polder model," a model characterized by ongoing and constructive dialogue between employers, unions, and the government.[13] The polder model—sometimes referred to as the *overlegeconomie* (the consultation economy)—is credited for reducing government debt, lowering the overall tax burden, and strengthening the market economy (see www.nrc.nl /evj/ artikel/800000904.html).

According to the Netherlands Foreign Trade Agency, the polder model has created a "smooth running and stable economy, marked by a long-standing international orientation and that is among the 15 largest economies in the world" (http://www.hollandtrade.com). Ewald Kist, former Chairman of the Board of ING, a large banking and investment firm in the Netherlands says,

---

13. A *polder* is a piece of land reclaimed from the sea by using a system of dykes and pumps.

One of the biggest competitive advantages of the Netherlands is the polder model. The unique cooperation between government and business allows us to maintain our place in the larger world. Every day we profit from the "polder model principle." I expect this model to spread and to be copied by other countries. (1998)

Kranenburg locates the history of the polder model in the Dutch inclination for consensus:

Consensus has been institutionalized in the Netherlands, where national identity is reflected in countless advisory and consultative bodies. Every issue bearing even the remotest risk of disagreement has a forum of its own in which all interested parties are represented, whether it be traffic issues, defence matters or education affairs.

The well known "Polder Model" was born in the early 80s. There were political plans to intervene in the country's wage levels: the government hoped to tackle the high rate of unemployment by sharply reducing labour costs. Facing the loss of their freedom of negotiation, unions and employers' organisations agreed to a voluntary wage restraint in return for a reduction in working hours . . . a trade off of interests that still lies at the heart of current socio-economic policy. (2001, 38)

But of course the history of the polder model extends back beyond the 1980s. The term itself was chosen because of its reference to the kind of cooperation needed to keep the polders dry. As Pleij notes, "The Netherlands owes its existence to the democracy of dry feet. We need each other literally in order not to drown" (quoted in Kranenburg 2001, 37).

Steenhuis (1998) noticed the roots of the polder model in a children's book series popular in the Netherlands in the 1950s and 1960s: the stories of the twin brothers Hielke and Sietse and their motorboat, the *Kameleon*.[14] The sixty books in the series describe the adventures of the twins as they come to the aid of stranded sailors and drowning children, modeling community spirit and personal responsibility. Steenhuis notes:

---

14. In 2002, a movie depicting the adventures of the Hielke and Sietse was made—*De Schippers van de Kameleon* ("The Skippers of the Kameleon"). See www.dekameleonfilm.nl for more information about the movie.

In her speech before the parliament the queen said: "Community spirit and personal responsibility are both needed to respond to the great questions and challenges of our time." For Dutch adults that grew up reading the books about Hielke and Sietse Klinkhamer and their boat the *Kameleon*—and that must be many, given that 13 million books have been sold—this will be "child's play" [*gesneden koek,* that is, "cut cake," or we Americans might say "a piece of cake"]. Because in these books Hielke and Sietse do nothing but fulfill the ideals of community spirit and personal responsibility. They solve problems in their community and help the unemployed and beggars in their village. When on the lake "Sunday sailors" or professional skippers find themselves in difficulty, Hielke and Sietse rush to their aid in their "lumbering but sturdy" motorboat the *Kameleon*. And they ask nothing for their life-saving activities.

It is no coincidence that the Netherlands is now reaping the benefits of the polder model . . . employees have agreed to moderate their salary demands so that Dutch corporations can better compete with foreign rivals. But in exchange for these concessions, employers have promised to create more jobs, giving opportunities for the unemployed. That is completely in the spirit of Hielke and Sietse: they themselves had no need of money or payment, instead they used their rewards to help the unemployed. The creation of the polder model is, at least in part, the result of the fact that when they were young both current employees and employers read the *Kameleon* books. (24)

But the polder model is not the simple result of this series of books written by Hotze de Roos, a Frisian carpenter. The readers of these books grew up in a "pillarized" society (see Chapter 4) that had to find a way to promote the larger good of the nation while seeing to the interests of each pillar. There is an interesting paradox here: How can solidarity emerge from a system of pillarization, with its inclination toward segregation?

Pettigrew and Meertens (1996) studied this puzzle. They asked, "How does a tolerant society emerge from pillarized social organization, where separate religious and social pillars (*zuilen*) distributed resources in a 'separate but equal' manner?" In order to answer this question, they examined both structural and cultural features of the Netherlands; two of their points about the Dutch are relevant here (6–7):

1. *A tradition of elite cooperation:* In the pillarized system, elites from each pillar developed a way to work together to balance the needs

of their pillar with the needs of other pillars and the nation, creating a tradition of compromise; and

2. *Conflict avoidance as a general Dutch characteristic:* They suggest that "Dutch tolerance may simply be part of a broader, more embedded characteristic of conflict avoidance. In a small land, with centuries of adapting to flood dangers and high population density, there have been good reasons to maximize cooperation and minimize conflict" (7–8).[15]

They conclude with this observation: "We suggest that an important part of the answer [to the puzzle of tolerance in a pillarized society] lies in a strong Dutch tradition of cooperation in pursuit of superordinate goals that benefit both the individual groups and the nation" (13).

The Vergadering: The Culture of Negotiation in Daily Life

If pillarization provided the historical backdrop for Dutch solidarity and the culture of negotiation, it is the Dutch idea of the vergadering (meeting) that sustains and recreates these values on a daily basis. Business people who travel to the Netherlands describe the Dutch as obsessed with meetings. The Dutch themselves speak of their vergadering culture—in fact, van Vree, a Dutch author, has gone so far as to name the Netherlands *vergaderland* (van Vree 1996). We need to take a closer look at the distinctive features of the Dutch vergadering if we are to understand the political system and the culture of negotiation that has sustained maternity policy in the Netherlands.

In her research on the Dutch/French differences in the relationship between the individual and the group, de Bony describes a typical Dutch vergadering:

> *"De vergadering"* proceeds through a well defined and structured series of steps . . . it begins with a go round the table in which each concerned individual has a chance to give his opinion. Then, after some possible negotiations, the group begins to elaborate a common decision. When everyone agrees on the decision, action points are defined and distributed. At the end there is a final tour which allows non-favored individuals to express their feeling in order to limit their frustrations." (2001, 3)

---

15. For more on the way the *waterschapbestuur* (water boards) worked and influenced Dutch culture see Bartstra and Banning (1948, 140–158).

Knowing that the Dutch place a high value on *both* the group and the individual, de Bony expected to find a high degree of tension at group meetings. She was "surprised" to find "an atmosphere of consensus and not a climate of friction" (2). She goes on: "The Dutch attitude toward situations of opposing interests looks peculiar to foreigners. Conflicts seem much more easily negotiated, escaped or denied" (2). As Benders and his colleagues put it, "The Dutch can state their opinions very strongly, but are aware that it is only an opinion and are prepared for a compromise" (2000).

De Bony traces the civility of the *vergadering* to lessons Dutch children learn early in their education: "Dutch social behavior is early implemented at the elementary school, which puts emphasis on self-consciousness, self-confidence and social interaction. These qualities are trained on a regular basis during the discussion circle [or] *het kringgesprek.*"

In order to give a picture of the *kringgesprek* (literally "circle speak"), de Bony cites Bessell:

> [The teacher] controls that the children listen to one another with patience and attention and that every child has his own turn. He encourages the contribution of each individual and strives in the first instance for the occurrence of a warm, tolerant, and sincere atmosphere in the group. The form of a circle adds its contribution to the process: [They] talk about the social magic of the circle. People feel physically a part of something. They are feeling more close together and less separate as individuals. (1979)

De Bony concludes her analysis with a comment on how the idea of the *vergadering* resonates through Dutch society: "Group cohesion is particularly important in the Dutch culture. Early implemented at school, it strongly appears in Dutch social life." She suggests that the Dutch word for society, *samenleving*—literally, "living together"—reflects the peculiar resolution of the tension between the individual and the group.

Bespreekbaarheid

Linked to Dutch notions of solidarity and the importance of negotiation is the widely shared view that when it comes to social policy, nothing should be outside the realm of discussion, everything should be *bespreeekbaar,* or "speakable." James Kennedy sees the Dutch desire to make everything bespreekbaar, as a key element in the controversial and often misunderstood Dutch policy on euthanasia:[16]

> Many Netherlanders think that a problem is half solved if they just make that problem bespreekbaar. For Americans this is a strange word, impossible to translate. In Sweden euthanasia has always been a taboo word, but in the Netherlands there has been a campaign—especially in the 1970s—to take euthanasia out of the arena of the taboo. Euthanasia might be good or it might be bad, but it is always bad if it is done secretly. . . . Netherlanders believe that as long as euthanasia is bespreekbaar, misuse will always come to light . . . [Netherlanders] have great trust in each other, perhaps because of their collective tendency to make everything bespreekbaar. They find themselves an empathetic, but also responsible and sober people . . . [and they] have faith in their institutions and their own good intentions. (2001)

It is easy to find evidence to support Kennedy's conclusion. When the Dutch discuss their law on euthanasia they never fail to mention their desire to "get the topic out in the open." In explaining their policy, the Web site of the Dutch embassy points out that euthanasia is practiced covertly in many countries but "the Dutch government does not turn a blind eye to the fact that euthanasia happens. The question of whether—and how—criminal liability for euthanasia should be restricted has been the subject of broad political and public debate for the past 30 years" (http://www.netherlands-embassy.org/). And the Dutch minister of health says, "I know there are misunderstandings. But I also know that

---

16. The evolving Dutch policy on euthanasia is a source of fascination for the foreign press, the subject of frequent news reports and ironically—or perhaps not—much misunderstanding. Most non-Netherlanders are surprised to learn that euthanasia *continues* to be an offense in a formal sense—Dutch law prohibits the taking of another person's life, even if it is at that other person's express request. The euthanasia law allows doctors who exercise "due care" in ending the life of another to escape criminal proceedings. The criteria for assessing whether a doctor has applied euthanasia with due care are:

a. Be satisfied that the patient's request is voluntary and well-considered;
b. Be satisfied that the patient's suffering is unbearable and that there is no prospect of improvement;
c. Inform the patient of his or her situation and further prognosis;
d. Discuss the situation with the patient and come to the joint conclusion that there is no other reasonable solution;
e. Consult at least one other physician with no connection to the case, who must then see the patient and state in writing that the attending physician has satisfied the due care criteria listed above under points a through d;
f. Exercise due medical care and attention in terminating the patient's life or assisting in his or her suicide.

there is much respect for the open, serious manner in which the Dutch deal with euthanasia. In other countries, the whole issue is shrouded in secrecy—which does not mean that euthanasia is never performed. What we want is for doctors to act in the open" (quoted in Rijk De Vries 2000).

Bespreekbaarheid is a product of Dutch notions of solidarity and their culture of negotiation, reflecting, as Kennedy says, the "great trust" the Dutch have in each other, in their institutions, and in their own good intentions.

The values that undergird the polder model, the vergadering, and bespreekbaarheid permeate Dutch life. For example, a 2001 study of the Dutch family concluded "in the modern gezin everything is negotiable . . . almost everything is bespreekbaar," leading one reporter to conclude the "polder model has infiltrated the gezin" (Schöttelndreier 2001).

These values play an important role in the persistence of midwifery and home birth. The emphasis on negotiation and on "hearing all sides" gives the profession of midwifery in the Netherlands a power and a voice it lacks elsewhere. A sense of solidarity, coupled with zuinigheid and a shunning of the heroic, sustains the choice of birth at home, away from the expensive interventions of high technology. Rather than a notion that birth is accomplished best with the latest and most expensive technologies, Dutch culture supports a view that insists a simpler approach to birth is best for everyone. Schut summarizes:

> In the . . . Dutch health care system, decision-making is the outcome of consensus policy. The Christian Democrats, who dominated politics throughout the twentieth century, deliberately rendered (or transferred) as much power as possible to representative organizations of providers, health insurers, employers, and employees. Those organizations are officially involved in the major advisory bodies and other quasi-governmental organizations, which play a determining role in the decision making process. Within this complex structure of checks and balances, neither the government nor any of the major interest groups has enough power to accomplish fundamental changes independent of the others. (1995, 646–648)

On the Web page that describes the philosophy that underlies the *Geboortewinkel* in Amsterdam that offers information and products for birth and parenthood, direct reference is made to the polder model: "Homebirth and the midwife play an important role [in the unique system of birth in the Netherlands], with the hospital and the gynecologist in the background for safety. The Birth Shop supports this Dutch polder model of midwifery" (http://www.degeboortewinkel.nl/).

Conclusion: Dutch Culture and Dutch Birth

Although the idea of a "national culture" is still held at arm's length by social scientists, it is clear that the Dutch have unique, historically situated notions about a variety of things—home, the family, roles of women, pain, the use of health services and medicines, thriftiness, heroes, and the relationship between the individual and the group (i.e., solidarity)—and that these ideas shape health care policy, indeed, *all* social policy. This collection of ideas has particular relevance for the unique maternity care policy of the Netherlands, helping us understand the why the Dutch have preserved a way of birth that seems old-fashioned elsewhere.

Others have noticed the link between cultural ideas and maternity care systems. The Dutch themselves have pointed to aspects of their culture that support their unique way of birth. Kloosterman (1966), although critical of the *British* use of Dutch culture to explain the persistence of home birth, offers his own cultural explanations of obstetrics in the Netherlands: He notes that the Dutch are inclined to be "domestic, sober, adverse to showiness, not fearful of pain and discomfort, and thrifty," which fits with their way of birthing. Writing in the journal of the association of Dutch midwives, Rottinghuis (1947) expresses a similar opinion: "Birth is a family event (*gezinsgebeuren*) and, given the high value placed on the family (gezin) in the Netherlands, it must occur in that context" (quoted in van Daalen 1988, 432–433).

In her discussion of the metaphors we use to talk about birth, Martin (1987) shows how English words—reproduction, labor, progress—reflect an industrial, capitalist mentality that demeans the experience of birth. Interestingly, the Dutch use *different* images when speaking of birth. Reproduction is *voortplanting,* literally "forward planting," an agricultural metaphor, and when a Dutch woman is in labor, she is *aan het bevallen,* "in the act of birthing." Labor pains are *weeën,* the same word found in *heimwee,* homesickness, or more literally, the "aching" (weeën) for home.

Having identified cultural ideas that lie behind the Dutch way of birth, it is fair to ask how much explaining we can we ask these ideas to do. Two caveats are in order. First, this portrayal of the role of culture in the shaping the Dutch obstetric system does *not* necessarily imply that Dutch society is homogenous or that all Dutch women have identical views of family, home, medicine, and the like. Indeed, Dutch society is increasingly multicultural, incorporating a number of peoples from former colonies in

Indonesia and South America as well as from Northern Africa, Turkey, and Eastern Europe. In the Netherlands, however, the majority of those who make policy are women and men who are steeped in the traditional ideas of Dutch culture, and the organization of maternity care there bears the marks of that culture; even in the midst of multiculturalization, nation-states continue to set important boundaries for discourse and practice.[17]

The Dutch government and midwives are aware that newcomers to their society must learn about the Dutch way of birth. More than one midwife told me about the need to point out the advantages of midwife-attended home birth to these women, many of whom see physician care in the hospital as a mark of being a modern, Western woman. The government has financed information campaigns for immigrants, using pamphlets and videos in several languages to familiarize new residents with the way birth is done in the Netherlands.

A second caveat about the explanatory power of culture: The influence of the cultural ideas described here must be seen in the context of several other features of society. Culture is not *the* explanatory variable: It is shaped by the structures of society even as it shapes those structures. The difficulty of measuring culture and parsing its influence, however, should not stop us from examining the important ways it shapes health care systems. Our timidity in this area has caused us to overlook the important ways health systems are produced by culture and has hampered efforts to create a more just distribution of health care.

* * * * *

What about Malpractice Insurance?

In discussing my research with other social scientists and medical professionals, I often heard that the real (and only) reason for the difference between obstetrics in the United States and in the Netherlands was the problem of malpractice. If obstetricians in the United States were not subject to so many malpractice actions, they would be free to behave more like gynecologists in the Netherlands. Malpractice, like medicine, is rooted in culture. The following excerpts from interviews with two different gynecologists highlight many of the cultural notions

---

17. This notion of the nation-state as a community of discourse and practice is especially true in the Netherlands—a small country with a high degree of centralization.

that inform health policy and medical practice. In these comments you will see how the medical system of the Netherlands—including its approach to malpractice—is the product of cultural ideas about solidarity, zuinigheid, a nonheroic approach to birth, pain, and the body:

> *I'm interested in hearing your reflections on malpractice. There was an article in* Vrij Nederland *a few weeks ago on the coming of malpractice to the Netherlands, and the* Algemeen Dagblad *had a piece encouraging people, saying "Hey, you can get* vergoeding *(reimbursement) for your damages." I thought "Oh, no; America is coming." What do you think?*

Luckily it's on a very low level, till now. And we have no insurance fees [for physicians] as you face.

You don't pay liability insurance?

We do . . . but being a private gynecologist I have been one to pay some thousands of guilders a year. But maybe a thousand is enough, that's all.[18]

You know, in the United States some doctors pay sixty or seventy thousand dollars or more.

And they even forbid you to do breeches in some states, vaginal birth for breeches. No, we have not that . . . I do a lot of advising in those [malpractice] cases, but I must say that even the number of cases are rather low.

Now how do you understand that; why is it, why are they low here?

It's of course the system of lawyers is quite different here. When I read in my paper that in American being a director and throwing some chocolates in the décolleté of a secretary may cost you 8 million dollars, we think you're quite mad. We always think you're quite mad when we're reading that kind of things.

In our eyes you have an amazing culture of justice and of lawyers . . . The whole circus. . . . of that sportsman who killed his wife [O.J. Simpson] on television, it's unbelievable. And the costs! We think that should be in court for two days, and the case is clear; shut him up in a cell for some years and it's over.

So I think the difference, the essence of the difference, is the culture in court and the culture with respect to lawyers. And that has influenced the public. And of course we all fear, we are all a little bit afraid of what we call "American situations," of course we're afraid of that sometimes. And of course, in our own practices we recognize a little

---

18. At the time of the interview a guilder was worth about $.60; he is suggesting that he paid between $600 and $1000 a year for malpractice insurance.

bit what we call "defensive medicine": in case of doubt, do something. But we don't like it. Because, in general in medicine, you should consider the possibility of "in case of doubt, don't." In case of doubt, the choice is to nature.

First do no harm, eh?

Yes; do not, so do no harm. Yes, you're right.

Certainly malpractice occurs, mistakes happen, you know. How is that handled? Do the patients just say "well, mistakes happen?"

We have a so-called *tucht*-court (a disciplinary council), you know that? That's a court from the [medical] specialty with some judges in it, not civil rights, so not for money, not punishments, but behavior. We call that *"tuchtrecht"* (disciplinary jurisdiction). In the majority of cases there is a behavior, communication problem. So I teach all my students, and all my assistants in training: "Be honest. When you make a mistake, be honest about your mistake. In most cases people will accept that."

And does it go farther? . . . there must be cases that . . .

There are some cases, and I advise . . . but in most cases, I must admit, it's rather a complication than a definite, absolute fault. People make the wrong choice between choices. When you consider the possibility of what you would have done yourself in those cases, you must admit that you could have made the same choice. You understand? And I think that's because we have not the practices from the court and insurance companies as you have. There is a common feeling, even among the public, that you must be able to make mistakes. As any one.

I'm curious what you think might explain the very low rate of cesarean section in the Netherlands. Or the very high rate in America.

Well, that must be due to defensive medicine. But there are interesting differences in [rates in] Holland as well, you must be aware of that. There are no American situations here, but there is a tendency in that direction . . . we are worried about the increase, and in Holland the increase now is due to eh . . . a little bit hastiness, a lack of patience, not to allow a first pregnancy under safe circumstances to wait one-and-a-half or two hours in second stage. That's one. [There is] a little bit of change in the attitude of the public as well. After one hour they say "here I am in the hospital and I had a first stage of one hour, and I think it's been enough, so do your job." Ja; a little bit. Eh . . . and also the false positive troubles of cardiotopography. Three-quarters of them are false, as you may know.

Our methods to know whether a child is in danger or not have a very low sensitivity. And more than half, yes I think three-quarters is false positive. And in hospitals where you have not the follow-up cardiotopography, for instance . . . blood samples to correct your impression, to objectify your impression, and in a lot of hospitals it's not in use any more, then you do a lot of cesareans.

We are a so-called third line care center, we have a lot of cesareans due to very little tiny children in danger.

You'd expect the third line to have more than the second line.

Yes. We are very worried. I think we have now 18 percent.

In the third line?

Yes.

I laugh, because you know, in the United States, nationwide it's twenty-two. And that's with everybody.

Ja; that's nonsense. That must be put down.

A second gynecologist gives his opinion about malpractice in the Netherlands and the United States:

Obstetricians in the United States would never feel comfortable saying what you've just said. They are paying sixty and seventy thousand dollars every year for malpractice insurance. Is malpractice becoming an issue in the Netherlands?

It raises; it raises extremely. Ten years ago we said we don't get American situations. No, not in Holland. But it's starting, and it's growing extremely.

And of course malpractice is important for understanding how American obstetricians work. Fear. Fear is, eh, like we say in Holland, "fear is a bad consultant." *"Angst is een slechte raadgever."* And that means, somebody who is pregnant now for six weeks, you can make a list of two papers of the extreme things which can happen to her. She can die in the eighth week because she has a miscarriage after an extrauterine pregnancy, she can die at delivery, she can die six weeks after delivery because of thrombosis, and we haven't given her something like anticoagulants. If you are afraid about that, you better go and sit in a corner, and be quiet. That's the difference between America and the Netherlands.

Do you think this is coming now though, this increase in malpractice?

Sure. And we can only be in front of this by making good regulations ourselves, good protocols, making it visible to politics and to lawmakers what we are doing.

A few months ago, it was in the papers, there were some gynecologists who made a serious error. Will they be sued?

Yes, I think so. They will be sued, yes. Because it has reached such a large public, they will be sued, yes, I think so. But I think that in the same period, in my hospital, the same complication has happened, but we are not sued. Because we have gone to the people who were involved. And we've said that we made a mistake, and it has such large implications, and why did we make a mistake, because it's no science, and we thought at that moment this was happening and that was happening, and we talked about it with the midwife and with the family doctor, and we talked about it with the couple, and again with the couple, and we've shown the baby, and we've made our apologies, and we've tried to get information about what kind of people were working.

It's not extreme that babies are dying. They're dying every day, in every hospital in Holland, but it's the way you inform people, and the way you work together with midwives. And a midwife which you don't see, and what you don't talk about, will say to the couples: "Well, to my opinion he has made a fault." A midwife which you see every month and with which you talk about things and you have nice contact with, will say to the same couple: "I have talked also with the gynecologist; he's so sorry, and he's made this fault and he has talked with you and he has a lot of questions to me, and . . ." Well, that's another way of dealing with it. So that's important. But things which happen in Helmond happen in Alkmaar, happen in Amsterdam, happen in Detroit, and everywhere where people deliver.

Sometimes it's the same like Zeeland, 1953. We had then a large disaster, with the sea overflowing the dunes and the dikes, and nobody had seen it coming, and thousands of people died and there was a lot of damage. But that's obstetrics. Sometimes a disaster happens, in a minute, in two minutes, and you can't see it coming. You know that it can happen, and that it can happen with every patient. That's the difference between American obstetrics. They see a sign "Oh Jezus, it can be an embolus of the amniotic fluid." In thousand situations it won't be and in thousand-and-one yes it is. In thousand-and-one situations we do a cesarean, "oh, let's do a cesarean, quick!" And then it wasn't an embolism. Well, okay.

But that's what I'm very curious about. You've described it exactly. Why is it that Dutch gynaecologen don't intervene?

Because they don't see their patients yet as enemies. Not yet.

In listening to these gynecologists talk we are forced to recognize that, yes, malpractice is an issue that distinguishes the Dutch and American ways of birth, but we also see that it will take more than tort reform to change the way American malpractice works. Birth in the Netherlands and malpractice in the Netherlands are different because of the many different values of the Dutch.

6   Two Sciences or No Science? Obstetric Research in the Netherlands

Obstetrics is wider and broader than pure medicine. It has to do with the whole of life, the way you look at life, making objective discussion difficult. You are almost unable to split the problem off into pure science; always your outlook on life is involved.

—Professor Jan Gerrit Kloosterman

WHEN I first arrived in the Netherlands, I assumed I would find a widely accepted science of obstetrics that "fit" their way of delivering care. I pictured gynecologists, midwives, health care researchers, and policymakers working together, doing research that supported the Dutch way of birth. In my earlier research, done in the United States, I observed obstetricians and supporters of midwives and home birth arguing from two *different* bodies of evidence. Each side was able to muster scientific research in defense of its position, even though the two positions were mutually exclusive. I did not expect to find this same scientific split in the Netherlands. It seemed reasonable to believe that, in the face of standard medical practices elsewhere, the odd system of maternity care found in the Netherlands would not survive without consensus about the wisdom of this approach to birth and a carefully constructed science that provided a foundation for their policies. If nothing else, I expected maternity caregivers to be united in their pride over their special way of birth—a way of birth that is the darling of alternative birth communities in other nations.

It came as something of shock, therefore, when I discovered a number of researchers—gynecologists and epidemiologists—who were unconvinced that this old-fashioned approach was the best way to bring babies into the world. I was not surprised to find quarrels over the way the system was administered, but I found it difficult to believe that there was—right there in the Netherlands—loyal opposition to the

180

Dutch way of birth. And yet, as I began to read the journals of Dutch medical professions, I found researchers and childbirth advocates engaged in serious, scientific debate about the safety and advisability of midwife-assisted birth at home.

It was a Dutch gynecologist who first told me about the two sciences of obstetrics in the Netherlands:

> At the Free University . . . obstetrics is: "there is a patient who is ill, who has to get a baby." And two kilometers away is the University of Amsterdam, where they say "Somebody who is pregnant is a very healthy woman. She has proved to be healthy because she's got pregnant. And she's only ill when she's proved to be ill." Do you know what I mean?

> *I do. But how did this happen? How is it that one university has one attitude about pregnancy and another, in the same city, has a completely different opinion?*

> The most important [reason] is that obstetrics is no science. Obstetrics is experience, is belief, is seeing wolves in the woods, is eh, depends on nature. But there are no . . . not many really, scientific papers about obstetrics. One of the nice examples is that there has been a controlled trial, a really good investigation, multi-center, in a lot of countries, about aspirin in pregnancy. In people with high blood pressure . . . about 7,000 people were involved in it, and what was the conclusion? Aspirin doesn't work! If you phoned to a university hospital [and said] I have that and that women [with high blood pressure] what would you do? [At] the Free University, they say "Well, I should try aspirin. I'm not happy with that investigation." Because it was not what they expected. At the other hospital (University of Amsterdam) they would say: "No aspirin. They've shown now that it's not effective"

> But it's not science.

> *You are convinced of that, eh?*

> Yes. And we're working on it; we're working hard on it. But why isn't it science? Because in obstetrics you can't do an investigation like in other [specialties]. You can't put a needle in the baby and give him a radio-diagnostic exam, and make photos of him, and put him out. . . . And I think that's the most important reason why such different opinions can exist.

He went on to detail the many roadblocks that hinder a thoroughgoing science of obstetrics. Not only is it difficult to get permission to do clinical studies of newborns, but also it is impossible to do randomized clinical trials. One cannot randomly assign pregnant women to experimental and control groups, demanding—with no regard for a woman's preference—that one mother birth her baby at home under the care of a midwife and another deliver at a hospital with physician assistance. Not only is this ethically unacceptable, but researchers are convinced that random assignment would affect outcome: Women assigned to a delivery method they do not prefer will have higher levels of anxiety, and this could complicate the course of delivery. And, he added, even if one *could* find a practical and ethically acceptable way to randomly assign women to different types of care there is the problem of sample size. Nearly all the researchers I interviewed mentioned this problem: Because women in Western societies are well nourished, well-educated, and well-housed, it would be necessary to enroll tens of thousands of women in a study in order to detect caregiver generated differences in morbidity and mortality rates at birth. This allows any study to be challenged:

> [A critic can always say] the figures are too small. It's not a real good investigation. It doesn't respond to the [experimental] criteria. So, if you want to talk about it, you have to have very large figures. And you can't go, . . . you can't work with this kind of figures.

This interview, conducted early in my research, disabused me of my idyllic and overly simple notions about Dutch obstetric science. I was forced to reconsider the relation between medical practice and medical science.

To be fair, the Dutch *have* generated a good deal of research confirming the safety of midwife-assisted birth at home, but the persistence of two sciences of obstetrics, where we might have expected gynecologists to speak with one voice to protect their maternity care system, suggests that Kloosterman is right: In creating a science of obstetrics, "always your outlook on life is involved." There seems to be something about birth that makes science especially difficult. Before we develop a sociology of obstetric science in the Netherlands, we must look more closely at the special problems that attend a science of obstetrics, wherever it is attempted.

The Difficulty of a Science of Obstetrics

Majorie Tew, an epidemiologist working in the United Kingdom, discovered the difficulties of doing obstetric science when she began her research on the safety of home and hospital birth. Her work in this area was serendipitous, the result of an assignment she devised for her students. As an epidemiologist with no special training, or interest, in maternity care, she assumed the shift to hospital birth that occurred in the first half of the twentieth century (in England and elsewhere) was based on solid medical grounds. Finding no published studies that confirmed this common-sense assumption, Tew assigned her students to do an epidemiological study of home and hospital birth. As their work as a class progressed, she was shocked to learn that there was *no* evidence that hospital birth was safer; in fact, the data seemed to suggest that *home* birth was the safer of the two options. In the preface to her "critical history of maternity care," Tew describes her and her colleagues' reaction to her surprising discovery:

> I was teaching students in the Department of Community Health in Nottingham University's young medical school how much they could find out about various diseases from the available official statistics. As part of these epidemiological exercises, I discovered to my complete surprise that the relevant routine statistics did not appear to support the widely accepted hypothesis that the increased hospitalization of birth had caused the decline by then achieved in the mortality of mothers and their new babies. At first, it seemed hardly possible that I could be right in questioning the justification for what the medical world and everyone else apparently believed, but my further researches only served to confirm my initial discovery. My pursuit of the subject was not encouraged in the Department. My temporary contract of employment was not renewed.
>
> Medical journals were not eager to publish an article presenting the results of my statistical analyses. I was dismayed that there was such formidable resistance to discussing openly honest, well founded criticism of the basis of established policies. Against all odds, I became determined to break through the resistance and to fight against the false use of statistics to support a system that was actually harming its proclaimed beneficiaries. (Tew 1995, viii–ix)

What struck Tew, and what strikes the readers of her work, is not only this large blind spot in the science of obstetrics, but the unwillingness (of scientists!) to correct it, or even *study* it. Research in this field goes on, with no systematic investigation of—indeed, with no *acknowledgement* of—the possible negative effects of its technological ministrations. Obstetricians claim the mantle of science even while they use custom and culture to protect their ways of practicing from scientific challenge.

One of the best illustrations of the way obstetric science is embedded in one's outlook on life is the story of Michael Klein's research on the value of episiotomies. After working with midwives in Ethiopia and the UK, who "rarely employed episiotomy and yet obtained apparently good results," Klein began to question the high rate of episiotomies in his native Canada; the rate at his hospital was in excess of 60 percent overall and greater than 80 percent for primiparous women. He decided to initiate a randomized clinical trial (RCT) to see whether episiotomy offered the benefits its supporters in North America believed it did: less pressure on the fetal brain, improved maternal soft tissue support and pelvic floor function, and decreased delayed morbidity, such as urinary incontinence.

Encouraged by the publication of a large, midwifery-based RCT in England, which showed *no* benefit from a policy of routine use of mediolateral episiotomy, Klein began organizing his research. But he failed to appreciate the inertia of established clinical practice. Not only did Klein and his colleagues have difficulty getting funded, they also had problems getting physicians to cooperate with the research protocol, and they struggled to get their results published.

Reviews of their research proposal were sharply divided. In one case two reviewers came to precisely opposite conclusions. One claimed, "The research questions are not relevant to clinical practice and the answers will not likely provide assistance in practice" while another asserted, "The research questions are relevant to clinical practice and the answers provided will be of assistance in the practice of obstetrics." The Medical Research Council of Canada denied funding even though three of four reviewers were supportive.

Klein and his team did eventually secure funding, but as their work progressed they found that certain physicians had difficulty following the research protocol: They were simply unwilling to assign women to the "restricted use" arm of the study. Even though all participating physicians had volunteered to be a part of the research and were well aware of its protocol, there were a number of doctors—most of whom looked favorably on episiotomies—who were quick to find reasons to exclude a subject from the study (and thus do an episiotomy).

In spite of a higher than expected use of episiotomy in the in the "restricted use" arm of the study, Klein and his colleagues were able to complete their research successfully. They discovered that routine use of episiotomy could not be justified: It did not prevent perineal trauma, reduce pain, or improve sexual and pelvic floor outcomes. Eager to get this news to widest possible audience they sent reports of their research to the leading journals in medicine, the *New England Journal of Medicine* and the *Journal of the American Medical Association (JAMA)*. But editors at these journals were unwilling to publish Klein's work. Both rejected three separate papers, and both editors sent only one of the three submissions out for external review. The paper sent by *JAMA* for external review garnered two positive reviews, a negative review that focused on statistical questions, and a strongly negative review that questioned the value of the study. This last reviewer accused Klein and his colleagues of having a "bias against episiotomy," and went on to use a very poorly constructed study—one that compared outcomes for 1,000 women who birthed in the 1930s with 1,000 women who gave birth in the researcher's clinic in the 1940s and 1950s (with no control for social, obstetric, and demographic factors)—to challenge the results of the paper.

Eventually, the authors were able to get the results of their work disseminated, but not in the better-known, more widely circulated medical journals. They were forced to settle for publication in specialty journals (Klein et al. 1992; Klein et al. 1994; Klein 1995), in the *Canadian Medical Association Journal* (Klein et al. 1995), and in the popular press (for example, the *New York Times, USA Today, Toronto Globe and Mail, Reader's Digest,* and *Parents Magazine*).

In reflecting on his experience with this research, Klein attributes the difficulties he encountered to the fact that he was challenging well-entrenched views about birth: "Getting funded and published proved to be difficult since we were questioning not only established views on episiotomy but also conventional views about birth. . . . Those who struggle with paradigm change must be prepared for a long fight" (Klein 1995, 483, 487).

Why did Tew and Klein face such difficulties in getting their research into the mainstream of obstetric science? The problems they encountered originate, in part, in the fact that science is a human enterprise and, as such, it is subject to the social forces that influence all human activities. In science and in medicine, ways of thinking and ways of practicing are based on *what we all know,* and *what we all know* takes a long time to change.

And yet obstetrics seems *especially* mired in tradition and culture, especially politicized. The pronounced presence of these nonscientific factors in the science of obstetrics is the result of the peculiar nature of the practice. As noted in Chapter 1, obstetrics is unique among medical disciplines:

- What is at stake in care at birth is not the survival of one patient, but the reproduction of society.
- Embedded in the care given to women at birth are ideas about sexuality, about women, and about families.
- Although all other medical specialties (with the possible exception of pediatrics) begin with a focus on disease, the essential task here is the supervision of normal, healthy, physical growth.

These observations help us make sense of the resistance of obstetrics to science. While their colleagues in other medical specialties are rooting out and treating pathology, obstetrician/gynecologists must, in most cases, stand by and simply watch a healthy event occur. A science that affirms that "less is more" in the supervision of birth—the type of science you might expect to originate from a practice that monitors a healthy process—will not help obstetricians strengthen their professional position. Furthermore, as a critical life event, it is important that birth be accompanied by the significant symbols of the culture: In modern societies this means a place must be made for the complex mechanical and electronic technologies of monitoring and intervention.[1]

Given these facts, we would expect the work of Klein and Tew to be marginalized: Obstetricians who work in countries where a technological science of obstetrics holds sway have no interest in a contrary science that challenges the need for the complicated technologies of birth. But what about the Netherlands? Dutch obstetric science offers us a unique case study, because it must find a way to take into account their low-technology approach to maternity care while remaining re-

---

1. In their movie, *The Meaning of Life*, the Monty Python troupe satirizes this tendency brilliantly. Machines and a number of gowned and masked attendants surround a woman giving birth in a hospital. As the time of birth approaches the supervising physician asks for the "machine that goes ping." The machine is wheeled in and the expectant mother asks what it does. The physician is forced to admit that he has no idea, but that he is comforted by its presence and its reassuring "ping."

spectable in the eyes of a larger scientific community that endorses a more medical view of birth.

A Sociology of Obstetric Science in the Netherlands

Most descriptions of maternity care in the Netherlands fail to mention the ongoing debate between the two sciences of obstetrics. Foreign visitors often assume, as I did, that a single, unified science supports the Dutch way of birth. This false assumption is seldom challenged because the presence of a lively, scientific debate about the safety and advisability of midwife-assisted birth at home complicates the otherwise simple story of Dutch obstetrics. But there can be no doubt that this debate exists. In my interviews, and in the professional literature of midwives, gynecologists, and epidemiologists, I continually discovered encounters between these two sciences.

One of the most interesting of these encounters occurred at the retirement party of Dik van Alten, a gynecologist who was an important contributor to the research literature on Dutch maternity care. This story, recounted for me by those who were there, gives us a glimpse behind the scenes of the more formal debates that occur in the pages of professional journals or at conferences.

In the Netherlands, when an academic of note retires, it is not enough merely to have a party; there must be a gathering where the work of the retiree is commemorated. In November of 1989 one such conference—an *afscheidssymposium* (farewell symposium)—was organized to celebrate the retirement of Professor Dr. van Alten, a defender of the Dutch way of birth. Van Alten's research, his presentations at professional meetings, his writing, and his support of the research of others form an important chapter in the story of obstetrics in the Netherlands; in order to acknowledge his contribution to the field, a number of researchers who were studying the Dutch maternity care system were invited to present summaries of their work. Among the invitees was Geert Berghs, a doctoral student whose dissertation research involved a comparison of outcomes of normal pregnancies supervised in both the *eerste* and *tweede* lines. It is particularly interesting that Berghs was invited to present at this symposium because his research—done together with Esmerelda Spaanjards (see Berghs and Spanjaards 1988)—was part of a larger research program undertaken by members of the loyal opposition to the Dutch way of birth. Berghs' study was designed to take a critical look at the persistence of midwife-assisted home birth in the Netherlands.

The suspicion of the sponsors of Berghs' research—that in spite of favorable outcomes, midwife-assisted birth at home was unsafe—was not unreasonable. Because the Obstetrics Indications List (VIL) separates physiological and pathological births, it is very difficult to discern the effects of caregiver and place of birth on morbidity and mortality. The problem of sample size, mentioned above, is amplified here: Women defined as healthy by the VIL have very few poor outcomes, regardless of where and with whom they birth.

In order to get around this problem, the team of researchers that employed Berghs and Spanjaards devised a research strategy that would allow comparisons to be made even when there was no overt morbidity and mortality. How was this to be done? Researchers would look for small but significant differences in the pH of blood taken from the umbilical cord: Lower pH values are suggestive of oxygen deprivation (acidosis) and, hence, less than optimal outcomes for the neonatal brain. In conjunction with measures of cord blood pH, researchers also assessed outcomes using a scale that measured the neurological condition of the newborn. Developed by Prechtl (1977), the scale involves observation of the body and reflexes of the newborn.[2] These close observations of the health status of the neonate introduced some variability into otherwise similar birth outcomes.

Armed with these finer measures, Berghs and Spanjaards (1988) followed 1,034 normal pregnancies (as defined by the VIL) attended by midwives ($N = 638$), *huisartsen* ($N = 128$), and gynecologists ($N = 268$). Using Prechtl's scale they discovered that 84.6 percent of newborns in their study were "Normal," 12.3 percent were "Suspect" (i.e., showed signs suggestive of neurological problems), and 3.1 percent were "Abnormal." When the researchers analyzed neonatal outcome by caregiver, however, they found *no* differences between the three groups. They concluded that there were no significant differences in the outcomes of normal births managed by midwives, huisartsen, and gynecologists. They *did* discover that the 268 women in the study who

---

2. There are various versions of the scale; Berghs and Spanjaards used a 60-item scale developed by Touwen et al. (1980).

chose the care of a gynecologist were more likely to have experienced a medical intervention during birth and that their infants had higher rates of morbidity, measured by Apgar scores (a caregiver assessment of newborn health) and eventual hospitalization.[3]

The directors of the research were taken aback by the findings of Berghs and Spanjaards: This was not what they expected. Earlier research using these same outcome measures showed that babies born at home under midwife care had less than optimal outcomes (see, for example, Lievaart and de Jong 1982). But now, one of their students was being asked to share findings from this larger project that *supported* the Dutch way of birth—and, no less, at a symposium honoring a champion of home birth, Dik van Alten.

Before the date of his presentation, the directors of the research, Drs. Eskes and Stolte invited Berghs to come in and discuss what he would say. Stolte advised him to emphasize that even though all mothers in the study were defined as having normal pregnancies, the population of women who chose care from gynecologists were, in fact, in poorer health. The research *did* show that the women under specialist care were more likely to smoke, were less educated, and had more medical interventions in pregnancy and birth. Stolte wanted Berghs to argue for the superiority of specialist care because neurological outcomes were the same in all groups, *in spite of* the presence of these background factors (although, according to the VIL, all women in the study were defined as "normal"). In the end, Berghs refused the requests of his supervisors and presented his data as they were reported in his dissertation.

A more recent encounter between the two sciences took place in the national media. In early 2001 a report about perinatal mortality in the Netherlands appeared in the Dutch Journal of Medicine (*Nederlands Tijdschrift voor Geneeskunde*). The study was part of a larger European research project designed to find ways to further reduce infant death. The Dutch portion of the study examined 332 cases of perinatal death that occurred in 1996 and 1997 in one region of the Netherlands. A panel of experts reviewed these cases: They concluded in that in 19 percent of the cases one or more substandard factors in care were "possibly" responsible for the death and that in 6 percent of the cases one or

---

3. See also Berghs et al. (1995).

more substandard factors in care were "probably" responsible for the death (Vredevoogd et al. 2001, 482–487).

Near the end of the article, the authors observed that the international nature of the study offered the opportunity to compare outcomes in the Netherlands with other countries in Europe. They concluded, "the percentage of possibly and probably preventable perinatal deaths is about the same in the Netherlands as in most other countries participating in the study" (486).

Looking for a *better* story, Dutch journalists gave the study a more sensationalist twist; media reports about the research mixed correct citations with improper and suggestive conclusions, the most misleading of which was "one-quarter of the deaths of newborn or unborn babies could have 'possibly' or 'probably' been prevented. These deaths were attributable to the negligent care of the medical personnel involved" (Koldenhoff 2001).

A flurry of stories followed the initial media reports. A professor of pediatrics from Groningen, Prof. Dr. P.J.J. Sauer, proclaimed in the *Metro*, a national newspaper distributed free at railroad stations throughout the country, that home birth is risky for the baby and that the safest place to give birth is in a large, specialized hospital. He went on to assert that the lower perinatal death rate in Sweden is the result of the fact that home birth is not permitted there and he accused the KNOV of perpetrating a "belief" in home birth in order to protect their interests (*Metro* 2001).

Defenders of the Dutch way of birth also responded. They contacted news agencies and insisted on more accurate descriptions of the research. A report in the *NRC Handelsblad* noted, "The research pointed out that the Dutch obstetric system is safe. The risk of infant death is not related to the place of birth or the accompanying caregiver" (14 February 2001). The article also affirmed the *expectant* approach to birth used in the Netherlands. After acknowledging that more could be done to reduce perinatal death in the Netherlands, Professor P. Verloove-Van Horick, one of the authors of the study, went on to say, "But then there exists the danger of *over*treatment because you will end up treating children where everything would have gone well. The not-optimal factors were probably also present in cases where babies were born with no health problems" (emphasis added).

The Royal Dutch Organization of Midwives (KNOV) played an important role as a defender of the Dutch way of birth in this controversy. Writing in their professional journal, the chair of the organization, M. van Huis (2001, 344–345) commented on the European study: "Based on this international research, it can be concluded that the typical Dutch phenomenon of home birth has no negative effect on the quality of care." In response to Sauer's observations, she quoted a statement released by Professor of Obstetrics (at Leiden) H.H.H. Kanhai and the head of section on reproduction and perinatology at the TNO-PG (*Nederlandse Organisatie voor Toegepast-Natuurwetenschappelijk Onderzoek'—Preventie en Gezondheid*, Dutch Organization for Applied Scientific Research—Prevention and Health), S. Buitendijk (344): "The pronouncements of Sauer have far less scientific support than the positive position [on home birth and midwifery] held by the KNOV and many others." Van Huis concludes by summarizing the evidence:

> Between 1977 and 1997 at least seven studies have been conducted [in the Netherlands] where the outcomes of pregnancy for women birthing at home were compared to the outcomes for women birthing in the hospital. Both groups had uncomplicated pregnancies. None of these studies discovered a difference concerning the outcomes for the baby. It did appear that women who birthed in the hospital had a greater chance of medical intervention. It also appears, from several other studies, that women value freedom of choice about the place of birth and that home birth is associated with higher levels of satisfaction. (344)

What are the sources of this continued debate about the Dutch way of birth? How can this society whose social structures and cultural values combine to produce a uniquely noninterventive maternity care system also support a highly medicalized view of birth?

Although it may shatter the image of the Netherlands as a "Mecca for midwives," we should not be surprised that two sciences of obstetrics exist in the Netherlands. We know the debate between the two sciences exists in other countries: The works of Tew and Klein confirm the presence of this same competition in the UK and Canada, and several studies describe a similar debate in the United States (see, for example, DeVries 1996; Goer and Creevy 1995). Furthermore, the assumption that the Dutch should have one, unified obstetric science is based on faulty logic. When we assume a single science of obstetrics in the Netherlands, we fail to recognize that science, unlike health care policy, cannot be contained within national borders. The science of obstetrics in the Netherlands must come to terms with the science of obstetrics as it exists elsewhere. Science may not be scientific, and it may be subject to social and political forces, but its pretense of objectivity must be taken seriously. Medical scientists around the world participate in a culture of science that transcends national boundaries, a culture that suggests an objective uniformity in bodies and therapies. Obstetric researchers in the Netherlands must reconcile their work to the larger field of obstetric science. This creates a special tension for Dutch scientists of obstetrics. Some researchers respond to this tension by "sticking to their guns," defending Dutch maternity policy, and challenging the taken for granted ideas of the field; others choose to ally themselves to the larger obstetric community and to expose the Dutch system as old-fashioned and out-of-date.

The presence of a debate between the two sciences of obstetrics in the Netherlands does not imply that the arrangement between these two sciences is the same there as it is elsewhere. In fact, the Dutch have reversed the position of the two sciences. In the Netherlands, mainstream obstetric science supports midwives and home birth, and the more marginal, alternative science is the one that suggests that these practices are dangerous. In the United States, hospital-oriented obstetricians exert a great deal of influence over maternity care policy, but in the Netherlands it is researchers whose work demonstrates the safety of midwife-assisted home birth who have the ear of the government and who help to shape policy.

Regardless of their position in this debate, Dutch researchers have long recognized that the Netherlands is one of the more interesting places to study care at birth. Because the Dutch system separates physiological and pathological births, it is the only place in the world where one can test the outcomes of treating birth as *normal* in the context of a highly technological medical system. So it is no surprise that the Dutch have done a good deal of evaluation research, assessing the safety of a maternity policy that:

1. Gives primary caregivers (i.e., midwives and huisartsen) the responsibility of sorting out physiological and pathological pregnancies, and
2. Assigns women expecting a physiological birth to the care of the eerstelijn.[4]

---

4. While most of this work focuses on the safety of this system, some researchers have also studied the factors that influence a woman's choice of birth place and caregiver (see Kleiverda et al. 1990, 1991; Wiegers and Berghs 1994).

There are, as we noted above, inherent difficulties with this research. Lacking the ability to do randomized clinical trials, researchers who are unwilling to devise new outcome measures must content themselves with the use of existing statistics or with prospective studies that analyze outcomes based on an "intention to treat" design. This design—where analyses are based on *planned,* rather than the *actual,* place of birth—is necessary because of the simple fact that most complicated births end up in the hospital; to simply compare home and hospital births builds in a negative bias toward the hospital and a positive bias toward home birth.

The peculiar nature of the debate between the two sciences of obstetrics in the Netherlands—where the definition of mainstream and alternative are flipped—coupled with the desire of the Dutch to produce a science that supports their maternity care policy while not isolating themselves from the larger obstetric community allows us special insight into the relationship between medical science and medical practice. In reviewing the work of obstetric researchers, we see science in action; we see how professional interests, health policies, funding decisions, and cultural values conspire to produce science. Like the maternity policy it supports, we will see that obstetrical science in the Netherlands is pushed, shaped, and bent by social structures and cultural ideas.

DOING OBSTETRIC SCIENCE IN THE NETHERLANDS 1: SUPPORTING THE SYSTEM

Mainstream obstetric science in the Netherlands confirms the safety of the Dutch way of birth and is used by policymakers to defend and encourage the use of midwife-assisted birth at home. Researchers have made their case in a variety of ways. Some have used existing statistics, others have used prospective studies that employ a variety of outcome measures; but in all cases, researchers whose findings support the Dutch way of birth recognize that their findings will generate some skepticism in the larger, international community of obstetric scientists.

Huygen's (1976) research is an example of a very simple study using existing statistics. He compared rates of hospital deliveries and perinatal mortality rates for the United Kingdom and the

Netherlands, showing higher rates of hospitalization and mortality in the UK. He also looked at changes in perinatal mortality rates *within* the Netherlands between 1953 and 1970 and discovered that "the perinatal mortality of hospital deliveries went down from 65.0 to 33.8 (almost halved), but for home deliveries it went down from 21.6 to 6.9 (being less than one-third the figure for 1953)" (245). He concludes, "Studies have proved that by good case selection and good prenatal care it is seldom necessary to rush emergencies to the hospital, and it is possible to obtain exceedingly low perinatal mortality figures . . . in home deliveries" (248).

In 1981, Damstra-Wijmenga carried out a prospective study examining all births in the municipality of Groningen, comparing outcomes for those who chose a home birth with those who chose a clinic birth. Her analysis, published in 1982, showed lower rates of morbidity for both mother and child among those who had *chosen* to give birth at home, irrespective of actual place of birth.

The best known, and most often cited prospective study of birth outcome in the Netherlands is the "Wormerveer research." This study followed the 7,980 women who booked at one of the practices of independent midwives in the Dutch town of Wormerveer between 1969 and 1983 (M. Eskes 1989; Van Alten et al. 1989; M. Eskes et al. 1993). The research showed that:

> the selection of pregnant women into groups at high and low risk is possible using the relatively modest means available to the midwife . . . the data available on perinatal mortality and infant morbidity warrant the conclusion that within the scope of the Dutch system of obstetric care it is possible to achieve very good results with midwifery care for selected women" (van Alten et al. 1989, 660, 662).

In spite of the fact that the loyal opposition sponsored their research, the study of Berghs and Spanjaards (1988), described earlier, proved supportive of the Dutch way of birth. In addition to their finding of no difference in outcomes between practitioners, they also discovered electronic fetal monitoring offered a less than reliable measure of fetal distress. Not only was there great variation in the interpretation of the readings produced by fetal monitors, but there was little correlation between actual fetal distress (measured by the pH of cord blood and the neonatal neurological optimality score) and distress predicted by reading the fetal monitor.

The research of Wiegers et al. (1996) looked at the outcomes of 1,836 births accompanied by midwives at home and in the polyclinic. Like the research of Damstra-Wijmenga, this was a prospective study comparing results on the basis of planned location of birth. To measure birth outcome, the researchers constructed a *perinatal outcome index* consisting of 22 items on childbirth, 9 on the condition of the newborn, and 5 on the condition of the mother after birth. They discovered that for women using midwife care, location of birth made no difference in outcome for primiparous women, when controlling for social and medical background. For multiparous women, perinatal outcome was significantly better for planned home births than for planned hospital births, with or without control for background variables.

Perhaps because of difficulties with the language, very few non-Netherlanders have studied the maternal and infant outcomes of the Dutch way of birth. The one notable exception is Marjorie Tew. Her work demonstrating the safety of home birth in England inspired her to look at the situation in the Netherlands and, in a detailed analysis of statistics provided by the Dutch *Centraal Bureau voor de Statistiek,* Tew and her colleague Damstra-Wijmenga demonstrated that "for the 98.2 percent of babies born after 32 weeks gestation, mortality is nearly 12 times lower if the birth takes place under midwives' care in hospital or at home than under obstetricians' care in the hospital." Higher mortality rates are, of course, associated with the fact that obstetricians see clients whose pregnancies are defined as pathological, but the authors assert that "excess risk might conceivably have been high enough to account for threefold or, at a stretch, a fourfold discrepancy between obstetricians' and midwives' perinatal mortality rates; it could not have been nearly high enough to account for the . . . discrepancy actually experienced" (Tew and Damstra-Wijmenga 1991, 59, 61; see also Tew 1995, 348–354).

These studies—the core of mainstream obstetric science in the Netherlands—present overwhelming evidence that Dutch obstetrics is safe. It is this research that provides the basis for Dutch obstetric textbooks and the creation of Dutch maternity care policy. But this research is at odds with obstetric science and practice outside the Netherlands. As Tew and Damstra-Wijmenga (1991, 55) point out, these studies "[contradict] the claims on which the organization of maternity services in most developed nations is now based, namely, that childbirth is made so much safer by the application of high technology that only this option should be provided." As such, these studies are not easily digested elsewhere.

Supporters of the Dutch system are constantly called on to defend their approach to birth against the prevailing wisdom of obstetrics that says, "birth is normal only in retrospect." Obstetricians are convinced that even with all their advanced monitoring equipment they cannot prospectively separate normal pregnancies from pathological ones. The researchers involved in the Wormerveer study were aware that their work would generate skepticism on the part of obstetricians elsewhere. Commenting on the research in *JAMA,* they note:

> Midwives were primarily responsible for the selection procedure, which was carried out with the relatively modest means available to them. More sophisticated methods of investigation, such as ultrasound and cardiotocography, were used not routinely but only occasionally, after request or referral of the midwife. *Some consider this a weak point of the system, because abnormalities are detected by professionals who are not, by their training and experience, experts in these abnormalities.* (Treffers et al. 1990, 2208, emphasis added)

The authors are quick to remind their readers, however, that their research evidence does not support these worries about the system: "The study demonstrates that it is feasible to distinguish between a group of pregnant women at high risk and a larger group at low risk. Moreover, the results indicate that midwives are fully competent to attend low-risk deliveries."

In discussing this same problem with me, Kloosterman had this to say:

> There are some gynecologists in this country who say "all deliveries have to take place in hospital." Like all German gynecologists say, like almost everywhere in the western world is said: "you never can tell what happens during delivery, they are only normal in retrospect, and therefore everybody has to go to hospital."

> This method of reasoning would be all right if there were no disadvantages of hospital delivery. We can show that by sending everybody to the hospital the number of cesarean sections rises, the number of prolonged labors rises, the number of inductions, of everything, rises. That is a negative influence of the hospital. So you must counterbalance these two things. I always can make up a case where a woman who was staying at

home could, as a result of her staying at home, have a disadvantage, because in the hospital they could have done a forceps delivery or a cesarean section immediately and now there is a delay of 20 minutes and that can be dangerous. So I can collect a few cases, 1 in 1,000, I think, where it is a disadvantage to stay at home.

I also know of one man who had a great embolism in the operating room of the surgery department in Amsterdam. He . . . lived another two years before he got the next embolism. If that man had been at home or in a small hospital, he would have died. So you always can give examples. People of my age would have to live in cardiological clinics because there is always the danger of an attack.

So if there would be no disadvantage of going to the hospital then I think I would agree completely that all deliveries should take place in the hospital. But I can show that there are disadvantages, and now we must make the disadvantage of staying at home as little as possible. In this country, the fact that a woman can stay at home if she likes to do so influences the attitudes in hospitals. Because a woman can always say "Now, I refuse to stay here, I'm going home," if she is healthy. And that makes the attitude of the nurses and the gynecologists in hospitals different.

The logic that underlies the Dutch system, eloquently explained by Kloosterman, is a logic that is not widely accepted outside of the Netherlands. In spite of the evidence reviewed here, the larger science of obstetrics casts a wary eye on the Dutch approach to birth; in other countries it is difficult to find obstetric researchers who will defend the possibility of prospectively separating physiological and pathological births. This skepticism emanating from *outside* the Netherlands has fueled a more critical science of obstetrics *within* the Netherlands.

DOING OBSTETRIC SCIENCE IN THE NETHERLANDS 2: CRITIQUING THE SYSTEM

Obstetricians and gynecologists who work outside the Netherlands continue to view Dutch maternity care as an anomaly. If pressed to explain its continued existence (and success), these practitioners and scientists might credit the peculiar geography of the Netherlands or its social homogeneity. For example, when asked to explain the differences in outcome between their system and the Dutch system, defenders of maternity care in the United States, where near total hospitalization of birth is accompanied by high rates of infant mortality and morbidity, will often say, "We would have equally good results if we only did not have all those poor outcomes associated with extreme poverty."

Dutch researchers who are part of the loyal opposition to their maternity care system ally themselves with the science of obstetrics practiced outside their country. They make their case against Dutch obstetrics using the same types of data used by the supporters of the system—data drawn from existing statistics or from prospective studies. As we might expect, the debate over the Dutch way of birth is waged far more intensely within the Netherlands than it is elsewhere. It is Dutch researchers who make the most pointed criticisms of their maternity care system, and it is Dutch researchers who rise to rebut these criticisms.

In the late 1970s, Hoogendoorn, a statistician at the *Centraal Bureau voor de Statistiek* (CBS) and a retired huisarts who had attended may births at home and in the hospital, issued a strong critique of Dutch maternity care, based on his analysis of existing statistics. In his article, "The Correlation between the Degree of Perinatal Mortality and the Place of Birth: At Home or in the Hhospital," published in the *Nederlands Tijdschrift voor Geneeskunde* (NTvG, Dutch Journal of Medicine), Hoogendoorn (1978) showed that provinces with high rates of hospitalized births also had the lowest rates of perinatal death, leading him to conclude: "there is some reason to expect that a further increase of the hospitalization of parturient women will result in a progressive decrease of perinatal mortality, especially in those provinces where the percentages of women who deliver in hospital are relatively small" (1177).

Hoogendoorn's article generated a number of responses. In an article in the same issue of the journal, Kloosterman (1978) suggested that this type of research suffers from the problem of spurious correlation: He agreed that there *is* a correlation between increased hospitalization and lower perinatal mortality, but pointed out that the inflation of the guilder is *also* strongly correlated with decreasing infant death. Kloosterman went on to look at the correlation between degree of hospitalization and perinatal mortality in the 13 largest cities in the Netherlands and found inconsistent results: Perinatal mortality decreased in cities where the percentage of hospital births declined and in cities where it increased. In the several months after the article was published, there were also numerous letters to the editors of the NTvG arguing in support and against Hoogendoorn's conclusions (see, for example, Treffers and Breur 1979; Citteur and Hoogendorn 1979).

In 1986 Hoogendorn published a second challenge to the safety of Dutch obstetrics in the NTvG. In this article, "Impressive but Nevertheless Disappointing Decline of Perinatal Mortality in the Netherlands," Hoogendoorn used existing statistics to compare the rates of *decline* in perinatal mortality in several European countries between 1970 and 1984. He concludes:

> After 1940 and especially after 1950 the perinatal mortality rate in the Netherlands has shown a remarkable decrease, to the extent that the rate for 1982 was only 25% of the 1940 figure. Since 1982, however, this rate has stagnated. The proportion of deliveries at home has also decreased progressively until approximately 1980, but since has remained constant. In virtually all European countries the perinatal mortality has decreased more than in the Netherlands, which country has lost its relatively high favorable position. Reconsideration of the problems of obstetrical care and particularly also the desirability of home vs. clinical delivery appears necessary. (1439)

This article—and especially Hoogendoorn's suggestion that the Dutch consider changing their maternity care policy from "birth at *home*, unless . . . " to "birth in the *hospital*, unless . . . " (1439, emphasis added)—created a heated debate in the media and in medical journals. For several months the "letters to the editor" pages of the NTvG were filled with responses to Hoogendoorn, most of which were critical of his analysis.[5] Many critics pointed out, as they had with his first article, that correlation does not imply causation. Verdenius and Groeneveld (1986) noted that if the disappointing decline was indeed the result of place of delivery then the trend would have to be completely attributable to the low risk women who choose to deliver at home—a fact that had been shown to be false in several studies. Other critics suggested that Hoogendoorn's analysis was flawed for the following reasons:

- It failed to consider the varied definitions of perinatal mortality used in Europe (Kloosterman 1986; van Bavel 1986);
- It took no account of higher perinatal mortality rates among ethnic

5. In a letter to researcher Edwin van Teijlingen, sent in 1988, Hoogendoorn said that the editors of the *Nederlands Tijdschrift voor Geneeskunde* sent him a Christmas gift in acknowledgment of the fact that his article generated the largest number of letters to the editor in "human memory" (see van Teijlingen 1994).

minorities (Gelderman-Vink 1986; Cranendonk 1986);
- The analysis did not hold if one looked at other countries where total hospitalization of birth was associated with slowed declines in perinatal mortality (Verdenuis and Groeneveld 1986).

Hoogendoorn defended his analysis against these charges in a series of five letters. The debate was so intense that the editors of the NTvG felt compelled to explain their decision to publish the original article, claiming that Hoogendoorn's analysis was done carefully and responsibly. They went on to express some surprise that so few letter writers had challenged Hoogendoorn's central premise—that the perinatal mortality rate in the Netherlands was lagging behind other European nations. Most responses focused on his suggestion that the "disappointing decline" was the result of home births, leading the editors to conclude that Dutch maternity care policy was based on emotional, not rational, grounds. The editors closed the pages of the journal to the debate in 1987, insisting that a half-year of discussion was enough.[6]

All studies that use existing statistics, whether supportive or critical of the practice of obstetrics in the Netherlands, are subject to the kinds of criticism faced by Hoogendoorn. In an effort to find a more scientific way of evaluating the Dutch way of birth, several researchers from the *Vrije Universiteit* and the *Katholieke Universiteit, Nijmegen,* two schools known for their critical stance towards home birth and midwifery, developed research designs that used more subtle outcome measures. This team—the one that included the then doctoral students Geert Berghs and Esmerelda Spanjaards—reasoned that in the absence of discernable *symptoms* of morbidity one might find *signs* of less than optimal outcomes, measurable by scientific instruments and scales.[7] As mentioned above, they settled on measures of umbilical cord blood pH and neurological scores. In a series of articles and papers, these researchers proposed, tested, and defended their choice of these measures as a fitting way to look more closely at the outcomes of home and hospital births (see de Jong 1975; Stolte et al.

---

6. See van Teijlingen (1994, 181–194) for a more complete discussion of the debate over Hoogendoorn's 1986 article.

7. According to one of my informants, this line of research (i.e., looking for differences in morbidity based on pH of cord blood and neurological assessment) received significant funding support because one of its advocates, Stolte, was chair of the *Preventiefonds*, a major source of research dollars for public health.

1979; Van den Berg-Helder 1980). It was their suspicion that the management of birth at home would result in more acidotic children. If proved true, this would be bad news for supporters of the Dutch system, because acidosis in fetuses is associated with growth retardation and damage to the central nervous system. In a paper presented at a conference in 1976, Stolte et al.—researchers advocating this new and more scientific approach to the study of the outcomes of Dutch maternity care—demonstrated a correlation between low pH values of umbilical cord blood and compromised neuromotor skills.

Throughout the 1980s several studies were done using these outcome measures, most of which showed specialist care in hospitals to be superior to birth at home with midwives: On average, babies born at home and/or under midwife care were more acidotic and had poorer neurological scores (see T. Eskes et al. 1981; Lievaart and de Jong 1982).[8] Research by Berghs and Spaanjards (1988), mentioned earlier, was a glaring exception to these findings. You will recall that, in seeking to understand these contrary results, Berghs and Spaanjards found that infants whose mothers had normal pregnancies displayed *no* differences in neonatal neurological optimality scores based on practitioner or location of care. Stolte and Eskes, directors of this project, claimed that a finding of "no difference" proved the superiority of specialist care because the population of women who choose care from gynecologists were more likely to smoke, were less educated, and required more interventions. In 1992 Eskes published an article formally making this argument, noting that there were no differences in neurological scores between groups "despite the lower socio-epidemiologic profile" of women under the care of gynecologists. Eskes explained his position in an interview:

> Finding no difference could obscure something. It could indeed obscure the fact that women who vote for [the hospital] do have some disadvantages, biologically, that they feel by intuition, for instance smoking. Because they feel by intuition that it's no good, that the fetus will be growth retarded, for instance and therefore they [prefer] to do delivery here. So the sociologic profile of the groups is not similar. There's where your profession (i.e., sociology) comes in. To make a clear-cut picture of women's profile in regard

---

8. These studies are among the few analyses of Dutch obstetrics to be published in English language journals. I discuss them in more detail in the next section.

to their choice of a clinical delivery. There's a need for a good scientific approach and description in this country. I think that that's very important because that came out of the Berghs and Spanjaards study.

You think that kind of study has not been done yet, I mean with the exception of Berghs and Spanjaards?

Yes, but we are no sociologists so what we just noticed was smoking habits, the lengths (i.e., heights) of women, so women who delivered here were shorter. That is associated with a smaller pelvis. So a small woman knows by instinct that she has a small pelvis and that the baby could have problems. . . . And also relative infertility, so for the women who delivered here [in the hospital], the wish to become pregnant and the actual realization, that time interval, was longer in the hospital group. So let's put it this way: there are some indications that you can describe a subset of women in the low risk group to be different when they choose for hospital delivery including with a midwife.

The internal arguments for and against the Dutch way of birth were summarized in 1980 when Professors T. Eskes and Kloosterman were invited to engage in a debate over the best place for birth in the pages of *Controversen in de geneeskunde* (Controversies in medicine, Querido and Roos 1980). Leaving no doubt about where he stood, Eskes opened his essay with the oft-quoted but unattributed epigram: "Labor is normal only in retrospect." In his "plea for birth in the hospital," Eskes went on to argue:

1. Home birth will be always be plagued by less than optimal monitoring;
2. Referrals from midwives to specialists during labor contribute significantly to the perinatal mortality rate;
3. Midwives and huisartsen are not skilled in recognizing "small size for gestational age" and "prematurity," both of which are major causes of perinatal morbidity; and
4. Electronic fetal monitoring should be used more regularly.

Kloosterman countered by making a "plea for the possibility of birthing at home," in which he claimed:

1. Selection and rapid and safe transfer to the hospital are possible;
2. The elimination of home birth would give a monopoly to the specialists and would allow technology to control the practice of obstetrics;

3. The elimination of home birth would create an "underground" of less well-trained practitioners;
4. Hospital births are more costly;
5. Unmedicated birth brings great advantage to mother, father, and family; and
6. Medication and other interventions bring risks that should not be introduced to all women.

It is fitting that this debate took place on the pages of a Dutch anthology about their medical care system. Most debates over the wisdom of the Dutch maternity care system have been confined to the Dutch language literature. Only rarely has the internecine arguing spilled over into English language journals, and on most of those occasions the arguments are typically limited to short articles or letters to the editor (see for example, Mascarenhas et al. 1994; Clarke et al. 1994). Given the position of Dutch obstetrics in the larger scientific community, it is instructive to look more closely at those rare occasions when English language medical and obstetrical journals published research on the maternity care system of the Netherlands.

Doing Obstetric Science in the Netherlands 3: The Reception of Dutch Obstetric Science *Outside* the Netherlands

English language reports and articles on the Dutch way of birth have appeared in a wide variety of professional journals and periodicals. The majority of these adopt either a neutral position—simply describing the Dutch system, its history, and its functioning—or positive stance (i.e., presenting evidence of the safety and success of the Dutch maternity policy). There are only a handful of English language articles that provide evidence that the system is *not* working well. However, favorable and unfavorable reports are not equally distributed across type of periodical. Most of the favorable reports are found in nursing journals, journals of social science or medical history, or health services journals, but *all* of the negative reviews of maternity care in the Netherlands are found in medical journals. There *are* a few positive reports found in medical journals, but these are limited to British journals, where there is a history of openness to well-designed research, regardless of the outcome[9] (see Treffers and Laan 1986; Wiegers et al. 1996), and to the *European Journal of Obstetrics, Gynaecology and Reproductive Biology* (the former Dutch language journal of obstetrics and gynecology). The *one* favorable description of the Dutch system found in an American medical journal—in *JAMA* (the Journal of the American Medical Association)—was not a scientific article. It was a review of various studies of maternity care in the Netherlands under the heading, "Letter from Amsterdam"(Treffers et al. 1990).

There are three scientific articles in the English language literature that challenge the safety of the Dutch way of birth. All three are based on the research method developed in Nijmegen under the supervision of Eskes and Stolte.

In 1981, Eskes et al. published their study comparing the pH of umbilical cord blood taken from births occurring at home and at the hospital in the *Journal of Reproductive Medicine* (an American journal). Six midwives and one huisarts agreed to participate; the 85 home births that they accompanied were matched (for parity, age, absence of medical indication, duration of second stage, no medication, and birth weight percentile) with 85 hospital births (28 primiparous women and 57 multiparous women). The researchers found significant differences between the groups, concluding, "It appears that delivery in the hospital with continuous fetal monitoring favors the birth of less acidotic children."

In 1982, the *American Journal of Obstetrics and Gynecology* published a similar study by Lievaart and de Jong. In this research the 85 first births accompanied by midwives (65 at home and 20 in the hospital) were compared to 27 first births accompanied by gynecologists in the hospital. Both groups were considered normal births according to the obstetric indications list. To evaluate outcomes, the pH of cord blood was tested, and the newborn was assessed using Prechtl's method of neurological examination. As with the study of Eskes et al. (1981), the babies born at home did not fair as well as their hospital-born counterparts. The infants born at home had poorer neurological scores and pH values. The authors concluded:

> The outcome advances more or less definite evidence that the obstetric system prevailing in the Netherlands, although concomitant with satis-

---

9. Recall that Klein was encouraged by articles from British periodicals that reported that episiotomies were overused.

fying neonatal mortality figures . . . is not adequate from the point of view of neonatal morbidity. The morbidity of the newborn infants delivered under the care of midwives of pregnancies deemed by them as normal is without any doubt much higher than expected on the basis of the philosophy of the underlying system of obstetric care. The fallacy of the system is not rooted in the place to be born, e.g., home or hospital. It is also not preponderantly related—at least not in the present study—to the lack of capability of the midwives to select abnormal pregnancies among those pregnancies originally thought to be normal. The better outcome of infants born in the hospital under the care of a gynecologist is most probably (also) due to the tools of surveillance used in the supervision of deliveries, i.e., electronic monitoring and determination of fetal scalp blood pH and the capability of performing a cesarean section. (385)

This study, in the best-known American journal of obstetrics, presented a clear challenge to the Dutch way of birth. Treffers and his colleagues responded in a letter to the editor. Published nearly a year later, they criticized Lievaart and de Jong for:

- Making conclusions about "the system prevailing in the Netherlands" based on so few cases from one region;
- Misreporting the results of studies available only in Dutch;
- Sloppiness in their research: pH values were given for only 81 of the 85 cases in the midwife group and 26 of 27 cases in the gynecologist group; there was no control over when the cord was clamped or how long the blood was stored before pH analysis was done—midwives are more likely to clamp late, and late clamping lowers the cord blood pH, as does prolonged storage of the blood;
- Biased selection of cases.

The authors closed their letter with this statement (Treffers et al. 1983, 872): "We conclude that the evidence produced by [Lievaart and de Jong] is insufficient to support their pretentious statements and that the system they are propagating implies a very high level of active intervention, which, in itself, could have undesirable consequences."

Lievaart and de Jong (1983) defended their research in a reply published in the same issue. In most cases they responded adequately to the critique, but their response to the criticism of how they collected and handled the cord blood contains a suspicious non sequitur:

The laboratory housing the Corning 175 automatic pH and blood gas system were [sic] alongside the delivery rooms used by the midwives and the
gynecologists. The acid-base measurements were performed by the same
technicians immediately after the arrival of the blood. Consequently, the
time intervals between the sampling of the cord blood and the assay did
not differ between the gynecologist group and the midwife ambulatory
group. Since the acid values in the cord blood of the neonates delivered by
the midwives in the hospital ambulatory unit did not differ from the values determined in the cord blood of the neonates delivered by the midwives at the patients' homes we can safely assume that the influence of different transport and storage times was of minor importance.

Simply having the laboratory at the same distance from the delivery
room does not ensure that the time intervals did not differ between the
two groups. In fact, the similarities found in pH values for home and
hospital deliveries of midwives are likely to be the result of the fact that
midwives practice the same way at home and in the hospital. In defending themselves in this way, by not reporting the actual time intervals for
midwives and gynecologists, Lievaart and de Jong seem to acknowledge
that they did not keep adequate records of clamping and storage times.

Unhappy with this study, Treffers and his colleagues replicated the
research, paying careful attention to the collection and storage of cord
blood. In one study the researchers measured the effects of various techniques of collecting and storing cord blood. They discovered slight variations in the time and temperature associated with storage had significant effects on pH levels, and they concluded that the only reliable way
to measure the pH of cord blood is to puncture the cord immediately
after birth, store the samples on ice and test them within 30 minutes. In
a second study they used these findings to repeat the work of Lievaart
en de Jong. When researchers took pains to assure that cord blood samples from the clients of midwives and gynecologists were treated in an
identical manner, the results were opposite to those reported by
Lievaart and de Jong: Women attended by midwives had significantly
higher values for their cord blood pH. The researchers concluded, "this
study shows, with respect to umbilical pH values, that there is no cause
for concern about the Dutch obstetric system in which midwives take
care of pregnant women and deliveries" (Knuist et al. 1987, 364).

Eager to get these results to the readers of *American Journal of
Obstetrics and Gynecology*, Treffers and his colleagues attempted to get
this research published there, but neither study was accepted for pub-

lication. Instead, the first was published in the *Journal of Perinatal Medicine* (Pel and Treffers 1983), an English language journal published in Germany, and the second was accepted by the NTvG, the Dutch Journal of Medicine (Knuist et al. 1987).

The third English language article that challenged the Dutch way of birth was published in the *International Journal of Gynecology and Obstetrics,* the official journal of the International Federation of Gynecology and Obstetrics. This article, by T. Eskes (1992), presented no new data; it was a review of 18 existing studies: 8 in Dutch and 10 in English. It is in this article that Eskes defends the larger Nijmegen study against the research claim of Berghs and Spanjaards—that there was no difference in morbidity between practitioners—asserting that the clients of gynecologists had a "lower socio-epidemilogic profile" (167).

Supporters of the Dutch way of birth see the publication decisions of editors of English-language medical journals, especially in the case of Lievaart and de Jong's research, as an act of prejudice against the maternity care system in the Netherlands. In seeking to get their studies supportive of the Dutch way of birth published in English-language medical journals, Dutch researchers encountered the same problems experienced by Klein and Tew. Apparently, editors accept scientific research only when it agrees with the practices espoused by the journal's readership.

Idealized accounts of science suggest that it stands outside of custom, that it is not influenced by "the way things have always been done." But here we see that accepted definitions of what is normal in pregnancy determine what is accepted as good science. Reviewers for the *American Journal of Obstetrics and Gynecology* accept the work of Lievaart and de Jong and reject the work of Treffers because of what they assume to be true about birth. They are unwilling to let research evidence influence their belief that "birth is normal only in retrospect."[10] Van Teijlingen points out that in the Netherlands the same process is at work, but it brings opposite results. He quotes one of his interviewees:

---

10. One of my interviewees told me that the *American Journal of Obstetrics and Gynecology* refused to publish an article by Berghs and Spanjaards based on their research that showed extremely low inter-observer agreement about the interpretation of electronic fetal monitoring recordings taken during the second stage of labor (see Berghs and Spanjaards 1988, 129–140). The letter of refusal stated that it would be "immoral" to publish these results.

Eskes argued that Lievaart and de Jong's article was rejected [for publication] in the Netherlands for ideological reasons and accepted in the US for scientific reasons. Whilst Kloosterman maintained that it was rejected in the Netherlands for scientific reasons and accepted in the US for ideological reasons. (van Teijlingen 1994, 180)

Dutch gynecologists who favor a hospital-based maternity care system feel their colleagues do not take their work seriously and that they are often excluded from discussions about maternity care policy. In an interview, one such gynecologist told me he was asked to review a recently published anthology about Dutch maternity care, *Successful Home Birth and Midwifery* (Abraham-van der Mark 1993). I asked him why he was not asked to write for that book. He replied,

> They always invite Treffers from Amsterdam and his previous man Kloosterman . . . what they do not do is invite people who have quite another obstetrical training. Now you might argue what my training is, but my training was at Case Western, a research university in Cleveland, which is in the US, where I as a youngster did my Ph.D. on physiology, during my specialization, and that gives you a rather hard scientific attitude towards your profession.

> [When I look at scientific work I want to know] what study you did, and what was the outcome of the study. So that everybody can judge that what you *feel* is exactly the *truth*. I will read that book [i.e., *Successful Home Birth and Midwifery*] with that eye and if there are no facts and figures then I have seriously to consider [if I will] review that book.

CONCLUSION: CULTURAL IDEAS AND THE STRUCTURE OF SCIENCE—SUPPORTING AN ALTERNATIVE SCIENCE OF BIRTH

The two sciences of obstetrics in the Netherlands provide a mirror image of the two sciences of obstetrics that exist in other modern medical systems. For the Dutch, mainstream obstetric science supports a noninterventive approach to birth; in other modern medical systems, mainstream research in obstetrics demonstrates the need for intervention. The very presence of two sciences of obstetrics—in any medical system—suggests that the gynecologist quoted at the outset of the chapter is correct: Obstetrics is "no science."

But of course, no science is truly scientific. When we recognize that science rests on a nonscientific foundation, we can begin to look more closely at the forces that shape the scientific enterprise. In my analysis of the way obstetric science gets done in the Netherlands, and elsewhere, we find a close association between science and practice. Mainstream obstetric science follows mainstream obstetric practice: An expectant approach to birth produces a science that proves intervention to be unnecessary, and an interventive approach to birth generates a science that demonstrates the need for monitoring and intervention. The assumed relation between science and practice is turned on its head: Practice is not based on science, rather science is based on practice.

Consider the research of Pel and Heres (1995). In their study of obstetric intervention rates, they discovered that physician intervention in birth was best predicted not by the clinical condition of the mother, but by characteristics of the gynecologist and by hospital policies. They found that, controlling for the signs and symptoms presented by the mother, the likelihood of interventions increased when electronic fetal monitoring was used routinely and decreased in units that employed midwives. If obstetric practice was governed by science, we would expect the condition of the mother—measured by signs and symptoms—to predict the use of interventions.[11]

Why is mainstream obstetric science in the Netherlands the opposite of mainstream obstetric science in other countries? In order to answer that question we must explain why the *practice* of obstetrics is so different there, we must look to the social structures that give rise to its maternity care system (Chapters 3 and 4), and to the cultural values that generated and sustain those structures (Chapter 5). In seeking to understand the *rejection* of Dutch obstetric science in mainstream medical journals published outside the Netherlands, we must look to the social structures and cultural ideas that shape the practices in those societies.

---

11. Zondervan et al. (1995) arrived at similar conclusions in their study of the use of episiotomy. While fewer episiotomies are done in the Netherlands than surrounding countries, the risk of receiving an episiotomy there is not solely related to the condition of the mother and baby. After adjusting for possible confounding factors, gynecologists did more episiotomies than midwives and more episiotomies were done in large, nonuniversity hospitals than in university hospitals.

Hidden in the story of Dutch obstetric science is an important, but little studied question: what happens when the culture of science meets national culture? How is this confrontation settled? The practice and science of obstetrics have a universalizing quality: this is why nearly all obstetricians outside the Netherlands accept the idea that "birth is normal only in retrospect." How have the Dutch resisted this essential premise of obstetrics? It is true that this idea did not fit with their practice policies, but that was true elsewhere as well. In those places the new technologies of monitoring and intervention were accepted and helped to generate the belief that birth is essentially risky. This did not happen in the Netherlands. I believe an important reason for the failure of the culture of obstetrics to overwhelm the culture of the Dutch was the presence of the *zuilen* in Dutch society.[12] The campaign of obstetric science to hospitalize and medicalize birth occurred in the 1910s, 1920s and 1930s, a time when Dutch society was strongly pillarized. In this pillarized society, the authority of science was weakened. The proclamations of science, and especially of medical science, had to be filtered through the institutions of the different zuilen, through their educational systems, their hospitals, their "Cross Associations," and their media. In other societies science could enter unmediated, but in the Netherlands science had to be worked into the identity and organizations of these different pillars. In the case of birth, the rituals and customs that attended the event created even more resistance to a standardizing science that had no room for the core values of each pillar.

The Dutch case also forces us to think about the interplay between political systems and science. In the Netherlands, the health care system is not as subject to the political power of professions and the health care industry. Unlike the United States, where the free-market system encourages the expansion of health care markets *and* of costs, there is a built-in incentive for managing costs in the Netherlands. In a health care system that is based on the free market, science can be used to sell products and services; when the health care system is steered by the government, science is subsumed in larger goals.

---

12. See Chapter 4 for a more complete explanation of the zuilen.

The story of obstetric science in the Netherlands allows us to see how culture and structure are implicated in the creation of health care. The debate over home birth in the Netherlands gives us a clear picture of the way cultural ideas shape the questions researchers ask and the methods they use to answer those questions. Under the guise of science, the knowledge generated by these researchers becomes the objective data that support health policy.

IV. RE-FORMING

IN THE preface I mentioned that the Dutch way of birth has two stories to tell. Much of this book has been concerned with the first story: the story of the unique maternity care system in the Netherlands. The second story—the story of how health systems are structured and maintained—has been implicit in the telling of the first tale: Our tour of maternity care in the Netherlands has shown the undeniable and important role of cultural ideas in the forming and re-forming of health systems. Any effort to change health systems—be it to make them more efficient, more just, more compassionate, less costly, or less prone to error—must consider the way culture is implicated in the current organization of care.

Social scientists and health policy analysts have given almost no attention to the role of culture in the development of health care systems. As noted in Chapter 5, medical sociologists and anthropologists *do* pay attention to the connection between culture and health care delivery, but in a very limited way. When they look at culture, they look for the influence of culture on the behavior of patients, imploring caregivers to heed the varied cultural backgrounds of clients. When looking at health systems, sociologists and anthropologists focus on structure, exploring forms of payment, the institutions health care delivery, political systems, and organizational forms.

This unwillingness to use culture to analyze and explain health care structures is understandable. Culture is difficult to measure and, when looking at large health systems, it is nearly impossible to isolate the effect of culture on health policy. But to ignore the way medical systems are influenced by culture—by ideas about the body, about men and women, about the value of medicine, and about the abilities of physicians and other caregivers—thwarts needed efforts to improve health care delivery. In Part IV we look at how our analysis of a small part of a health care system located in a small country in Europe offers a new and important vision of how health care systems operate. We begin by recognizing the dynamic nature of culture, looking at how culture is re-shaping current practices in Dutch maternity care and how the government is attending to both structure and culture in developing policy for the maternity system. We conclude with suggestions for using cultural analysis to re-form health systems.

7   Is All This Suffering Still Necessary?
Pressure to Change the Dutch Way of Birth

WHEN I left for the Netherlands I was well-versed in the feminist position on childbirth. Over the course of the twentieth century, patriarchal physicians had developed a number of interventions that slowly but surely separated women from the experience of childbirth. Twilight sleep, episiotomies, forceps, scopolamine, cesarean sections, epidurals: All of these technologies moved the mother from center stage and made the obstetrician the new "star" of the birth process. In the Netherlands, my feminist friends told me, everything was different. Because the Dutch practice an expectant approach to birth, mothers in the Netherlands remain at the center of the event. Dutch physicians and their assistants have not taken over the birth process.

I was surprised, then, when shortly after I began my research I discovered an article on epidural anesthesia in *Opzij*—a monthly magazine that is the rough equivalent of *Ms.* magazine in the United States—that asked, "Is all this suffering still necessary?" The author of the article, Anke Manschot (1993), suggested that it is the *Dutch medical system* that is acting in a patriarchal fashion by *denying* women access to epidurals. In making her point to a Dutch audience she recounted a well-known "parable about pain" offered by the Dutch author Multatuli:

> A seaman develops a gangrenous leg. It is amputated without any anesthesia. The man does not utter a sound. During the bandaging of the stump, the nurse pricks his skin with a safety pin. The man screams. "But sir," says the shocked nurse, "first you were so brave and now you scream at a little pinprick." To which the man replies indignantly, "This pain was not necessary!" (30)

In response to the claim made by some Dutch feminists that weathering the pain of childbirth *is* necessary to a woman's identity and faith in herself, Manschot said,

> When it comes to an appendectomy or the drilling of a tooth, no one suggests that these should take place in your cozy home, with your favorite

214

music playing, without anesthesia, in order to realize your own power [or] . . . to recover our self-confidence on a deeper level. The only argument that should count for or against painless birth is the degree to which an epidural can be damaging for mother and child. (31)

She went on to criticize the current arrangement for pain relief at birth in the Netherlands:

There appear to be few medical reasons to refuse anesthesia to a woman during birth. Nevertheless this happens in our country. Recently an acquaintance of mine was reprimanded in an Amsterdam hospital when she begged for pain relief during the birth of her first child. She was induced, which leads to painful and strong contractions and she had to endure "the torture" to the bitter end "on her own strength." (31)

Manschot's article inspired a heated exchange of letters in the next two issues of *Opzij*. On the one side were those who claimed the widespread use of epidurals would result in the end of home birth (it is not feasible to administer epidurals at home) and the loss of control over the experience that comes with birthing in one's own environment; on the opposite side were those who congratulated Manschot for breaking the taboo on this topic and who labeled those who deny pain relief at birth as "sadists." The issue clearly struck a nerve with readers: The editor of *Opzij* told a mutual friend that she had never received more mail on a single article.

This article, and the responses it generated, presaged change in the Dutch way of birth. And indeed, in the years since 1994, when I began my research, I have seen significant changes in the way birth is approached in the Netherlands, changes that suggest that the pillars that support the Dutch system are weakening. In November 1999, I sat down with a well-known Dutch health researcher to discuss the future of midwifery and home birth in the Netherlands. He is a strong supporter of the Dutch obstetric system and an advocate for home birth, and he told me, "In five years it is over . . . there will be no home birth in the Netherlands." To support his prediction he quoted a quip attributed to the German poet Heinrich Heine: "If the world should perish, I will move to the Netherlands because everything there happens fifty years later." He went on to say that Heine was right: Other nations had abandoned home birth 50 years ago and now the Dutch were finally following that lead. Five years earlier, near the end of my first year of research, we had discussed this same quote and its relationship to Dutch maternity care. Back then he had been far more optimistic: He insisted that Heine was *wrong;* he expressed great confidence that the Dutch system would not only persist, but that it would serve as a model for others.

This policy analyst is not alone in his concern for the future of the Dutch way of birth. Although it appears that the percentage of births occurring at home has leveled in the low 30 percent range, various groups in the Netherlands are worried about further declines. The government and health insurance companies fear that the shift to short-stay hospital births will drive up the cost of maternity care with no consequent improvement in outcomes. Midwives are concerned that the disappearance of home birth will diminish the autonomy of their profession. Organizations representing the users of maternity care fear that the choices offered Dutch women will be limited. In fact, it was not until the late 1990s that an organization was formed to promote and protect consumer interests in birth care. The *Stichting Perinatale Zorg en Consumenten* (Foundation for Perinatal Care and Consumers) was created largely because of concern that the declining rate of birth at home would eventually eliminate this choice for Dutch women.

Will home birth and autonomous midwifery survive in the Netherlands? The answer to this question is to be found by examining the structural and cultural supports of Dutch maternity care. The Dutch way of birth is not being challenged by direct opposition but by subtle and gradual change in society and culture, reminding us once again that health policies are grounded in both the *organizations* and *ideas* of a society. Let us begin with a brief look at the structural factors that are influencing the contemporary shape and the future of Dutch birth.

STRUCTURE

Several features of Dutch society, including new government policies, changes in the labor market, change in the way midwives are organizing their practices, and changes in medical education have conspired to change the way birth care is delivered.

Policy analysts in the Netherlands often attribute the sharp decline in home births that occurred in the 1970s (see Figure 7-1) to a government decision to allow healthy women to give birth in the *polikliniek* (i.e., a short-stay hospital birth). Ironically, the government made this decision in an effort to forestall the decline of births in the *eerstelijn*. Government

FIGURE 7-1

Home Births in the Netherlands (as a Percentage of All Births), 1955–2000

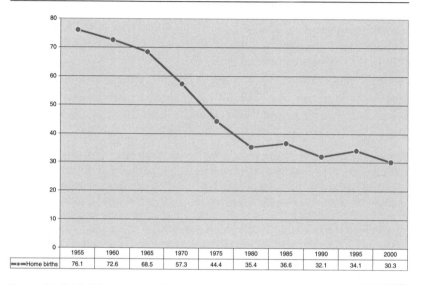

	1955	1960	1965	1970	1975	1980	1985	1990	1995	2000
Home births	76.1	72.6	68.5	57.3	44.4	35.4	36.6	32.1	34.1	30.3

Source: See Table 2-1.

officials believed that the growing popularity of gynecologist-assisted hospital births was the result of women inventing complications because they wished to be in a hospital. These officials reasoned that if women with no complications were allowed to choose a hospital birth, more of them would stay under the care of midwives and general practitioners. This decision did not have the desired effect: Coupled with other changes in Dutch society, it resulted in a rapid decline in the number of births at home and a rise in the number of births accompanied by specialists.

In spite of a general pride in the Dutch way of birth, some obstetric specialists continue to speak out against a care system that appears so outdated, calling for policy changes that would hospitalize birth. In his inaugural speech, *"De foetus verdient meer"* ("The fetus deserves more"), celebrating his appointment as Professor of Obstetrics at the Universiteit Maastricht, Jan G. Nijhuis (2000) argued that the Dutch way of birth has become too expensive. After pointing out the high rates of transfer from the *eerste* to the *tweedelijn*, Nijhuis claimed:

This makes obstetrics very expensive, because a large percentage of mid-wifery care, and care during the birth, is now billed twice, by the midwife and the *vrouwenarts* (gynecologist). These extra costs are estimated at around 65 million guilders (€29.5 million) per year. (17)

Nijhuis goes on to suggest that both midwives and their clients might be better off if birth moves to the hospital, where the relationship between caregivers can be better organized and a good perinatal audit can be "better realized." According to Nijhuis, the move of birth to the hospital will allow "the Netherlands to measure itself against the results of neighboring countries" (18). His conclusion points toward a medicalized future for birth in the Netherlands:

> I hope that I have made it clear to you that the fetus deserves more. *Perhaps not more home birth,* but certainly a good perinatal audit, more pre-conceptual research, more prenatal diagnostics, preferably not invasive, more research and care for the protection of the fetal condition, more attention to what the fetus hears and feels, more care around birth, more research on the cause of handicaps, and more research on the fetal factors that can influence the quality of the fetus's later life. (19, emphasis added)

Recent policy decisions strengthening the profession of midwifery suggest that Nijhuis's words are out of synch with the government's plans for maternity care, but his speech and his appointment as professor (i.e., chair) of obstetrics remind us of the continued pressure to medicalize birth.

Health policy alone does not explain the choices of childbearing women; other trends in society shape the choices women and midwives make. One of the more important correlates of the general decline in birth at home in the Netherlands over the past few decades is an increasing level of participation in paid labor by Dutch women, a trend noted in Chapter 5. Although Dutch women participate in the paid labor force at lower rates than women in other industrialized countries, it is also true that their participation rate has risen rapidly over the past 20 years. This upward trend has several consequences for decisions about care at birth, many of which incline toward a preference for hospital birth (see Figure 7-2). Working women are more likely to postpone or forgo childbearing, bringing an increase in older mothers (with a greater likelihood of complications) and a decrease in fertility. When both partners work, a woman's place in the family and the home is renegotiated, and, for many working women, the hospital seems a convenient choice for birth, a respite from the duties of their jobs and the chores of housekeeping.

FIGURE 7-2

Labor Force Participation and Percentage of Births at Home, the
Netherlands, 1960–2000

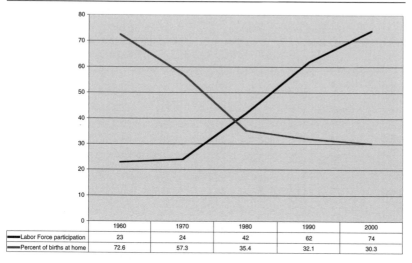

	1960	1970	1980	1990	2000
Labor Force participation	23	24	42	62	74
Percent of births at home	72.6	57.3	35.4	32.1	30.3

Source: See Table 2-1 and Figure 5-2.

The working patterns of midwives are also changing rapidly. In just
20 years the predominant organizational form for Dutch midwives has
changed from solo practice to group practice (i.e., three or more midwives in one practice); in 1980 nearly 75 percent of midwives worked
alone, by 2003 less than 10 percent were in solo practice (see Table 7-1).
Group practice is kinder to midwives: When midwives practice in a
group they can reduce the heavy demands of their profession by sharing
hours on call and by giving each other regular days off. But group practice also brings subtle change in the relationship between client and caregiver: The *gezelligheid* of home birth with *your* midwife is threatened by
the rationality and efficiency of a modern organization. This small step
toward a more rationalized relationship between mothers and midwives
is a step in the direction of the even more rational and efficient hospital,
where one midwife can tend to several laboring women at once.[1]

---

1. Nijhuis, Professor of Obstetrics in Maastricht, suggests that "The midwife no
longer wishes a work week of 80–100 hours and is seeking group practice, *or better yet*, a
position in a hospital with a normal work week" (Nijhuis 2000, 17, emphasis added). He
cites no evidence for his claim.

Table 7-1

Independently Established Midwives by Type of Practice,
1980–2003 (as of 1 January)

	Working in Solo Practice		Working in Duo Practice		Working in in Group Practice		Total	
	N	%	N	%	N	%	N	%
1980	409	74.2	112	20.3	30	5.4	551	100.0
1985	360	56.3	234	36.6	45	7.0	639	100.0
1990	287	37.5	288	37.6	191	24.9	766	100.0
1991	271	33.4	290	35.8	250	30.8	811	100.0
1992	248	29.8	295	35.5	289	34.7	832	100.0
1993	227	26.7	271	31.9	351	41.3	849	100.0
1994	212	24.2	279	31.9	384	43.9	875	100.0
1995	186	20.5	294	32.4	427	47.1	907	100.0
1996	177	18.9	285	30.4	475	50.7	937	100.0
1997	154	15.8	271	27.8	551	56.5	976	100.0
1998	153	15.3	267	26.7	581	58.0	1,001	100.0
1999	141	13.4	246	23.5	662	63.1	1,049	100.0
2000	132	12.2	242	22.3	712	65.6	1,086	100.0
2001	119	10.4	237	20.6	792	69.0	1,148	100.0
2002	109	9.2	238	20.1	837	70.7	1,183	100.0
2003	113	9.3	215	17.8	880	72.9	1,208	100.0

Source: Hingtsman and Kenens 2002; Kenens and Hingstman 2003.

Changes in the educational system also have an effect on the Dutch way of birth. Professor Kloosterman is concerned that gynecologists have little or no experience with home birth in the course of their training:

> But there is one great danger, and that is [true] also in our country, all kinds of gynecologists have during their education, now that is six years, no experience with home confinements, not at all . . . and therefore there is now coming up a generation of gynecologists who know very much about obstetrics and about deliveries, but only in the hospital situation. And our general practitioners have less experience than in the past.

Professor Klomp echoes this concern:

> I am quite sure that residents in training and young obstetricians don't know anymore about normal deliveries. They get such a lot of all advanced technology in gynecology and obstetrics that it's hardly possible that they still know what a normal delivery is.

This development in the educational curriculum for Dutch gynecologists will gradually alter the way these practitioners view birth.

Gynecologists in training are, of course, aware of the unique charac-teristics of birth in the Netherlands, but if their only experience with birth is in the hospital, with women who have been referred to the tweedelijn, they cannot help but learn to distrust the birth process. In my research with midwives in the United States I saw a similar pat-tern in midwifery education. Home-birth midwives who decided to get formal training as nurse-midwives would often tell me that they were now horrified at the great "risks" they took when attending birth at home. They had learned, from their time in the hospital, that birth is fraught with danger (see DeVries 1996). Recall the words of Dutch midwife, first quoted in Chapter 3:

> There are also a lot of gynecologists who haven't met midwives in their training, who are not familiar with this profession, this group of professionals.
>
> So they think: "It's weird, those people are doing some things at home. Oooh, it's dangerous, they don't have a CTG [ultrasound scans]." And then, what they remember is those people going from home to the hospital; those situations where you can say: "Hmmm, could have been better." And they say: "You see, those midwives, they are doing irresponsible work." So I think it's very important that every gynecologist is doing a traineeship in a midwifery practice. So that they can see how midwives are working, how they are doing it, what their knowledge is.
>
> And you see also in the recent promotion [i.e., dissertation] research . . . they see that those hospitals who have midwives working there, that there the interfering rate of the gynecologists is lower than in other hos-pitals. So, it has an influence.
>
> I think that the two professions must more work together, and must learn from each other.

As we learned in earlier chapters, these structural changes are closely associated with changes in the way birth is regarded. This is a reciprocal and dynamic relationship: Change in structure brings change in cultural ideas, and changes in cultural ideas result in the modification and/or creation of structures.

CULTURE

The link between structure and culture can be clearly seen in the increasingly normal use of echograms (ultrasound scans) during pregnancy.[2] Pasveer and Akrich (2001) point out that this seemingly harmless technology—many parents have an ultrasound done merely to have a souvenir for the baby book—brings significant change in the way a woman experiences her pregnancy, undermining her confidence in her ability to give birth at home away from the expertise and equipment of the medical clinic:

> New technologies do much more than offer a better view of a given unchanging process. They change the very ontology of pregnancy: they change trajectories, they change pregnancies and their markers, and they change the content and distribution of competencies. Prenatal trajectories that consist of visits to a series of caregivers, of examinations by a variety of people and apparatuses residing in different and rather unconnected places, and a number of dossiers that contain crucial information about the pregnancy but that are not "owned" by the pregnant woman are different from trajectories that consist of visits to a midwife, examinations within her practice, and a dossier that is carried around by the woman herself. The first kind of trajectory makes for a referent—the pregnancy—which is distributed over a number of actors who are related, but not physically attached, to the woman. The second kind of trajectory makes for a pregnancy that remains in the body, that loads the body with abilities, knowledge, and confidences that come in handy at home birth. In this trajectory the midwife is the [only] external informant, and she is present at the birth.

Indeed, interviews with expectant parents show that Dutch attitudes toward birth are becoming more like those in other countries. When asked why they chose a *polikliniek* birth, many parents expressed an attitude toward home and technology more like those in surrounding lands. The most common reasons for not staying home for birth are *te veel rommel* (too much mess) and the desire to have *alles bij de hand* (emergency equipment readily available; see Wiegers 1997). Increased trust in high-technology maternity care is also seen in the growing demand for a routine *echo* (sonagram—a picture of the fetus taken with sound waves) during pregnancy (*NRC Handelsblad* 2003).

One way to better understand the relationship between culture and birthing preferences is to examine changes in the maternity care choices of Dutch women across time and across levels of education. We know that cultural ideas change across time and that varied levels of education are associated with differing tastes and, in our case, with dif-

---

2. The *Ziekenfondsen* will reimburse for two echograms during pregnancy.

fering ideas about a proper birth. When we examine the relationship between level of education and the choice of where and with whom to give birth, we find that women with lower levels of education are more likely to get a baby at home and to be accompanied by a midwife. Figure 7-3 presents data from the Dutch National Survey of General Practice (NIVEL 1995)—an interview survey done in the late 1980s that included over 13,000 subjects.[3] The data represented in this figure are for the first births of respondents—births that occurred between 1916 and 1988 (N = 16,745)—grouped by level of education. Note that for this 72-year time period, as the level of education rises, the percentage of births at home and the percentage of births with midwives declines.

We discover an interesting trend, however, when we break these data down by ten-year time periods:[4] In the period that extends from

FIGURE 7-3

Percentage of Births at Home and Percentage of Births Accompanied by a Midwife, by Level of Education, the Netherlands, 1916–1988

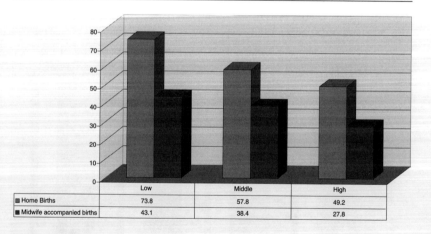

	Low	Middle	High
▦ Home Births	73.8	57.8	49.2
■ Midwife accompanied births	43.1	38.4	27.8

Source: NIVEL 1995.

---

3. Survey participants reported where their children were born and who was in attendance, which provides a picture of birth practices in the Netherlands for the greater part of the twentieth century.

4. The survey was done in 1988; thus the last time period covers only the three years 1986–1988.

the mid-1950s to the late-1980s, the relationship between educational level and birth preference reverses itself. In these four decades the *structural* features of the health care system were the same for all women, but *ideas* about a proper birth changed over time and by level of education (Figures 7-4 and 7-5).

The patterns we find here are similar to patterns seen in breastfeeding in the United States. In the 1950s middle- and upper-class women saw breastfeeding as old-fashioned, a practice for poor women who could not afford the "benefits" of formula. A few decades later these attitudes had changed. Women in higher social classes were returning to breastfeeding, having seen the results of scientific research demonstrating its benefits, while women in the lower classes were abandoning the breast for what they took to be the more sophisticated use of formula. A gynecologist comments on the changing fashion in birth preferences in the Netherlands:

FIGURE 7-4

Percentage of Births Attended by Midwives by Level of Education, the Netherlands, 1956–1988.

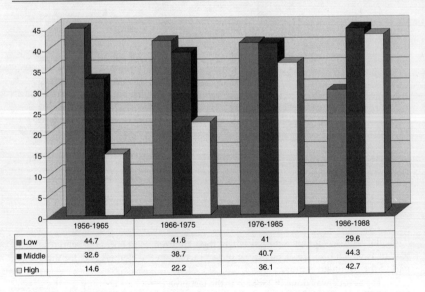

	1956-1965	1966-1975	1976-1985	1986-1988
■ Low	44.7	41.6	41	29.6
■ Middle	32.6	38.7	40.7	44.3
□ High	14.6	22.2	36.1	42.7

Source: NIVEL 1995.

FIGURE 7-5

Percentage of Births at Home by Level of Education, the Netherlands, 1956–1988

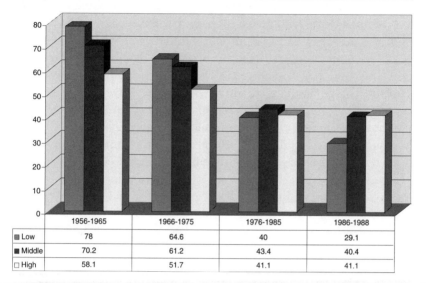

	1956-1965	1966-1975	1976-1985	1986-1988
■ Low	78	64.6	40	29.1
■ Middle	70.2	61.2	43.4	40.4
□ High	58.1	51.7	41.1	41.1

Source: NIVEL 1995.

But you see [variation in birth preferences] even in our small country. It's changing of course, it's getting more uniform, but with the progressive population of the west, and the rural population of the east and south, we still have differences in polyclinic (i.e., short-stay) deliveries. First they started here (i.e., in the west) to go to hospital for deliveries, and in the east they wanted to stay at home, whether it was medically advisable or not. And then here the more educated people started wanting to have home deliveries, but then in the east they started to go to the hospital . . . Turkish and Moroccan women started here to stay at home. . . . Now you see the Turks wanting to go to hospital. It's a status symbol. While Dutch women want to stay at home.

EFFORTS TO PRESERVE THE DUTCH WAY OF BIRTH INCLUDE BOTH STRUCTURE AND CULTURE

There can be no doubt that the unique Dutch way of birth is threatened by developments inside and outside of the Netherlands. Today all the forces that have shaped midwifery in other countries exist in the Netherlands: The rationality of medicine and the efficiency of the hospital can be (and are being) used to achieve the (professional) goals of medical specialists and to meet the needs of a new generation of clients. And yet there are also features of Dutch culture and the structure of health care in the Netherlands that deflect the drive toward medical rationality. Most important is active government support of midwifery and home birth, the result of the "democracy of interests" in the Netherlands and peculiar Dutch ideas about *zuinigheid* and heroism. The government continues to take an active role in defending and promoting the profession of midwifery and its jurisdiction over home birth; interestingly, the policies pursued by the government recognize the need for both structural and cultural interventions.

On the structural side the government has (1) increased funding for the training of midwives; (2) opened up more spaces for first-year midwifery students; (3) improved the working conditions of midwives by raising their salaries and reducing their workloads; and (4) lifted the *primaat*, allowing *huisartsen* to assume some of the workload of eerstelijn births. On the cultural side, the government is aware that ideas about birth shape decisions about care, leading them to initiate campaigns to promote home birth (see Chapter 1) and to acculturate immigrant women to the Dutch way of birth. The decision to add a fourth year to the midwifery curriculum was, to a certain extent, a culturally informed decision. It was a recognition of the cultural weight of science: Aside from the obvious benefits of a fourth year of training, midwives and policymakers knew that a scientific background would enhance the status of the profession.[5]

Midwives and their supporters are also well aware of how structures and cultural ideas conspire to support (or diminish) their profession and the choice for birth at home. In several of my interviews, without using the language of social science, midwives and others called attention to culture and structure and the way they interacted. In the following excerpts we see a sociological sensitivity in reflections about the future of the Dutch way of birth. In this first excerpt a midwife talks about how the experience of birth and *ideas* about birth are altered by the *environment* in which birth takes place; she goes on to

---

5. The policies of the government appear to be effective. In 2003, Coffie et al. reported that the home birth rate has remained essentially the same (slightly above 30 percent) over the 15 years and that "the fear of a decade ago that home birth . . . in the Netherlands would disappear as it has in other western European countries no longer exists" (315). See also Wiegers and Coffie 2003.

explain how she uses this knowledge to shape her clients' ideas about birth and thus to protect her profession:

The profession will disappear, if home births are eliminated. I'm totally convinced. And you know why? Because eh . . . when you do a home birth, what happens to you as a midwife, it's a completely different experience. You have a totally different profession if you work at home or if you work in a hospital, as a midwife. I've done so many births at home and in hospitals, and if I compare myself in that sense, the way I act . . . I am almost a different person.

When they call me in the middle of the night—I never get used to that—but automatically, you dress yourself, get in the car, and already you start to feel better, and . . . then you drive to the woman's house, and you come there, and there's the husband, and you see the wallpaper and the furniture, and she's screaming from the shower: "Take a cup of coffee, I can manage," and the grandmother's there, and the dog, and you all of a sudden dive into the center of the world, and you just leave out your personal melodrama.

You know, you don't care about yourself any more; you forget about yourself, which is very relaxing, and then all of a sudden you are part of the family for a while. And you really want to give them a very good special experience. Because you are there where the baby is made . . . And that makes [the midwife] get a real VIP-feeling. You're alone, and you're totally responsible. And she gets VIP-treatment. And because you're alone, you're very alert, and you listen to the heart very well. . . . At the same time you have to relax.

If you have to wait, maybe you even go to sleep in the house, but you're very alert because you're the only one responsible, and you don't have this so-called safety around you. You listen much more careful to the heart. . . . She is the only one you have to observe. And you are very patient. Because you are in a nice environment, you're not in a little room with this couple, and bored very quickly, but you can go out and do some shopping maybe, if it's in the daytime, and you come back. You take your time, and then, you know, when the birth is imminent, you know . . . and it's so important and you get very inventive, to do anything of your midwifery art to make her do it.

All women, all midwives and all doctors have this existential fear around birth. You know, it's the same fear people have when someone dies. It's a mystery; you don't know where this baby comes from—even if you're religious—it's madness that there is all of a sudden a baby between those legs . . . it scares you; it scares everybody. That's why midwives at home have those rituals; that you put your birthstool always on one side, and your scissors on the other side, you know? That's to control your nerves; which you always have, unconsciously.

And then when the baby finally is born, and you go to this climax with those people who really love her, and the baby's out, there is this enormous euphoria. Not only for the woman, because the pains are over, but also for the midwife, enormous . . . especially when the placenta is there. You see, the midwife will be happy when the placenta is there. And this enormous euphoria, that makes that you go on wings back home, even if you were up all night. And you will always remember this woman, because you know her furniture, you know her address, and you've talked about their love history maybe.

And if I do a hospital birth, it's totally different. The woman is on the phone and she says "Ja, I want to give birth in the hospital," and very often the midwife will say: "Go to the hospital, I'm coming as well." We changed this in our practice. We always go to the woman's house now, because of this reason. But very often, most midwives in Holland will say "Okay, I'm coming to the hospital as well."

When you come in the hospital, you come into this boring little room . . . And the nurse comes in and she says: "Hey . . . are you back from holidays? How was it?" And you start talking over [the mother's] head, and you think "Oh, I think I'm going to have a coffee with the nurses," because you get very bored. You forget to listen to the heart, because you think "Oh, we're in the hospital now. Everything is fine." You don't pay as much attention, [the mother] doesn't get a VIP-treatment, because nurses do those births all the time. The midwife is bored: "How long is this going to take? Shit, this is not going fast enough." She cannot go shopping, because it's always outside the big medical center . . . And she is getting very bored.

I take books with me, and I have to force myself to go inside to listen, to force myself not to do too many internal vaginal examinations.

Just for something to do, eh?

Ja. You know, and then I'm more inclined to go and get medical help early, because . . . you know, for then something is happening. Midwives are more inclined to medicalize birth in a hospital. Speed it up, because you don't want to wait too long. At home it's a totally different story. So, finally maybe she gives birth, and you think: "I want to go home." Weigh the baby and get out of there.

You know, it's dull in the hospital. The work in a hospital is dull, it's anonymous; you're less alert; you're less afraid, because you think you're safe as a midwife, and you're not. So that euphoria is less . . . You have less adrenalin, but the euphoria afterwards is less too. So what happens to the woman in the hospital happens to the midwife as well.

The interest of the midwife is always the interest of the woman. The happiness of the midwife is the happiness of the woman. . . . And the problem is, she doesn't get a VIP-treatment. Even if I'm home, and there's a problem for instance, and during the labor I have to go to the hospital, I call the obstetrician. [The mother] comes into the hospital with me and she is immediately the VIP again. You know what I mean? Because she is a special case. And immediately all the attention is there . . . and she's something special again.

So I think in this home birth system you get the best. You get the best at home, from the midwife, and if you need to be referred you get the best of hospital care, and you're not a routine number. So that's why in our practice we've changed the protocol. Now everybody starts at home, everybody. If they want to give birth in a hospital, fine, but they have to start at home. Then you have the advantages of the home environment. The labour will go easily . . . And if the birth is easy we stay at home.

Even if the woman says "I want a poliklinische birth?"

Very often she says "I don't want to go any more." That's the trick. She doesn't want to go to the hospital.

It is a trick?

Ja. It is a trick; but we explain the tricks. We say: "Listen, our experience is that if you stay at home and you don't have to worry about going to the hospital, your labour will really go better. So you make your decision to go to the hospital during labour, not now. You don't have to worry about decisions. We decide during labour. If it goes very quickly, you'll probably decide to stay home. And that's fine, you're safer. If there are problems, you go to the hospital, and you'll get even better treatment, because then you're a special case. If you go to the hospital because you want to, for a normal birth, you get a routine treatment, and that's not what the hospital's for."

Do you find women are resisting this? Saying "I really want to be in a hospital?"

No. Really they want to stay home. They want to go to the hospital because they think it's safer. But for dilation they are very good to stay home; you know what I mean? And we promise them: "If you want, you always go. No problem."

Do you find resistance from the fathers, or the partners?

No. They, the partners can also see that for dilation home is the best place. It's better to be on your own toilet. So there's no discussion any more. Since we have this rule we have 96 percent home births in [our practice], and we have a very happy clientele, because they make their own decisions.

And 96 percent are choosing to stay at home, or 96 percent are delivering at home?

When they first come to the birth centre about 66 percent choose for a home birth immediately. We ask the first time "What do you want?" but we don't discuss then. We say "What do you want?" and we say "That's fine, but we start at home. Everybody starts at home. Even if you want to give birth in a hospital, we come to your home." Then during all the courses, of course, a lot of women already change their minds, but then during birth a lot of people change their minds as well. We have had this policy since three years now, and it works incredibly.

And the thing is that since we have this policy of not polarizing any more, so I never say any more "Home is better," or whatever. I never polarize any more. I say that in Holland we have the best of two worlds, and this system is best. We should not polarize this system. It's not home birth or hospital birth, it's this cooperation between hospital and home that is so perfect in Holland, and we should not lose the cooperation. Do you know what I mean? That's a totally different approach than home against hospital. No, it's perfect harmony between home care and hospital care.

Sensitive to the changes in women's lives in the Netherlands, a group of midwives in Amsterdam created the *Geboortecentrum* (birth center). It is not a center where birth occurs—midwives already have a great deal of autonomy in home births and polyclinic births—it is rather a center that collects all the various services related to pregnancy and birth under one roof: a prenatal clinic, pregnancy, postpartum and parenting courses, a bureau to arrange postpartum care, once-a-week consultations with an obstetrician, a shop with articles for pregnancy and birth, a clinic for care of the newborn, and day-care services (see http://www.geboortecentrum.nl). The idea behind this structural intervention is to strengthen the position of the midwife, putting her in control of various services associated with birth, keeping women in the eerstelijn. And, of course, if women continue to have good experiences in the first line, the idea of home birth and midwifery as safe and desirable alternatives is maintained. The following excerpt shows that midwives recognize the need to do more than make their services attractive, they understand that they must build institutions:

[We need to] make our service so attractive to women that we have a natural flow, in the future, to midwives. And now we are complaining that pregnant women go to the tweedelijn, and directly to the hospitals. Whereas if you make the midwifery care attractive, and I mean not only cozy, but also high quality of care, but also attractive to woman, "gezellig," everything together in one street, service, then the tweedelijn, the hospitals can never compete. The hospital can never compete with this institute. Women love it. It's high quality of care; it's *kleinschaligheid* [small scale], it is cozy, they meet each other, they make friends; it's an institute of the *eerstelijns verloskundige zorg* [first-line midwifery care].

What I feel is needed for midwifery care in Holland is that midwifery, eerstelijns verloskunde, becomes an institute like the tweedelijn. But now the tweedelijn has an institute, has buildings; midwives don't. They have only maybe a private practice themselves. When a woman in Holland is pregnant, she first goes to the GP, then she might go to the midwife. For maternity care she has to go to the *kruisvereniging* [the cross association], for ultrasound she has to go somewhere else. If there is a problem she has to go to the hospital for an obstetrician. Then when the baby is born she has to go to the *consultatiebureau* [for well baby care] somewhere. She is shuttled around; there's no service for a pregnant woman. So what I thought, as an experiment, "How can I make, create, an institute where the midwife is the queen?" She is the hub, she is absolutely in charge. And you bring her together with her natural friend, the maternity care assistant, then you make a very strong bulwark against the ramparts of the second line. And then, if you take the pre- and postnatal courses, and you get your hands on the information, and you take workshops with us, just to make it attractive, to give information, and you also take the children up to age four [for well baby care], then you have a rampart of first-line care, against the big buildings outside . . . Right?

If you explain to women that to go to a midwife is just as safe, and you give her all those statistics, you lose many women. If you just make your care the best care there is, and the most attractive care, you don't have to discuss safety any more, they just come right here, for you give the best, low profile fun care there is.

This midwife went on to explain that the idea of a geboortecentrum also appeals to the interests of the government and of private insurers in keeping their costs down:

What I'm doing now is meeting these very important private insurance people. Because what did I think? In the thirties it was the *Ziekenfonds* that protected the midwives. Because of financial reasons . . . to provide good quality for the poor. Right? Now the *Ziekenfondsen* are going to the private sector, so now I have to go to the private insurance VIPs to propose to them the concept that it's cheap, much cheaper than the second line, and that it is a golden formula, and that it protects the midwives again, in the nineties.

A gynecologist who supports home birth and midwifery notes how the structural limitations placed on the practices of midwives, for example, limiting their use of the new technologies of birth, helped to create new ideas about the way birth should be accomplished:

And of course midwives, I've told them repeatedly, they are only humans. So, most of them would do [high-risk births] if they were allowed to. So I think it's a very good thing that there is a limitation of what they

may do. And now they are creating *a whole ideology about doing nothing.*
And I think that's excellent. (Emphasis added.)

She goes on to say that midwives are learning to use the language of medicine (i.e., science) to support their ideology of limited intervention in birth:

> And what they are starting to do, is to do more scientific work, and to limit their own sphere of practice. It was always limited by us, by doctors. But they should limit their own sphere of practice, and not listen too much to doctors any more. And that they are starting to do now.

> I do hope that within the next ten years or so we will have some midwives who write a thesis and get a doctorate in medicine. They are allowed to now. Our schooling system now allows them, with their midwifery training, to write a thesis and to get a doctorate at one of the universities. And then I hope we will get a few professors of midwifery, the normal physiology of pregnancy and delivery, who are midwives themselves.

> *I heard there was talk of trying to establish a chair in physiological obstetrics.*

> That must be a midwife. She must have a doctorate. There's discussion about it now. So that's what I see as a future. Chairs of physiological pregnancy and delivery at the universities, and then chairs by professors of midwifery who are trained midwives and have a doctorate in midwifery.

In speaking about the threats to her profession, a Dutch midwife concurs with these ideas about the usefulness of science to the cause of midwives:

> Threats are midwives themselves that, eh, refer a lot. Who are not so sure about their own knowledge. You see that the referral rate is rising, and that's also one of the reasons why we have to take care, and to do research with our own material: how does it come that the referral rate, during the first stage of labor, why is it so high? Is the human uterus not working any more? How come?

The "ideology of doing nothing" will not survive the "ideology of intervention" of modern obstetrics if policymakers do not attend to the cultural pillars that support this unique way of birth. Those who tinker with the structure of health care systems must constantly ask themselves how the changes they propose fit with the ideas and values of those who use the system.

8   Re-Forming Health Care: Culture and Health Policy

Most Americans are shocked when told about the Dutch way of birth. They find it difficult to believe that there is a modern country that still endorses birth at home (with no doctor present!). In order to understand this peculiarity we have been forced to push beyond typical explanations of the structure and operation of health care to see that the organization of obstetrics in the Netherlands could not survive if it did not match the cultural ideas of the Dutch. By looking at one small part of the health care system of a small country, and thus avoiding the problems of the "detailer" and the "tourist," we discovered that culture forms and re-forms health practices, a discovery that not only offers a new way of thinking about the organization of health systems, but also presents policymakers with the possibility of a fresh approach to the development and promotion of innovative health policies.

Learning from Failures Large and Small

Careful study of health policies that have failed is a necessary first step toward successful health care reform. When we understand why health reforms do *not* work, we can fashion reforms that will succeed. In the past, culture was seen as irrelevant to the process of health reform; cultural assumptions were taken for granted and no one bothered to ask how new policies fit, or did not fit, cultural understandings and cultural expectations about health and medicine. This oversight led to improper conclusions about the failure of health policies. Three brief examples illustrate how lack of attention to culture doomed or delayed reform.

Hospice Care
In the mid-1960s the British began experimenting with hospice care for dying patients. The idea made a lot of sense. Dying had become an industrial, medical event. Patients approaching death experienced

relentless interventions, separated from their loved ones by a thicket of paraphernalia and drugs. Hospice care was a reasonable and humane alternative. Recognizing the inevitability of terminal illnesses, the hospice offered pain relief, palliative care, counseling to patients, and support to their families. The practicality and the simplicity of the idea made it irresistible: Here was a form of care that was both *more* satisfying to patients and *less* costly. Health care workers from around the world began to make their way to the United Kingdom to learn more about hospice care. In the United States, would-be reformers found their efforts to humanize dying thwarted by doctors and insurance companies. The hospice idea—so popular in Europe—was fiercely resisted in the United States. Only after a decade of lobbying and consumer pressure did insurance companies begin to cover hospice care.

Electronic Fetal Monitoring (EFM)

Electronic fetal monitoring (EFM) is a process that uses computerized equipment to oversee and record fetal heartbeats and the strength of uterine contractions during labor. EFM became a popular alternative to simple auscultation (i.e., listening with a stethoscope) 35 years ago. Not only was it believed to be more reliable—sensitive equipment was regarded as more trustworthy than the ear of a nurse—but it promised cost savings; with EFM one nurse could watch several laboring women simultaneously. Interestingly, as EFM became more common, the number of cesarean sections increased. Intrigued by this natural correlation, several researchers set out to explore the relationship between EFM and cesarean sections. Two questions drove this research: Did EFM cause the rise in cesarean sections? Do EFM and cesarean sections reduce morbidity and mortality? Study after study showed the same thing. EFM had one, and only one, striking effect: It raised the rate of cesarean sections. It had no effect on the health of mothers and babies. The evidence was so overwhelming that the American College of Obstetricians and Gynecologists formally recommended that routine EFM be discontinued. This advice has had little effect: Today EFM accompanies over 80 percent of births in America.

The Inefficiencies of American Health Care

The American health care system is one of the most inefficient in the world. We spend over one trillion dollars each year on health care, about 15 percent of our gross domestic product (GDP), and over 40 million Americans have no health insurance. Although nearly everyone agrees that our way of delivering health care is seriously flawed—with one in seven Americans lacking health insurance, it is likely we all know at least one person who is soldiering along with only limited access to medical services—any effort to change the system is inevitably stymied. The frustration we Americans feel with our health care system has boiled over into a Hollywood film cum exposé of the injustice, the maldistribution, and the inefficiencies that attend medical care in the United States. *John Q.*—the person and the film (New Line Productions, 2002)—gives voice to the complaints of a silent majority of Americans who have suffered without health insurance or with insurance plans that have a numbing array of restrictions and limitations.

Other countries spend far less while offering universal coverage; the Netherlands spends about 9 percent of its GDP on health care, the United Kingdom about 7 percent. In those countries, infant mortality rates are lower and the citizens are healthier and have longer life expectancies. In spite of the models offered by these other countries, legislators in the United States have been unable to move their country toward a more just, more efficient, health care system. The last serious attempt to reform American health care was in 1993, when the Clinton administration offered a plan to provide universal coverage. If enacted, the Clinton legislation would have guaranteed a basic package of benefits to all Americans; it would have also reduced the startling array of insurance companies and policies that crowd the American market, consuming 30 percent of the dollars spent on health care. In spite of a strong desire for health care reform on the part of the population, the Clinton plan failed. More recently, an attempt to create a patient's bill of rights met the same fate as the Clinton plan, and even modest attempts to achieve reform by changing the practices of clinicians are routinely stalled or sidetracked, leaving the free market in control of health care.

The Cultural Source of Health Policy Failures

These three examples—hospice care, EFM, and the failure of health care reform in the United States—give us the impression that Americans prefer more expensive, less satisfying, more interventive, and more complicated medicine. What is the source of this seemingly irrational resistance to reform? What is the thread that ties these failures together? In each case, reform was resisted *not* because it was (medically or economically) irrational, but because the change being proposed did not fit with *cultural ideas* about medicine and health.

The big failures in health reform have received plenty of attention (the defeat of the Clinton plan for universal coverage has been analyzed and reanalyzed in articles, books and essays) and yet, in spite of all these details, we learned little about how to accomplish reform. Part of our problem is this tendency to focus our attention on the large and public failures, where structural and political issues stand out and where the role of culture is easily overlooked. Only when we step back and look for the common features of failed reform efforts, both large and small, will we begin to see how culture is implicated and learn how to do health reform better.

The conventional wisdom is that the Health Security Act proposed by Clinton failed because of nepotism and overly complicated regulations. These are undeniably the *overt* reasons for the demise of the act, but these political and structural problems can do only part of the explaining. The Clinton plan failed because it was flawed at its foundation, giving no consideration to the cultural ideas that animate and support medical systems. The proposed reforms required Americans to rethink their ideas of the physician-patient relation, their notions of responsibility for the health of others, their use of technological solutions for health care problems, and their understanding of the power and efficacy of medicine. Medical special interests were able to play on the cultural uneasiness created by the health reform proposal, using a well-crafted ad campaign to defeat the bill, in spite of the fact that the majority of Americans favored reform.

Similarly, the overt explanation for our slowness to adopt the hospice model and our continued use of EFM focuses on the "politics of reimbursement," but the machinations of those with vested interests in these practices would not be possible if their interests did not match our cultural ideas about technology. At birth and death we Americans are comforted by technology, by—as Monty Python reminded us in *The Meaning of Life*—"machines that go ping."[1]

---

1. See Chapter 6, footnote 1.

Seen in this light, the repeated failure of health reform in the United States is not the simple consequence of the politics of health care or the structural difficulties of change, it is the result of insufficient attention to the important and inextricable links between cultural ideas and the structure of health care delivery systems. Health policymaking in the United States proceeds as if structural features are all that matter. Health care reformers believe that with enough tinkering they will find the perfect balance of incentives and disincentives to create an affordable and just way of delivering medical care. This is not true. Only when we look closely at the ways culture shapes health care delivery we will be able successfully to re-form health systems.[2]

USING CULTURE: TOWARD MORE EFFECTIVE REFORM

Social scientists of all stripes will agree that, although culture changes, it is extremely difficult, if not impossible, to engineer that change. Thus, the challenge of employing cultural ideas in health policy work is to (1) identify the relevant cultural assumptions of the society in which a reform is proposed, and (2) to find a way to link the proposed reform to some commonly held value.

Analysis of any society will uncover a plethora of values, many of which contradict others. To the extent that the film reflects American values, *John Q.* offers an apt example. In the film a man argues for more solidarity in health care by "heroically" intervening and threatening to kill someone if his son does not get life-saving surgery. Here we see two values in conflict: Americans love the "cowboy" hero who asserts himself and takes what he needs, but they are also sympathetic to notions of fairness and solidarity. Reformers must speak to these cultural contradictions, allowing citizens to appreciate and understand the conflict, and to decide which value is more important to them.

Bringing these contradictions to the surface is preferable to ignoring them and allowing a vague uneasiness and confusion to be exploited by the well-placed advertising of vested interests. In the United States this will require true dialogue about what it would take to have a more

---

2. By identifying six myths used by stakeholders to thwart health reform in the United States Geyman (2003) points to importance of ideas for the success or failure of reform efforts.

just health care system. Rather than the emotional rush of watching a lone hero conquer an evil medical system, we need to ask each other if we are willing to improve medical access for the poor even if it would require us to wait for nonelective surgery.

Culturally informed health reformers must look for models of successful reform both at home and abroad. Most interesting will be health legislation that brings value conflicts to the surface (e.g., laws on euthanasia in Oregon or in the Netherlands) because these situations offer the opportunity to see how cultural ideas can be used to support or undermine reform efforts. The passage of the laws on euthanasia required public discussion of the proper ends of medicine, the meaning of life, and the value of suffering (Kennedy 2002). Ongoing debates about the use of stem cells (cloned or otherwise) offer a similar opportunity. In this case conflicting notions about the definition of life, the value of science, and the meaning of suffering are used either to defend or criticize proposed policies.

Americans have assumed, for far too long, that they can change their approach to the allocation of the precious resource of health care without attending to the habits of their hearts. Health reform will not succeed until cultural analysis becomes a routine part of health policy work. How can policymakers use cultural analysis? I close with an example of how culture can inform the reform of childbirth in the United States.

CHANGING THE AMERICAN WAY OF BIRTH

The American way of birth changed markedly at the beginning of the twentieth century, when midwives and home births were replaced by physicians and hospital birth (see Declercq et al. 2001). However, since that time, birthing practices in the United States have proved remarkably resistant to change.[3]

Birth practices in the United States rode a wave of culture through the twentieth century. In the 1920s, suffragists, fresh from their success in gaining the right to vote, turned their attention to birth and demanded—and won—the right to "twilight sleep," a cocktail of drugs that promised to relieve the pain of birth. These women were responding to a cultural ideal that celebrated the new and the modern, and the

---

3. See Wertz and Wertz (1977) for a thorough history of childbirth in America.

ability of science to conquer the ills that plagued humanity. Seen in this light, a hospital birth was a better birth.

In their rush to take on the values of their new country, to become true Americans, immigrant women adopted this new and modern view of birth, abandoning the old-fashioned practice of birth at home with a midwife. As a result, midwifery in America, which had been kept alive in ethnic enclaves, disappeared: "In the end midwifery, practiced by immigrant, working class women, remained rooted in the cultural life of traditional ethnic communities. When these communities began to assimilate and adopt American ideas, there was no place for the midwife" (Borst 1989, 48).[4]

Over the next decades some of the women who had argued for "modern" obstetrics realized they had made a devil's bargain, gaining some pain relief but losing the experience of birth. Beginning in the 1950s, with a *Ladies' Home Journal* exposé of abuses in maternity wards (Shultz 1958), American obstetrics has faced a steady, but ineffective, stream of criticism.

Picking up on the values of the counterculture, the alternative birth movement emerged in the 1960s, calling for a return to birth at home under the care of midwives without the use of anesthesia (De Vries et al. 2001, 245–248). The movement was fueled by several books that made a compelling case for a less medicalized birth: Suzanne Arms's *Immaculate Deception: A New Look at Women and Childbirth in America* (1975) described how maternity care in the United States abused women, ignoring their needs and separating them from their babies, and Barbara Katz Rothman's *In Labor: Women and Power in the Birthplace* (1982) presented an outline of the glaring inequalities of power in the maternity wards of American hospitals. With the exception of a few cosmetic changes, however, this countercultural criticism did little to change the delivery of maternity care (De Vries 1996).

---

4. Wilson (1995) provides further confirmation of the role of culture in the fading fortunes of female midwives. He concludes his study of the rise of man-midwifery in England with this observation: "Male practitioners were turned into midwives not by their own desire, but through the choices of women . . . the making of man-midwifery was the work of women" (192). His work rests on an analysis of the role of fashion in shaping medical practice: "Fashion was in general the symbolic reflection of a new culture of class; in the world of women, for which childbirth was so crucial, fashion dictated the need for the man-midwife . . . fashion offered a bridge by which those of intermediate or ambiguous status could symbolically climb the ranks" (191).

The cultural fit, and consequent staying power, of the status quo in American obstetrics are well-illustrated by the plight of a group of midwives in New York City. In that city's public hospitals, nurse-midwives provide a majority of the care for birthing women. Midwives were brought into the system (in the late seventies) because they were less expensive than physicians. This move was part of a larger trend in health care where the *business* of medicine was gaining control over the *practice* of medicine (Starr 1982). More and more medical decisions were being made not by MDs, but by MBAs. In the case of maternity care, midwifery offered cost-conscious health care managers an alternative to high-tech, high-cost obstetrics: an alternative as safe (or safer) than obstetric care (Goer and Creevy 1995) with the extra benefit of high levels of client satisfaction. To birth reformers it seemed only a matter of time before obstetricians would be hoisted by their own petard of excessive, costly intervention: The clinically irrational resistance of physicians to midwives (i.e., midwives are opposed, not because they are unsafe, but because of fear of competition) could not survive the cool rationality of business managers.

An early assessment of the work of the nurse-midwives in New York City showed them to be providing high-quality care. The perinatal mortality rates for the midwifery service were lower than the average in New York City and in the nation, in spite of the fact that their clients had little or no prenatal care and inadequate nutrition (see Haire 1981; Goer 1999). Proponents of alternative birth saw their success as further proof of the wisdom of changing our system of childbirth. If nothing else, here was compelling evidence for administrators who were being pressured to cut the cost of care.

This evidence notwithstanding, in 1995, a team of investigative reporters for the *New York Times*, looking to explain poor perinatal outcomes in New York City, turned their gaze to that which seemed out of place in American medicine: midwives (Baquet and Fritsch 1995). In a three-part exposé, the authors maligned midwives and the insufficient use of obstetric technology as the culprits for poor obstetric results. When the maternity care system is not functioning well, it is not the system that is to blame, rather it is the insufficient application of the system. Too many perinatal deaths? In a culture that values technology, the solution must be *more* technology, *more* intervention. Following this logic, the authors faulted the midwives for their low rate of cesarean sections, 12.9 percent, and asked why it was not closer to the city average of 23.1 percent.

In a letter of response to the exposé, an epidemiologist offers another way to think about the problem:

> Among other causes for [the high number of perinatal] deaths, you blame insufficient use of birth technologies such as electronic fetal monitoring and Caesarean section, and midwives who do not function properly. These are . . . complaints of American obstetricians who wish to divert blame from themselves. . . underlying New York's maternity care crisis is an *unfounded faith in birth technology*. In your . . . article is the statement that "a fetal monitor malfunctioned, making it impossible to determine the baby's condition." Before there was a monitor there was a stethoscope. The monitor should only complement the stethoscope. (Wagner 1995, emphasis added)[5]

Using evidence from European countries, where both cesarean section and perinatal mortality rates are low, the letter-writer characterizes the problems in New York City as the result of an *over*dependence on technology, rather than too little use of technology. He argues that the proper use of technology requires the careful separation of healthy and high-risk mothers, reserving technological solutions for difficult cases. In New York City, misplaced faith in technology results in too little care in the selection of cases (if all births are high risk it makes no sense to separate them) and the improper use of obstetrical support (private patients get more attention from specialists than public patients).

Even as physicians in other specialties continue to lose control to administrators, childbirth in the United States remains in the hands of obstetricians. American obstetrics survived the alternative childbirth movement and managed care essentially unchanged: Today, more than 26 percent of all births in the United States are accomplished surgically; in spite of research suggesting negative effects, epidural anesthesia is increasingly popular and is used routinely by healthy women (a trend that has led to a new specialty in obstetric anesthesiology); and episiotomy and electronic fetal monitoring remain the norm. Midwives have found a niche working in inner cities and in rural locations—medically under-served areas—but they attend less than 9 percent of the nation's births.

---

5. See also Marsico (1995).

The door to the medicalization of birth, opened by the suffragists some 80 years ago, now seems impossible to close. Culture is at work here: As Davis-Floyd (1992) suggests, American obstetric practices fit well with American culture. Americans, she points out, value, among other things, technology, the control of nature, and patriarchy; birthing rooms in the United States, dominated by men and by technological devices that impose their timing and regulation on the natural process of birth, merely reflect these values. In spite of structural and economic pressures and a continuing stream of criticism (Mitford 2000; Wolf 2002) a pleasing birth in the United States is one that is an expensive, high-technology, medical experience.

Is there any hope of changing maternity care in the United States? Independent midwifery and home birth survived in the Netherlands because the cultural soil there sustained them. The cultural soil in the United States is not nearly as hospitable, but there *are* themes in American culture that are consistent with a less-interventive birth, themes that can be emphasized and used to change the American way of birth. Three are particularly salient: American beliefs about pain, nature, and money.

In general, Americans view pain as something to be avoided at all costs. Unlike the sailor in the Multatuli story (see Chapter 7), Americans view *all* pain as unnecessary—witness the explosive growth of pharmacological solutions for the pain of grief, anxiety, and shyness. The avoidance of pain at birth is evidenced by the increased demand for epidural anesthesia and elective cesarean section.[6] But there is also a cultural theme that *values* pain, which sees pain as worth suffering for some greater good. This is most visible in the American penchant for exercise and dieting. No one would suggest that the pain of vigorous exercise should be dulled by narcotics; rather, pain is seen as "worth the gain" it brings in health and feelings of well-being.

American attitudes about nature are inconsistent. On the one hand, Americans want to rearrange the natural world for their benefit and comfort; but on the other hand, there is an important American tradition of preserving nature (think of John Muir and Teddy Roosevelt), of

---

6. Although the notion that cesarean section is less painful than vaginal delivery is often misguided: The postnatal recovery period after surgery is often protracted and painful.

valuing nature and the wilderness for its restorative value. American birth tends to emphasize the first theme and ignore the second. When it comes to labor and birth there is an impatience with natural processes and a desire to schedule birth to fit in with busy schedules. Emphasis on the latter view of nature—as good, beautiful, and regenerative—supports a more patient approach to birth.

When it comes to money, Americans are not quite as thrifty (*zuinig*) as the Dutch, but Americans are greatly concerned with the runaway cost of their health care. American individualism makes it difficult to implement system-wide savings—the general attitude seems to be that costs should be cut on services to others, but *my* care should be the best and most costly—however, American thriftiness leaves them open to rational arguments about the cost of unneeded interventions in birth. Eliminating medically unnecessary cesarean sections, anesthesia, and episiotomies would save billions of health care dollars a year.

Apart from making direct appeals to these latent cultural themes, reformers must also seek to create incremental structural changes that will support alternative views of birth. Cultural ideas are given credence by structural arrangements. Freestanding childbirth centers—an American equivalent of the *geboortecentrum* (see Chapter 7)—can play an important role here. Although they have not caught on as quickly as some had hoped, these childbirth centers serve to alter ideas about pain, nature, and expensive interventions in birth. Birth centers are inherently countercultural, emphasizing nonmedical approaches to pain relief and giving women the freedom to labor and birth as they wish (not on a medically prescribed timetable). Women who birth in these centers often become advocates of a less medical approach to birth.

Data from other countries can also be used to make a case for midwives and noninterventive birth. Statistics demonstrating the safety of low-technology birth will appeal to American's rationality—showing the success, safety, and economy of more natural approaches to birth. The Netherlands is the most obvious case in point, but changes taking place in Canada and the United Kingdom are moving those systems toward less technological birth. In 1993, the British government released its report, *Changing Childbirth*, which recommended that the National Health Service move to a model of maternity care where midwives serve as lead professionals. The province of Ontario recently introduced a model of midwifery care based on that found in the

Netherlands, using Dutch midwives as consultants to set up education programs and practice guidelines. These programs, in other English-speaking countries, are generating evidence of the efficacy of midwifery (in English language journals) that can be used to show the folly of costly, interventionist obstetrics and help redefine birth as a normal and healthy life event.

THE PROMISE OF CULTURALLY INFORMED REFORM

Among the benefits of a culturally informed approach to health reform is the opportunity to learn new things from the ways other societies organize health care. It is not unusual to look to other countries when searching for ways to improve health care systems, but we unwisely limit our search to the *structure* of care, weighing the wisdom of things like payment plans, clinical arrangements, or health promotion programs. An appreciation of the influence of culture in other health systems allows us to see things we simply ignored before: We see that the practice of medicine is not only improved by new and better science or by better systems of incentives, but by attention to the values and ideas that are at play in the structure and delivery of health care.

The practice of obstetrics in the Netherlands embodies cultural values that might well be adapted to general medicine elsewhere. For example, the stubborn disinclination of Dutch doctors to play the hero can go a long way toward humanizing care in all medical specialties. Admittedly, there are times when caregivers must act heroically, but to assume this stance at all times can be costly and, in some cases, dangerous.[7]

Similarly, the Dutch insistence that obstetrics be *watchful and reactive* rather than active and interventive has something to teach caregivers in a variety of fields. This approach is based on the idea that everything is normal until evidence suggests otherwise—rather than the other way around—and it enriches the quality of birth, both medically and experientially. It is often said that when physicians in the United States hear hoof beats, the first thing they think is "zebras!"—that is,

---

7. We see the same attitude in the Dutch approach to euthanasia. One need not agree with the Dutch policy in order to see that many of the heroics at the end of life are unneeded and harmful (Kennedy 2002).

American doctors are always looking for, and expecting, the unusual diagnosis. Unlike their American counterparts, when Dutch doctors hear hoof beats they think "horses," and as a consequence patients are not subjected to a battery of unnecessary and costly tests.

The case of Dutch maternity care makes clear that all health policy rests on cultural foundations and that policy proposals that do not match cultural ideas are doomed to failure. Whether it be the search for a pleasing birth—a birth with a minimum of fear and pain, in the company of supportive family, friends, and caregivers, a birth that ends with a healthy mother and baby gazing into each other's eyes—or for a more just and loving system of health care, we must account for the role of culture in the form and reform of health systems.

Glossary

begeleiden: To accompany.

bevallen: To give birth or to please.

bevalling: A birth.

EAC (external advisory commission): EACs are created by the government to offer advice on new initiatives or revisions of existing regulations; EAC members include representatives of interest groups as well as civil servants and academics considered to be experts in the policy area under consideration.

eerstelijn: The "first line" of medical care, what we in the United States might call "primary care." However, in the Dutch system the first line acts as a gatekeeper for access to specialist care (the second line, see **tweedelijn**): In order to see a specialist, a referral must be given by a caregiver in the first line, most notably a midwife or a general practitioner (see **huisarts**).

gezellig: Cozy, homey, comfortable, friendly, warm.

gezin: Nuclear family. The Dutch language is unique in having a single word that distinguishes the nuclear family.

gynecoloog: Gynecologist. This is the most commonly used term for a medical doctor who specializes in the care of women. On occasion the term *obstetricus* is used, as is *vrouwenarts*, but in general these specialists are called *gynecologen* (pl. of *gynecoloog*).

HBO (Hoger Beroeps Onderwijs): Higher Occupational Education. HBO is required for midwives, accountants, managers, teachers, and other professionals and requires five years of secondary school.

huisarts: House doctor. Typically translated as "general practitioner," these caregivers, members of the eerstelijn, act as gatekeepers to specialist care. In many cases the offices of *huisartsen* (pl.) are connected to their homes.

KNOV (Koninklijk Nederlandse Organisatie van Verloskunigen): The Royal Dutch Organization of Midwives.

kraam: Literally a stall or booth, but when coupled with other words, kraam refers to the postpartum period; for example, a *kraamvrouw* is a woman who has just given birth and a *kraambezoek* is a postpartum visit.

kraamverzorgenden: A postpartum caregiver, formerly a *kraamverzorgster.*

LHV (Landelijke Huisartsen Vereniging): The National Huisartsen Association.

MBO (Middelbaar Bereops Onderwijs): Middle Occupational Education. MBO prepares one to do police work, carpentry, plumbing, and the like and requires four years of secondary education.

NIVEL: This was the acronym for *Nederlands Instituut voor Onderzoek van de Eerstelijnsgezondheidszorg* (Dutch Institute for Research on First Line Health Care). In 1996 the mission of the NIVEL was broadened to include research on all sectors of the health care system. The organization changed its name to *Nederlands Instituut voor Onderzoek van de Gezondheidszorg* (Dutch Institute for Research on Health Care), but held on to the acronym.

NOV (Nederlandse Organisatie van Verloskundingen): The Dutch Organization of Midwives. In 1998 the organization became the "Royal" Dutch Organization of Midwives, see **KNOV.**

NVOG (Nederlandse Vereniging voor Obstetrie en Gynaecologie): The Dutch Association for Obstetrics and Gynecology.

polikliniek: Polyclinic. When used together with "birth," as in "polikliniek bevalling," it refers to a short-stay (i.e., less than 24 hours) hospital birth.

primaat: A preference for midwives, formerly part of the health regulations. When the primaat was in effect, a healthy woman seeking care for pregnancy and birth was obliged to use the services of a midwife, if one was working in her neighborhood. This meant that if a midwife had a practice nearby, a woman could not choose the care of her huisarts.

thuis: Home.

thuisbevalling: Home birth.

TNO (Nederlandse Organisatie voor Toegepast-Natuurwetenschappelijk Onderzoek): The Netherlands Organization for Applied Scientific Research.

toeter: A wooden fetoscope widely used by midwives in the Netherlands.

tweedelijn: The "second line" of health care. Specialist care, which one can receive only after referral from the **eerstelijn.**

verzuiling: Pillarization. The division of Dutch society into separate "pillars," based on religious or political affiliation. Between the 1920s and the 1970s, when the Netherlands was highly pillarized, there were separate schools, hospitals, media, and social services for each pillar.

VIL (Verloskundige Indicatielijst): Obstetric Indications List. A list of indications that defines a physiological birth and a pathological birth, creating the boundaries for care in the first and second lines.

vrouwenarts: Literally "women doctor," an old-fashioned term for *gynecoloog.*

welzijn: Well-being. Often mistranslated as "welfare," bringing with it—for Americans at least—connotations of the "undeserving poor."

WO (Wetenschappelijk Onderwijs): Scientific Education (i.e., university education). For admission to WO, a student must have six years of preparation (in gymnasium, athenaeum, or lyceum).

VVAH (Vereniging van Verloskundige Actief Huisartsen): Association of Obstetrically Active Huisartsen.

VWS (Ministerie van Volksgezondheid, Welzijn, en Sport): The Ministry of Public Health, Well-Being, and Sport.

Ziekenfonds: Sick fund. Often mistranslated at "sickness fund." The Dutch term conveys the notion of funds for *people* who are sick, not funds for the treatment or study of sickness. The government program that mandates health insurance coverage—paid for through a combination of employee and employer contributions—for those making less than a specified sum per year. The government determines a standard package of benefits and sets prices on health care services; private insurance companies compete to enroll clients within this framework.

Ziekenfondsen: Sick funds. The collection of private companies that offer insurance under the provisions of the Sick Fund Law.

zuinigheid: Thriftiness.

References

Abbott, A. (1988). *The System of Profession: An Essay on the Division of Expert Labor.* Chicago: The University of Chicago Press.

Abraham-Van der Mark, E. (Ed.). (1993). *Successful Home Birth and Midwifery: The Dutch Model.* Westport, CT: Bergin and Garvey.

Ackermann-Liebach, U., Voegeli, T., Gunter-Witt, K., Kunz for Zurich Study Team. (1996). Home versus hospital deliveries: Follow up study of matched pairs for procedures and outcome. *British Medical Journal, 313,* 1313–1318.

Adamson, G., and Gare, D. (1980). Home or hospital births? *JAMA, 243,* 1732–1736.

Adviescommissie. Kloosterman. (1989). *Regeringsstandpunt Adviescommissie Kloosterman* [Government Standpoint on the Kloosterman Advice Commission]. Ministerie van Welzijn, Volksgezondheid en Cultuur. SDU-uitgeverij 's Gravenhage.

Akrich, M., and Pasveer, B. (1996). *Comment la Naissance Vient aux Femmes* [How Birth Goes for Women]. Paris: Les Empêcheurs de Penser en Rond.

Amelink, M., and van Leent, C. (1994). Een goede keuze bevalt beter [A good choice means a more pleasing birth]. *Tijdschrift voor Verloskundigen, 19(7/8),* 343–346.

American Medical Association. (1977). *Statement on Parent-Newborn Interaction.* Chicago: American Medical Association.

Andeweg, R. B., and Irwin, G. A. (1993). *Dutch Government and Politics.* New York: St. Martin's Press.

Arestad, F. H., and McGovern, M. A. (1950). Hospital service in the US. *JAMA, 143(1),* 25–37.

Arms, S. (1975). *Immaculate Deception: A New Look at Women and Childbirth in America.* Boston: Houghton Mifflin.

Arney, W. R. (1982). *Power and the Profession of Obstetrics.* Chicago: University of Chicago Press.

Bakker, R. H. C., Groenewegen, P. P., Jabaaij, L., Meijer, W. J., Sixma, H. J., de Veer, A. J. E. (1996). "Burnout" among Dutch midwives. *Midwifery, 12,* 174–181.

Baquet D., and Fritsch, J. (1995, March 5–7). New York's public hospitals fail, and babies are the victims. *New York Times.*

Barstra, J. S., and Banning, W. (1948). *Nederland Tussen de Natien, II* [The Netherlands between Nations, II]. Amsterdam: Ploegsma.

Beaver, H. (1987, July 5). Healthy, wealthy, and worried too. *New York Times,* Section 7, 1.

Benders, J., Noorderhaven, N. G., Keizer, A. M., Kumon, H., and Stam, J. (Eds.). (2000). *Mirroring Consensus: Decision Making in Japanese-Dutch Business*. Utrecht: Lemma.

Benoit, C., Davis-Floyd, R., Teijlingen, E., Sandall, J., and Miller, J. F. (2001). Designing midwives: A comparison of educational models. In R. De Vries, C. Benoit, E. van Teijlingen, and S. Wrede (Eds.), Birth by Design: Pregnancy, Maternity Care, and Midwifery in North America and Europe (pp. 139–165). New York: Routledge.

Berger, P. L. (1963). *Invitation to Sociology: A Humanistic Perspective*. Garden City, NY: Doubleday.

Bergsjø, P. (1988). A perspective on childbirth at home and in hospital. *Nordisk Medicin, 103*, 97–101.

Berghs, G., and Spanjaards, E. (1988). De Normale Zwangerschap: Bevalling en Beleid [The normal pregnancy: birth and policy]. Ph.D. thesis, Catholic University, Nijmegen.

Berghs, G., Spanjaards, E., Driessen, L., Doesburg, W., and Eskes, T. (1995). Neonatal neurological outcome after low-risk pregnancies. *European Journal of Obstetrics, Gynecology, & Reproductive Biology, 62*(2), 167–71.

Berkelmans, I. (2000). Het spel en de knikkers. [The game and the marbles]. *Tijdschrift voor Verloskundigen* [Journal for Midwives], 25(5), 334–339.

Bessell, A. (1979). *Het Kringgesprek: Emotional and Social Opvoeding op School, deel 1* [The Circle Speak: Emotional and Social Upbringing at School, Part 1]. Lemniscaat.

Bleker, O. P. (1997). Thuis bevallen. Herwonnen ideaal of anachronisme? [Home birth ideal regained or anachronism?]. *Nederlands Tijdschrift voor Obstetrie en Gynaecologie, 110*, 409–411.

Bleker, O. P. (2000). Verloskundigen zorg [Midwife care]. *Medisch Contact*, 55(35).

Borst, C. (1989). Wisconsin's midwives as working women: Immigrant midwives and the limits of a traditional occupation. *Journal of American Ethnic History, 8*(2), 24–59.

Borst, C. (1995). *Catching Babies: The Professionalization of Childbirth, 1870–1920*. Cambridge, MA: Harvard University Press.

Borst-Eilers, E. (1997). Health policy in the Netherlands. In A. J. P. Schrijvers (Ed.), *Health and Health Care in the Netherlands* (pp. 15–19). Utrecht, the Netherlands: De Tijdstroom.

Borst-Eilers, E. (2000a, February 9). *Voortgang Kraamzorg: Brief aan de Voorzitter van de Vaste Commissie voor Volksgezondheid, Welzijn, en Sport* [Progress in Postpartum Care: Letter to the Chair of the Permanent Committee for Public Health, Welfare, and Sport]. Den Haag: Ministerie van Volksgezondheid, Welzijn, en Sport.

Borst-Eilers, E. (2000b, July 3). *Brief aan de Voorzitter van de Vaste Commissie voor Volksgezondheid, Welzijn, en Sport. Onderwerp: Verloskunde* [Letter to the Chair of the Permanent Committee for Public Health, Welfare and Sport. Subject: Obstetrics]. Den Haag: Ministerie van Volksgezondheid, Welzijn, en Sport.

Borst-Eilers, E. (2000c, October). *Notitie Modernisering Verloskunde: Standpunt op het eindrapport van de Stuurgroep Modernisering Verloskunde* [Notes on Modernizing Obstetrics: Standpoint on the Final Report of the Steering Committee for the Modernizing of Obstetrics]. Den Haag: Ministerie van Volksgezondheid, Welzijn, en Sport.

Borst-Eilers, E. (2000d, November 7). *Brief aan de Voorzitter van de Vaste Commissie voor Volksgezondheid, Welzijn, en Sport. Onderwerp: Verloskunde* [Letter to the Chair of the Permanent Committee for Public Health, Welfare, and Sport. Subject: Obstetrics]. Den Haag: Ministerie van Volksgezondheid, Welzijn en Sport.

Bourgeault, I., Benoit, C., and Davis-Floyd, R. (2004). Reconceiving midwifery in Canada. In I. Bourgeault, C. Benoit, and R. Davis-Floyd (Eds.), *Reconceiving Midwifery* (pp. 3–13). Montreal: McGill-Queen's University Press.

Brief van huisarts [Letter from huisarts]. (1963). *Medisch Contact*, 18, 91, 95.

British Department of Health. (1992). *Health Committee Second Report, Maternity Services*, Vol. 1 (Winterton Report).

British Department of Health and Social Security. (1970). *Domiciliary Midwifery and Maternity Bed Needs* (Peel Report).

British Department of Health Expert Maternity Group. (1992). *Changing Childbirth*. Part I. London: HMSO.

British Medical Journal. (1977, September 3). Editorial: Helping mothers to love their babies, *British Medical Journal.*

British Ministry of Health. (1959). *Report of the Maternity Services Committee* (Cranbrook Report).

British Ministry of Health. (1960). *Report on Confidential Enquiries into Maternal Deaths in England and Wales 1955–1957.*

Bruning, G., and Plantenga, J. (1998). *Ouderschapsverlof en emancipatiebeleid: ervaringen uit 8 Europese landen. Tijdschrift voor arbeidsvraagstukken* [Parental Leave and Emancipation Policy: Experiences of 8 European Countries], 4, 343–355.

Bultman, J. (1999, January). Oprichting van het Werkoverleg Verloskunde [The Creation of the Obstetric Work Consultation Group]. Appendix 1 in *Ziekenfondsraad, Vademecum Verloskunde: Eindrapport van het Werkoverleg Verloskunde van de Ziekenfondsraad* [Final Report of the Sickness Funds Council Work Group on Obstetrics]. Amstelveen, the Netherlands: Ziekenfondsraad.

Campbell, R., and Macfarlane, A. (1990). Recent Debate on the Place of Birth. In J. Garcia, R. Kilpatrick, and M. Richards (Eds.), *The Politics of Maternity Care.* Oxford University Press.

Campbell, R., and MacFarlane, A. (1994). *Where to Be Born?* 2nd ed. Oxford: National Perinatal Epidemiology Unit.

CBS [*Centraal Bureau voor de Statistiek*]. (Various years through 1993). *Geborenen naar Aard Verloskundige Hulp en Plaats van Geboorte* [Births by Source of Obstetric Help and Place of Birth]. Voorburg, the Netherlands: CBS.

CBS. (1998). *Vademecum Gezondheidsstatistiek 1998* [Vademecum of Health Statistics of the Netherlands 1998]. 's-Gravenhage: Sduuitgeverij.

CBS. (1999). *Vademecum Gezondheidsstatistiek Nederland* [Health Statistics of the Netherlands]. Voorburg, the Netherlands: CBS.

Central Raad voor de Volksgezondheid. (1972). *Advies Inzake de Verstrekking van Verloskundige Hulp* [Advice on the Provision of Obstetric Care]. Rijswijk, the Netherlands: Central Raad voor de Volksgezondheid.

Central Raad voor de Volksgezondheid. (1977). *Advies Inzake de Verstrekking van Verloskundige Hulp* [Advice on the Provision of Obstetric Care]. Rijswijk, the Netherlands: Central Raad voor de Volksgezondheid.

Chalmers, I. (1986). Minimizing harm and maximizing benefit during innovation in health care: Controlled or uncontrolled experimentation? *Birth, 13*, 155–164.

Chalmers, I., Enkin, M., Keirse, M.J.N.C. (Eds.). (1989). *Effective Care in Pregnancy and Childbirth*. Oxford University Press (National Perinatal Epidemiology Unit).

Chamberlayne, P., Cooper, A., Freeman, R., and M. Rustin (Eds.). (1999). *Welfare and Culture in Europe: Towards a New Paradigm in Social Policy*. Philadelphia: Jessica Kingsley Press.

Citteur, C.A.W., and Hoogendoorn, D. (1979). Ingezonden: De relatie tussen de hoogte van de perinatale sterfte en de plaats van bevalling: Thuis, dan wel in het ziekenhuis [Letter: The correlation between the degree of perinatal mortality and the place of birth: At home or in the hospital]. *Nederlands Tijdschrift voor Geneeskunde* [Dutch Journal of Medicine], *123*(24), 1039–1040.

Clark, P., Toms, A., Hamfield, T., and Jones, S. (1994). Dutch model of maternity care: Midwifery led service is safe. *BMJ, 308*, 1102.

Coffie, D., Wiegers, T., and Schellevis. (2003). Het Gebruik van Verloskundige Zorg en Kraamzorg [The use of midwive care and postpartum care]. *Tijdschrift voor Verloskundigen, 28*(6), 315–320.

Cranendonk, E. (1986). Ingezonden [Letter to the editor]. *Nederlands Tijdscrift voor Geneeskunde* [Dutch Journal of Medicine], *130*, 1715.

Créybas, A. (1990). De kraamzorg: Enkele historische data [Postpartum care: Some historical data]. *Tijdschrijft voor Verloskundigen, 15*(12), 370.

Croon, M. (1998). Koninklijk en in verandering [Royal and changing]. *Tijdschrift voor Verloskundigen, 23*(7), 493.

Croon, M. (1999, May 4). Routinematige ruggenprik is onverantwoord [Routine epidurals are irresponsible]. *NRC Handelsblad*, 9.

Damstra-Wijmenga, S. M. I. (1982). Veilig bevallen: Een vergelijkende studie tussen thuis en de klinische bevalling [Safe birthing: A comparative study between home and clinic birth]. Ph.D. thesis, Groningen University.

Davies, J., Hey, E., Reid, W., and Young, G. (1996). Prospective regional study of planned home births. *British Medical Journal, 313*, 1302–1306.

Davis-Floyd, R. (1992). *Birth as an American Rite of Passage*. Berkeley: University of California Press.

De Baena, D. (1975). *The Dutch Puzzle*, 5th edition. The Hague: L. J. C. Boucher. First published 1966.

De Bony, J. (2001, April). Decision making process in the Dutch and French cultures: Differences in the relationship between the individual and the group.

Presented at the conference, Comparing Cultures, Tilburg, the Netherlands.

Declercq, E. (1998). "Changing Childbirth" in the UK: Lessons for US health policy. *Journal of Health Politics, Policy, and Law, 23*(5), 833–860.

Declercq, E., and Viisainen, K. (2001). The politics of numbers: The promise and frustration of cross-national analysis. In R. De Vries, C. Benoit, E. van Teijlingen, and S. Wrede (Eds.), *Birth by Design: Pregnancy, Maternity Care, and Midwifery in North America and Europe* (pp. 267–279). New York: Routledge.

Declercq, E., De Vries, R., Viisainen, K., Salvesen, H., and Wrede, S. (2001). Where to give birth? Politics and the place of birth. In R. De Vries, C. Benoit, E. van Teijlingen, and S. Wrede (Eds.), *Birth by Design: Pregnancy, Maternity Care, and Midwifery in North America and Europe* (pp. 7–27). New York; Routledge.

De Haan, H., and van Impe, M. (1983). *Hoe Bevalt Nederland?* [How Does the Netherlands Birth?] Utrecht, the Netherlands: Spectrum.

De Haan, J., and Smits, F. (1983). Home deliveries in the Netherlands: Present situation and sequelae. *Journal of Perinatal Medicine, 11*(3), 3–8.

De Jong, P.A. (1975). The neurological investigation of the newborn according to Prechtl-Beintema as a yardstick for obstetrical care. Ph. D. thesis, Free University, Amsterdam.

De Melker, R. A. (1997). The family doctor. In A. J. P. Schrijvers, (Ed.). *Health and Health Care in the Netherlands* (pp. 60–72). De Tijdstroom, Utrecht, the Netherlands.

De Miranda, E. (1996). Moet de huisarts de thuisbevalling redden? [Must the huisarts save home birth?]. *Tijdschrijft voor Verloskundigen, 21*(3), 13–16.

De Snoo, K. (1930). *Leerboek voor Verloskunde* [Textbook of Obstetrics]. Groningen: Wolters.

De Telegraaf (1994). Thuis bevallen mag in Engeland [Home birth possible in England]. *De Telegraaf,* October 19.

De Telegraaf (1995). Zo bevalt Europa [How babies are born in Europe]. *De Telegraaf,* July 22.

De Vries, R. (1984). Humanizing childbirth: The discovery and implementation of bonding theory. *International Journal of Health Services Research, 14,* 89–104.

De Vries, R. (1985). *Regulating Birth: Midwives, Medicine, and the Law.* Philadelphia: Temple University Press.

De Vries, R. (1996). *Making Midwives Legal.* Columbus: Ohio State University Press.

De Vries, R. (2001). Midwifery in the Netherlands: Vestige or vanguard? In R. Davis-Flyd, S. Cosminsky, and S. L. Pigg (Eds.), *Daughters of Time: The Shifting Identities of Contemporary Midwives. Medical Anthropology, 20*(2–4), 277–311.

De Vries, R. (2003, April 11). The ethics of professional rivalry. Presented at the University of Minnesota Center for Bioethics.

De Vries, R., and Barroso, R. (1997). Midwives among the machines: Reinventing midwifery in the 20th century. In H. Marland and S. Rafferty (Eds.), *Midwives, Society, and Childbirth: Debates and Controversies in the Modern Period.* London: Routledge.

De Vries R., Salvesen, H., Wiegers, T., and Williams, A. S. (2001). What (and why) do women want? The desires of women and the design of maternity care. In R. De Vries, C. Benoit, E. van Teijlingen, and S. Wrede (Eds.), *Birth by Design: Pregnancy, Maternity Care, and Midwifery in North America and Europe* (pp. 243–266). New York: Routledge.

De Vries, Rijk. (2000). Q & A Euthanasia 2001. Online at http://www.min-buza.nl/default.asp?CMS_ITEM=MBZ413077.

De Wit, L. (2003, February). Vroedvrouwenschool komt in September 2004 naar Randwijck [Midwife school comes to Ranwijck in September 2004]. *M*, 14–15.

Donegan, J. B. (1978). *Women and Men Midwives: Medicine, Morality, and Misogyny in Early America.* Westport, CT: Greenwood Press.

Donnison, J. (1977). *Midwives and Medical Men: A History of Inter-Professional Rivalries and Women's Rights.* New York: Schocken Books.

Dreiser, T. (1913). *A Traveler at Forty.* New York: Century Company.

Drenth, P. (1998). *1898/1998: 100 Jaar Vroedvrouwen Verenigd* [1898/1998: 100 Years of Midwives United]. Bilthoven, the Netherlands: Nederlandse Organsatie van Verloskundigen.

Eskes, M. (1989). *Het Wormeveer Onderzoek* [The Wormerveer Study]. Amsterdam: University of Amsterdam.

Eskes, M., van Alten, D., and Treffers, P. E. (1993). The Wormerveer study: Perinatal mortality and non-optimal management in a practice of independent midwives. *European Journal of Obstetrics & Gynecology and Reproductive Biology, 51,* 91–95.

Eskes, T. K. A. B. (1980). Pleidooi voor bevallen in het ziekenhuis [A plea for hospital birth]. In A. Querido and J. Roos (Eds.). *Controversen in de geneeskunde* [Controversies in Medicine] (pp. 180–190). Utrecht, the Netherlands: Uitgeverij Bunge.

Eskes, T. K. A. B. (1987, March 20). Naar een nieuwe vorm van verloskundige zorg [Toward a new form of obstetric care]. *Medisch Contact, 12,* 372–374.

Eskes, T. K. A. B. (1992). Home deliveries in the Netherlands: Perinatal mortality and morbidity. *International Journal of Gynecology and Obstetrics, 38,* 161–169.

Eskes, T. K. A. B., Jongsma, W., and Houx, P. C. W. (1981). Umbilical cord cases in home deliveries versus hospital-based deliveries. *Journal of Reproductive Medicine, 26,* 405–408.

European Communities. (2000). *Science Policies in the European Union: Promoting Excellence through Mainstreaming Gender Equality.* Luxembourg: Office for Official Publications of the European Community.

Gelderman-Vink, M. (1986). Ingezonden [Letter to the editor]. *Nederlands Tijdscrift voor Geneeskunde* [Dutch Journal of Medicine], *130,* 1714–1715.

Geyman, J. P. (2003). Myths as barriers to health care reform in the United States. *International Journal of Health Services, 33*(2), 315–329.

Giaimo, S. (2002). *Markets and Medicine: The Politics of Health Care Reform in Britain, Germany and the United States.* Ann Arbor, MI: University of Michigan Press.

Giesen, P. (1999). *Nederland bestaat!* [The Netherlands exists!]. *de Volkskrant, 17 December, 23.*

Gladdish, K. (1991). *Governing from the Center: Politics and Policymaking in the Netherlands.* Dekalb, IL: Northern Illinois Press.

Goer, H. (1999). *The Thinking Woman's Guide to a Better Birth.* New York: Perigee.

Goer, H., and Creevy, D. (1995). *Obstetric Myths versus Research Realities.* Westport, CT: Bergin and Garvey.

Goudsblom, J. (1967). *Dutch Society.* New York: Random House.

Grootscholte, M., Bouwmeester, J. A., and de Klaver, P. (2000). *Evaluatie Wet op het ouderschapsverlof* [Evaluation of the Parental Leave Law]. Den Haag: *Ministerie van Sociale Zaken en Werkgelegenheid.* Elsevier.

Haire, D. (1981). Improving the outcomes of pregnancy through increased utilization of midwives. *Journal of Nurse-Midwifery, 26,* 5–8.

Hiddinga, A. (1987). Obstetrical research in the Netherlands in the 19th century. *Medical History, 31,* 281–305.

Hiddinga, A. (1993). Dutch Obstetric Science: Emergence, Growth, and Present Situation. In E. Abraham-Van der Mark (Ed.), *Successful Home Birth and Midwifery: The Dutch Model* (pp. 45–76). Westport, CT: Bergin and Garvey.

Hiddinga, A. (1998). Verloskunde in Nederland: Vroedvrouwen en de thuisbevalling [Obstetrics in the Netherlands: Midwives and home birth]. In R. van Daalen, and M. Gijswijt-Hofstra (Eds.), *Gezond en Wel: Vrouwen en de Zorg Voor Gezondheid in de Twintigste Eeuw* [Safe and Sound: Women and Health Care in the Twentieth Century]. Amsterdam: Amsterdam University Press.

Hingstman, L. (1994). Primary care obstetrics and perinatal health in the Netherlands. *Journal of Nurse-Midwifery, 39*(6), 379–386.

Hingstman, L., and Kenens, R. (2002). *Cijfers uit de Registratie van Verloskundigen: Peiling 2002* [Numbers from the Registry of Midwives: 2002]. Utrecht, the Netherlands: NIVEL.

Hingstman L., Foets M., and Riteco J. (1993). Thuis of in het ziekenhuis bevallen. Meningen van de consument [Home or hospital birth: Opinions of consumers]. *Tijdschrift voor Verloskundigen, 2*(18), 66–73.

Hingstman L., Pool, J. B., and Barentsen, R. (1992). *Behoeftebepaling Gynaecologen/Obstetrici* [Determining Need for Gynecolgists/Obstetricians]. Utrecht, the Netherlands: NIVEL.

Hingstman L., Pool, J. B., and Barentsen, R. (1994). Behoefteraming voor Gynaecologen/Obstetrici tot het jaar 2005 [Estimating the need for Gynecolgists/Obstetricians through 2005]. *Nederland Tijdscrift voor Geneeskunde* [Dutch journal of medicine], *138*(19), 969–973.

Hofstede, G. (2001). *Culture's Consequences: Comparing Values, Behaviours, Institutions, and Organizations across Nations.* London: Sage.

Honigsbaum, F. (1979). *The Division in British Medicine.* London: Kogan Page.

Hoogedoorn, D. (1978). De relatie tussen de hoogte van de perinatale sterfte en de plaats van bevalling: Thuis, dan wel in het ziekenhuis [The correlation between the degree of perinatal mortality and the place of birth: At home or in the hospital]. *Nederlands Tijdschrift voor Geneeskunde* [Dutch Journal of Medicine], *122*(32), 1171–1178.

Hoogedoorn, D. (1986). Indrukwekkende en tegelijk teleurstellende daling van de perinatale sterfte in Nederland [Impressive but still disappointing decrease in perinatal mortality in the Netherlands]. *Nederlands Tijdschrift voor Geneeskunde* [Dutch Journal of Medicine], *130*, 1436–1440.

Hooker, M. T. (1999). *The History of Holland.* Westport, CT: Greenwood Press.

House of Commons Health Committee. (1992). Second Report, Maternity Services, Vol. 1. London: HMSO.

Houtzager, H. L. (1997). Introduction. In H. L. Houtzager, and F. B. Lammes (Eds.), *Obstetrics and Gynaecology in the Low Countries: A Historical Perspective* (pp. 3–5). Ziest, the Netherlands: Medical Forum International.

Huisarts (1963). Uit de praktijk: Arts en vroedvrouw [From the practice: Doctor and midwife]. *Medisch Contact, 18* (7, 15 February), 95.

Huisjes, W. (1987, June 26). De nieuwe verloskundige indicatielijst [The new obstetrics indications list]. *Medisch Contact, 26*, 813.

Huygen, F. (1976). Home deliveries in Holland. *Journal of the Royal College of General Practitioners, 26*, 244–248.

InterNetKrant. (2000, September 14). *Nederlanders het Zuinigst van Europa* [The Dutch Are the Thriftiest in Europe]. Online at http://www.ics.ele.tue.nl/ink/.

Jabaaij, L., Winckers, M., Hingstman, L., and Meijer, W. (1994). *De Vrijgevestigde Verloskundige in Nederland: Werk en Werkdruk* [The Independent midwife in the Netherlands: Work and Workload]. Utrecht, the Netherlands: NIVEL.

James, H. (1972). *Transatlantic Sketches.* Freeport, NY: Books for Libraries Press. First published 1875.

Jordan, M. (2001, June 14). For Brazilian women caesarean sections are surprisingly popular. *Wall Street Journal,* A1, A8.

Keirse, M. (1980). *De Betekenis van Hakjes* [The Meaning of Parentheses]. Leiden, the Netherlands: Universitaire pers Leiden.

Kenens, R., and Hingstman, L. (2001). *Cijfers uit de Registratie van Verloskundigen: Peiling 2001* [Numbers from the Registry of Midwives: 2001]. Utrecht, the Netherlands: NIVEL.

Kenens, R., and Hingstman, L. (2003). *Cijfers uit de Registratie van Verloskundigen: Peiling 2003* [Numbers from the Registry of Midwives: 2003]. Utrecht, the Netherlands: NIVEL.

Kennedy, J. (2001, April 7). Euthanasie komt voort uit verheven zelfbeeld. [Euthanasia the result of positive self-image]. *NRC Handelsblad,* 9.

Kennedy, J. (2002). *Een Weloverwogen Dood: Euthanasie in Nederland* [A Well-Considered Death: Euthanasia in the Netherlands]. Amsterdam: Bert Bakker.

Kerssens, J. (1991). *Het Oordeel Kraamvrouwen over Thuiskraamzorg* [The Opinion of Postpartum Women about Postpartum Care at Home]. Utrecht, the Netherlands: NIVEL.

Keyfitz, N., and Flieger, W. (Eds.). (1990). *World Population Growth and Aging: Demographic Trends in the Late Twentieth Century.* Chicago: University of Chicago Press.

Kirejczyk, M. (2000). Beleidsculturen en menselijke embryo's: Een historische vergelijking van de beleidsontwikkeling betreffende embryo-onderzoek in Nederland en het Verenigd Koninkrijk [Policy culture and human embryo's: An historical comparison of policy developments regarding embryo research in the Netherlands and the United Kingdom]. *Beleidswetenschap, 14*(3), 203–228.

Kist, E. (1998). Het poldermodel wordt straks gekopieerd [The polder model is soon to be copied]. VNO-NCW: http://www.vno-ncw.nl/infromatie/publicates/jr_1998/kist.htm.

Klaus, M., and Kennel, J. (1981). *Parent-Infant Bonding.* St. Louis, MO: Mosby.

Klein, M. (1995). Studying episiotomy: When beliefs conflict with science. *Journal of Family Practice, 41*(5), 483–488.

Klein, M., Gauthier, R. J., Jorgenson, S. H., Robbins, J. M., Kaczorowski, J., Johnson, B., et al. (1992, July 1). Does episiotomy prevent perineal trauma and pelvic floor relaxation? *Online Journal of Current Clinical Trials,* Document 10.

Klein, M., Gauthier, R. J., Robbins, J. M., Kaczorowski, J., Jorgenson, S. H., Franco, E. D., Johnson, B., Waghorn, K., Gelfand, M. M., Guralnick, M. S., Luskey, G. W., and Joshi, A. K. (1994). Relationship of episiotomy to perineal trauma, sexual dysfunction, and pelvic floor relaxation. *American Journal of Obstetrics and Gynecology, 171*(3), 591–598.

Klein M., Kaczorowski, J., Robbins, J. M., Gauthier, Gauthier, R. J., Jorgenson, S. H., and Joshi, A. K. (1995). Physicians' beliefs and behaviour during a randomised controlled trial of episiotomy: Consequences for women in their care. *Canadian Medical Association Journal, 153*(6), 769–779.

Kleiverda, G. (1990). Transition to parenthood, women's experiences of 'labour'. Ph. D. thesis, University of Amsterdam.

Kleiverda, G, Steen, A. M., Andersen, I., Treffers, P. E., Everaerd, W. (1990). Place of delivery in the Netherlands: Maternal motives and background variables related to preferences for home or hospital confinement. *Eur J Obstet Gynecol Reprod Biol, 36,* 1–9.

Kleiverda, G, Steen, A. M., Andersen, I., Treffers, P. E., Everaerd, W. (1991). Place of delivery in the Netherlands: Actual location of confinement. *Eur J Obstet Gynecol Reprod Biol, 39,* 139–146.

Klomp, J. (1994). *De Jaren Zestig: De Vroedvrouwen Bijna Verdwenen, Leve de Vroedvrouw* [The Sixties: Midwives Nearly Disappear, Long Live the Midwife]. Bilthoven, the Netherlands: Catharina Schrader Stichting.

Kloosterman, G. J. (1961). De Toekomst van de Nederlandse Vroedvrouw [The future of the Dutch midwife]. *Tijdscrijft voor Sociale Geneeskunde, 39*(20), 627–629.

Kloosterman, G. J. (1966). De bevalling aan huis en de hedendaagse verloskunde [The birth at home and contemporary obstetrics]. Nederlands *Tijdschrift voor Geneeskunde* [Dutch Journal of Medicine], *110,* 1808–1816.

Kloosterman, G. J. (Ed.). (1973). *De Voortplanting van de Mens: Leerboek voor Obstetrie en Gynaecologie* [Human Reproduction: Textbook for Obstetrics and Gynecology]. Haarlem, the Netherlands: Uitgeversmaatschappij Centen.

Kloosterman, G. J. (1978). De Nederlandse verloskunde op de tweesprong [Dutch obstetrics at the crossroads]. *Nederlands Tijdschrift voor Geneeskunde* [Dutch Journal of Medicine], *122*(32), 1161–1171.

Kloosterman, G. J. (1980). Pleidooi voor de mogelijkheid tot de bevalling thuis [Plea for the possibility of birthing at home]. In A. Querido, and J. Roos (Eds.), *Controversen in de geneeskunde* [Controversies in Medicine] (pp. 191–197). Utrecht, the Netherlands: Uitgeverij Bunge.

Kloosterman, G. J. (1986). Ingezonden [Letter to the editor]. *Nederlands Tijdschrift voor Geneeskunde* [Dutch Journal of Medicine], *130*, 1714.

Kloosterman G. J., and Thiery, M. (1977). Begeleiden tijdens de baring [Accompaniment during the birth]. In G.J. Kloosterman (Ed.), *De Voortplanting van de Mens: Leerboek voor Obstetrie en Gynaecologie* [Human Reproduction: Textbook for Obstetrics and Gynecology]. Haarlem, the Netherlands: Uitgeversmaatschappij Centen.

Kloosterman, M. D., and Vervest, H.A.M. (1991). Letter to the Chairman of the Sick Funds Council. 31 October, Utrecht.

Knuist, M., Eskes, M., and van Alten, D. (1987). De pH van het ateriele navelstrengbloed van pasgeborenen bij door vroedvrouwen geleide bevallingen [The pH of umbilical cord blood of newborns at midwife-accompanied births]. *Nederlands Tijdschrift voor Geneeskunde* [Dutch Journal of Medicine], *131*(9), 362–364.

Kojo-Austin, H., Malin, M., and Hemminki, E. (1993). Women's satisfaction with maternity health care services in Finland. *Social Science and Medicine, 37*(5), 633–638.

Koldenhoff, R. (2001, February 13). Babysterfte blijkt vaak vermijdbaar [Infant death appears to be often avoidable]. *Haagsche Courant.*

Kooiker, S., and Van der Wijst, L. (2003). *Europeans and Their Medicines: A Cultural Approach to the Utilization of Pharmaceuticals.* The Hague, the Netherlands: Social and Cultural Planning Bureau.

Kranenburg, M. (2001). Polder Model. In *NRC Handelsblad* (Eds.), *The Netherlands: A Practical Guide for the Foreigner and a Mirror for the Dutch* (pp. 35–39). Rotterdam, the Netherlands: Prometheus.

Kuhn, T. S. (1962). *The Structure of Scientific Revolutions.* Chicago: University of Chicago Press.

Kutulas, J. (1998). Do I look like a chick? Men, Women, and Babies on Sitcom Maternity Stories. *American Studies, 39*(2), 13–32.

LVT/NOV (Landelijke Vereniging Voor Thuiszorg/Nederlandse Organisatie van Verloskundigen) [National Association for Home Care/Dutch Organization of Midwives]. (1997). *Concept Zwartboek Kraamzorg. Hoe Slecht Gereguleerde Marktwerking de Kraamzorg in Gevaar Komt* [Black Book of Postpartum Care: How Poorly Regulated Market Forces Endanger Postpartum Care]. LVT, Bunnik.

Lapré, R. M. (1972). Aspecten van marktanalyse met betrekking tot verloskundige diensten in Nederland [Aspects of market analysis with regard to obstetric services in the Netherlands]. Nijmegen, Dekker, en Van de Vegt. Ph. D. thesis.

Leavitt, J. W. (1986). *Brought to Bed: Childbearing in America, 1750 to 1950.* New York: Oxford University Press.

Lems, A. A., Groenveld, A., and Verdenius, W. (1987). Naar een nieuwe vorm van verloskundige zorg [Toward a new form of obstetric care]. *Medisch Contact, 12*(20 March), 371–372.

Lewis, J. (1980). *The Politics of Motherhood.* London: Croom Helm.

Lieburg, M. (Ed.). (1984). *C. G. Schrader's Memory Boeck van de Vrouwens* [C. G. Schrader's Memory Book of the Women]. Amsterdam: Rodolpi.

Lievaart, M., and de Jong, P. A. (1982). Neonatal morbidity in deliveries conducted by midwives and gynecologists: A study of the system of obstetric care prevailing in the Netherlands. *American Journal of Obstetrics and Gynecology, 144,* 376–386.

Lievaart, M., and de Jong, P. A. (1983). Reply to Monagle and Treffers et al. [Letter] *American Journal of Obstetrics & Gynecology, 146*(7):872–874.

Lijphart, A. (1968). *The Politics of Accommodation: Pluralism and Democracy in the Netherlands.* Berkeley: University of California Press.

Lijphart, A. (1975). *The Politics of Accommodation: Pluralism and Democracy in the Netherlands,* 2nd edition. Berkeley: University of California Press.

Litoff, J. (1978). *American Midwives: 1860 to the Present.* Westport, CT: Greenwood Press.

Litoff, J. (1986). *The American Midwife Debate: A Sourcebook on Its Modern Origins.* Westport, CT: Greenwood Press.

Loudon, I. (1992). *Death in Childbirth.* Oxford: Clarendon Press.

Mander, R. (1995). The relevance of the Dutch system of maternity care to the United Kingdom. *Journal of Advanced Nursing, 22,* 1023–1026.

Manschot, A. (1993, December). Is al dat lijden nog wel nodig? [Is all that suffering still needed?]. *Opzij,* 28–31.

Manshanden, J.C.P. (1997). De keuze van nulliparae; wanneer, waarom? [The choice of nulliaprous women: When, why?]. *Tijdschrift voor Verloskundigen,* (22), 34–40.

Marland, H. (Ed.). (1987). *Mother and Child Were Saved: The Memoirs (1693–1740) of the Frisian Midwife Catharina Schrader.* Amsterdam: Roldopi.

Marland, H. (1993a). The guardians of normal birth: The debate on the standard and status of the midwife in the Netherlands around 1900. In E. Abraham-Van der Mark (Ed.), *Successful Home Birth and Midwifery: The Dutch Model* (pp. 21–44), Westport, CT: Bergin and Garvey.

Marland, H. (1993b). The *burgerlijke* midwife: The *stadsvroedvrouw* of eighteenth-century Holland. In H. Marland (Ed.). *The Art of Midwifery Early Modern Midwives in Europe* (pp. 192–213). New York: Routledge.

Marland, H. (Ed.). (1993c). *The Art of Midwifery Early Modern Midwives in Europe.* New York: Routledge.

Marland, H. (1995). Questions of competence: The midwife debate in the Netherlands in the early twentieth century. *Medical History, 39,* 317–337.

Marland, H., and Rafferty, A. M. (Eds.). (1997). *Midwives, Society, and Childbirth: Debates and Controversies in the Modern Period.* New York: Routledge.

Marsico, T. (1995). All the news that's fit to print: The ACNM sets the record straight. *Journal of Nurse-Midwifery, 40*(3), 253–255.

Martin, E. (1987). *The Woman in the Body: A Cultural Analysis of Reproduction.* Boston: Beacon Press.

Martin, J., Smith, J., Haddad, S., Walker, J., Wong, A. (1992, July 25). Women prefer hospital births. *British Medical Journal, 305,* 255.

Martin, J. A., Hamilton, B. E., Ventura, S. J., Menacker, F., Park, M. M., Sutton, P. D. (2002). *Births: Final Data for 2001. National Vital Statistics Reports, Vol 51, No. 2.* Hyattsville, MD: National Center for Health Statistics.

Mascarenhas, L., Biervliet, F., Gee, H., and Whittle, M. (1994). Dutch Model Limits Choice. [Letter]. *BMJ, 308,* 342.

Medical Birth Registry of Norway. (1997). *Medical Birth Registry of Norway 1967–1996. Births in Norway through 30 years.* Bergen, Norway: University of Bergen.

Mehl-Madrona, M., and Mehl-Madrona, L. (1993). The future of midwifery in the United States. *NAPSAC News, 18*(3-4), 1–32.

Metro. (2001, February 16). Bevallen in ziekenhuis veiliger: Hoogleraar Sauer wijst op risico thuisbevallingen [Birth in the hospital safer: Professor Sauer points to the risk of home birth.]

Mills, C. W. (1959). *The Sociological Imagination.* New York: Oxford University Press.

Ministerie van Volksgezondheid, Welzijn, en Sport. (1998, July 15). Knelpunten kraamzorg worden aangepakt [Bottlenecks in postpartum care will be dealt with]. News brief number 67. Den Haag: Ministerie van Volksgezonheid, Welzijn, en Sport.

Ministerie van Welzijn, Volksgezondheid, en Cultuur. (1987). *Verloskundige Organisatie in Nederland: Uniek, Bewonderd en Verguisd* [Obstetric organization in the Netherlands: Unique, Admired, and Reviled]. Final report of the Midwifery Advisory Commission. Rijswijk: Ministerie van Welzijn, Volksgezondheid, en Cultuur.

Ministerie van Welzijn, Volksgezondheid, en Sport. (2001). *Zorgnota, 2002* [Care Budget, 2002]. Den Haag: Sdu Uitgevers.

Ministerie van Welzijn, Volksgezondheid, en Sport. (2002). *Zorgnota, 2003* [Care Budget, 2003]. Den Haag: Sdu Uitgevers.

Mitford, J. (1992). *The American Way of Birth.* New York, NY: Dutton.

Mundy, P. (1925). *The Travels of Peter Mundy in Europe and Asia, 1608–1667, Vol. 4, Travels in Europe, 1639–1647,* R. C. Temple (Ed.). London: Hakluyt Society.

National Center for Health Statistics (U.S.). (1980, April 28). *Monthly Vital Statistics Report, 29*(suppl. 1).

Nederlands Dagblad. (2000, October 19). Thuisbevalling gaat verdwijnen. [Home birth will disappear].

Nederlandse Vereniging voor Obstetrie en Gynaecologie (NVOG). (1987). *Commentaar op het eindrapport van de werkgroep bijstelling Koostermanlijst* [Commentary on the final report of the work group for the revision of the Kloosterman list]. Nederlandse Vereniging voor Obstetrie en Gynaecologie.

Nijhuis, J. G. (2000). *De Foetus Verdient Meer: Inaugurele Rede*. (The Fetus Deserves More: Inaugural Speech.) Maastricht, the Netherlands: Universiteit Maastricht.

NIVEL (Netherlands Institute for Health Care Research). (1995). *Dutch National Survey of General Practice: A Portfolio*. Utrecht, the Netherlands: NIVEL.

NIVEL (Netherlands Institute for Health Care Research). (1998). *Pas Afgestudeerde Verloskundigen* [Recently Graduated Midwives]. Utrecht, the Netherlands: NIVEL.

NIVEL (Netherlands Institute for Health Care Research). (1999). *Praktizerende Verloskundigen* [Practicing Midwives]. Utrecht, the Netherlands: NIVEL.

NMPMSCG (Northern Region Perinatal Mortality Survey Coordinating Group). (1995). Collaborative survey of perinatal loss in planned and un-planned home births. *British Medical Journal, 313*, 1306–1309.

NRC Handelsblad. (1968, October 15). *Opleiding vroedvrouwen: Alleen verpleegsters naar examen* [Education of midwives: Only nurses allowed to sit for exams].

NRC Handelsblad. (2000, Janurary 3). De eerste Millenniumplacenta [The first millennium placenta].

NRC Handelsblad. (2001a, February 14). Babysterfte bij geboorte kan 6 pct lager zijn [Baby death at birth be reduced by 6 percent].

NRC Handelsblad. (2001b). *The Netherlands: A Practical Guide for the Foreigner and a Mirror for the Dutch*. Rotterdam, the Netherlands: Prometheus.

NRC Handelsblad (2003, December 4) Ik wil een 20-weken echo hebben, [I want a sonagram at 20 weeks].

NRC Weekeditie. (1996, January 2). Zwangere vrouw mag kiezen voor huisarts [Pregnant women may choose general practitioner], 3.

Oakley, A. (1980). *Women Confined: Towards a Sociology of Childbirth*. Oxford: M. Robertson.

Oakley, A. (1984). *The Captured Womb: A History of Antenatal Care in Britain*. New York: Blackwell.

Oppenheimer, C. (1993). Organising midwifery led care in the Netherlands. *British Medical Journal, 307*, 1400–1402.

Pasveer, B., and Akrich, M. (2001). Obstetrical trajectories: On training women/bodies for (home) birth. In R. De Vries, C. Benoit, E. van Teijlingen, and S. Wrede (Eds.), *Birth by Design: Pregnancy, Maternity Care, and Midwifery in North America and Europe* (pp. 229–242). New York: Routledge.

Payer, L. (1988). *Medicine and Culture: Varieties of Treatment in the United States, England, West Germany, and France*. New York: Henry Holt.

Pel, M., and Heres, M.H.B. (1995). OBINT: A study of obstetric intervention. Ph. D. thesis, University of Amsterdam.

Pel, M., and Treffers, P. E. (1983). The reliability of the result of the umbilical cord pH. *Journal of Perinatal Medicine, 11*, 169–174.

Pettigrew, T., and Meertens, R. (1996). The verzuiling puzzle: Understanding dutch intergroup relations. *Current Psychology, 15*(1), 3–13.

Phaff, J. M. L. (1986). The organisation and administration of perinatal services in the Netherlands. In J. M. L. Phaff (Ed.), *Perinatal Health Services in Europe*.

Searching for Better Childbirth. London, Sydney, Dover, New Hampshire: Croom Helm.

Pilote, L., Califf, R. M., Sapp, S., Miller, D. P., Mark, D. B., Weaver, W. D., Gore, J. M., Armstrong, P. W., Ohman, E. M., Topol, E. J., the GUSTO-1 Investigators. (1995). Regional variation across the United States in the management of acute myocardial infarction. *New England Journal of Medicine, 333*(9), 565–572.

Porter, M., and Macintyre, S. (1984) What is, must be best. *Social Science and Medicine, 19*(11), 1197–1200.

Pott-Buter, H. (1993). *Facts and Fairy Tales about Female Labor, Family, and Fertility.* Amsterdam: University of Amsterdam Press.

Prechtl, H. F. R. (1977). *The Neurological Examination of the Full-Term Newborn Infant. Clinics in Developmental Medicine, Number 63.* London: Heinemann.

Press, N., and Browner, C. (1997). Why women say yes to prenatal diagnosis. *Social Science and Medicine, 45*(7), 979–989.

Putnam, R. D. (2000). *Bowling Alone: The Collapse and Revival of American Community.* New York: Simon and Schuster.

Querido, A., and Roos, J. (1980). *Controversen in de Geneeskunde* [Controversies in Medicine]. Utrecht, the Netherlands: Uigeverij Bunge.

Radio Nederland Wereldomroep. (1999, December 31). Korte staking vroedvrouwen in Amsterdam [Short strike by midwives in Amsterdam].

Raju, T. (1999). Ignac Semmelweis and the etiology of fetal and neonatal sepsis. *Journal of Perinatology, 19*(4), 307–310.

Ridderbeck, R. (1990). Bevallingen en kraamzorg, GE 1987/1988 [Deliveries and maternity care, GE 1987/1988]. *Maandbericht Gezondheidsstatistiek CBS* [Monthly Briefing on Health Statistics CBS], *9*(4), 4–13.

Riteco, J. A., and Hingstman, L. (1991). *Evaluatie Invoering Indicatielijst* [Evaluation of the Implementation of the Indications List]. Utrecht, the Netherlands: NIVEL.

Riteco, J. A., and Hingstman, L. (1992a). De verloskundige indicatielijst: How denken huisartsen, verloskundigen en gynaecologen erover? [The obstetric indications list: What do general practitioners, midwives and gynecologists think about it?] *Medisch Contact, 47*(5), 151–158.

Riteco, J. A., and Hingstman, L. (1992b). De verloskundige indicatielijst: How gaan huisartsen, verloskundigen, en gynaecologen ermee om? (The obstetric indications list: How are general practitioners, midwives, and gynecologists using it?) *Medisch Contact, 47*(5), 151–158.

Rochon, T. T. (1999). *The Netherlands: Negotiating Sovereignty in an Independent World.* Boulder, CO: Westview Press.

Rooks, J. (1997). *Midwifery and Childbirth in America.* Philadelphia: Temple University Press.

Rothman, B. K. (1982). *In Labor: Women and Power in the Birthplace.* New York: Penguin.

Rothman, B. K. (1993). Going Dutch: Lessons for Americans (pp. 201–211). In E. Abraham-Van der Mark (Ed.), *Successful Home Birth and Midwifery: The Dutch Model.* Westport, CT: Bergin and Garvey.

Rottinghuis, H. (1947). De verloskunde nu en in de toekomst [The midwife now and in the future]. *Nederlands Tijdschrift voor Verloskunde, 68,* 377–389.

Rybczynksi, W. (1986). *Home.* New York: Penguin.

Sandall, J., Bourgeault, I., Meijer, W., and Schuëcking, B. (2001). Deciding Who Cares: Winners and Losers in the Late Twentieth Century. In R. De Vries, C. Benoit, E. van Teijlingen, and S. Wrede (Eds.), *Birth by Design: Pregnancy, Maternity Care, and Midwifery in North America and Europe* (pp. 117–138). New York: Routledge.

Schama, S. (1988). *The Embarrassment of Riches: An Interpretation of Dutch Culture in the Golden Age.* Berkeley: University of California Press.

Scheerder, R. (1997). The Financing of the Dutch Health Care System. In A. Schrijvers (Ed.), *Health and Health Care in the Netherlands* (pp. 163–170). Utrecht, the Netherlands: De Tijdstroom.

Schellekens, W. (1987, May 15). De nieuwe verloskundige indicatielijst [The new obstetrics indications list]. *Medisch Contact, 20,* 619–623.

Schiet, M. (1994). Bevallen in het buitenland [Birthing in other countries]. *In Verwachting, 1,* 112–113.

Schöttelndreier, M. (2001, June 23). In modern gezin is alles onderhandelbaar [In the modern family everything is negotiable]. *Volkskrant,* Voorpagina.

Schultz, G. D. (1958). Cruelty in maternity wards. *Ladies Home Journal,* May, 44–45, 152–155.

Schut, F. T. (1995). Health care reform in the Netherlands: Balancing corporatism, etatism, and market mechanisms. *Journal of Health Politics, Policy, and Law, 20,* 615–652.

Senden, I. P., van du Wetering, M., Eskes, T. K., Bierkens, P., Laube, D., and Pitkin, R. (1988). Labor pain: A comparison of parturients in a Dutch and an American teaching hospital. *Obstetrics & Gynecology, 71*(4), 541–544.

Shelley, M., and Shelley, P. B. (1989). *History of a Six Weeks' Tour.* Oxford: Woodstock Books. First published 1817.

Shetter, W. Z. (1997). *The Netherlands in Perspective.* Utrecht, the Netherlands: Nederlands Centrum Buitenlanders.

Shultz, G. (1958, May). Cruelty in maternity wards. *Ladies' Home Journal,* 44–45, 152–155.

SIG (SIG Zorginformatie). (1990). *Results of Dutch Midwifery Care.* Utrecht, the Netherlands: SIG.

SIG (SIG Zorginformatie). (1992). *Jaarboek Verloskunde* [Obstetric Yearbook]. Utrecht, the Netherlands: SIG.

SIG (SIG Zorginformatie). (1996). *Verloskunde in Nederland: Grote Lijnen 1989–1993* [Obstetrics in the Netherlands: Major Trends, 1989–1993]. Utrecht, the Netherlands: SIG.

Sikkel, A. (1979). *De Verloskundige Organsatie in Nederland, 1979* [The Organization of Obstetrics in the Netherlands, 1979]. Rijswijk, the Netherlands: Ministerie van Volkjsgezondheid en Milieuhygiene.

Smal, J. A. (1997). Medical education (pp. 216–222). In A.J.P. Schrijvers (Ed.), *Health and Health Care in the Netherlands.* Utrecht, the Netherlands: De Tijdstroom.

Social and Cultural Planning Office of the Netherlands. (2000a). *The Netherlands in a European Perspective: Social and Cultural Report 2000.* The Hague: Social and Cultural Planning Office.

Social and Cultural Planning Office of the Netherlands. (2000b). *Van Arbeids-naar Combinatie-Ethos* [From Work- to Combination-Ethos]. Work Document 66. The Hague: Social and Cultural Planning Office.

Spanjer, J., de Haan, E., Dijk, H., Poortman, L., Gorter, A., de Waal, M., de Jong, M., and Hagens, H. (1994). *Bevallen en Opstaan* [Birthing and Uprising]. Amsterdam: Uitgeverij Contact.

Springer, M. P. (1987, May 15). Het verloskundig handelen van huisartsen [The obstetric care of general practitioners]. *Medisch Contact, 20,* 624–630.

Springer, M. P. (1991). *Kwaliteit van Verloskundig Handelen van Huisartsen* [Quality of Obstetric Care by General Practitioners in the Netherlands]. Utrecht, the Netherlands: Drukkerij Elinkwijk.

Springer, N., and Van Weel, C. (1996). Home birth: Safe in selected women, and with adequate infrastructure and support. *British Medical Journal, 313,* 1276–1277.

Starr, P. (1982). *The Social Transformation of American Medicine.* New York: Basic Books.

Steenhuis, P. (1998, September 29). *Wegbereiders van het poldermodel* [Preparers of the way for the polder model]. NRC Weekeditie, 24.

Stolte, L., van den Berg-Helder, A. F., De Jong, P. A., Van Kessel, H., Kurver, P. H. J., Njiokiktjien, C. J., and Voorhorst, F. J. (1976). Non-iatrogenic deleterious influences of pregnancy and delivery on neurological optimality of newborns. Paper presented at the Fourth International Congress of the International Society for the Scientific Study of Mental Deficiency, Washington, D.C.

Stolte, L., van den Berg-Helder, A. F., De Jong, P. A., Van Kessel, H., Kurver, P. H. J., Njiokiktjien, C. J., and Voorhorst, F. J. (1979). Perinatale morbiditeit als maatstaf voor de verloskundige zorg [Perinatal morbidity as a criterion of obstetric care]. *Nederlands Tijdschrift voor Geneeskunde* [Dutch Journal of Medicine], *123*(7), 228–231.

Stuurgroep Modernisering Verloskunde (SMV). (2000, August). *Meerjarenvisie op de Verloskundige Zorgverlening in de 21e Eeuw* [Multiple Year Vision of Obstetric Care in the 21st Century). Den Haag: VWS.

Sullivan, D., and Weitz, R. (1988). *Labor Pains: Modern Midwives and Home Birth.* New Haven, CT: Yale University Press.

Tasharrofi, A. (1987). Midwifery Care in the Netherlands. *Midwives Chronicle and Nursing Notes,* 286–288.

Ten Berge, M. (2001). Niet bang voor de fysiologische bevalling: Hang in there, Dutch midwifes (sic). [Not afraid of physiologic births: Hang in there Dutch midwives] *Tijdschrift voor Verloskundigen, 26*(7/8), 607–611.

Tew, M. (1995). *Safer Childbirth? A Critical History of Maternity Care.* London: Chapman and Hall.

Tew, M., and Damstra-Wijmenga, S. M. I. (1991). Safest birth attendants: Recent Dutch evidence. *Midwifery, 7,* 55–63.

TNO. (2002). *De Thuisbevalling in Nederland. Eindrapportage: 1995–2000* [Home Birth in the Netherlands. End Report: 1995–2000]. Leiden, the Netherlands: TNO-Preventie en Gezondheid.

Torres, A., and Reich, M. R. (1989). The shift from home to institutional childbirth: a comparative study of the United Kingdom and the Netherlands. *International Journal of Health Services, 19*(3), 405–414.

Touwen, B. C. L., Huisjes, H. J., Jurgens-van der Zee, A. D., Bierman van-Eendenburg, Smrkovsky, M., and Olinga, A. A. (1980). Obstetrical condition and neonatal neurologic morbidity: An analysis with the help of the optimality concept. *Early Human Development, 4*(3), 207–228.

Treffers, P. E. (1993). Selection as the basis of obstetric care in the Netherlands. In E. Abraham-Van der Mark (Ed.), *Successful Home Birth and Midwifery: The Dutch Model.* Westport, CT: Bergin and Garvey.

Treffers, P. E., and Breur, W. (1979). Ingezonden: De plaats van bevalling en de perinatale sterfte [Letter: The place of birth and perinatal mortality]. *Nederlands Tijdschrift voor Geneeskunde* [Dutch Journal of Medicine], *123*(20), 852–853.

Treffers, P. E., and Laan, R. (1986). Regional perinatal mortality and regional hospitalization at delivery in the Netherlands. *British Journal of Obstetrics and Gynaecology, 93,* 690–693.

Treffers, P. E., and Pel, M. (1993). The rising trend for caesarean birth: Britain could learn from the Netherlands. *British Medical Journal, 307,* 1017–1018.

Treffers P. E., van Alten, D., and Pel, M. (1983). Condemnation of obstetric care in the Netherlands? [Letter]. *American Journal of Obstetrics & Gynecology, 146*(7), 871–872.

Treffers, P. E., Eskes, M., Kleiverda, G., and van Alten, D. (1990). Home births and minimal medical interventions. *JAMA, 264*(17), 2203–2208.

Tweede Kamer. (1988–1989). *Regeringsstandpunt Adviescommissie Kloosterman.* (Government Standpoint on the Kloosterman Advice Commission).

Twentsche Courant. (2001, August 24) Thuis bevallen word teen stuk moeilijker. [Home birth becomes a bit more difficult].

Vallgarda, S. (1996). Hospitalization of deliveries: The change of place of birth in Denmark and Sweden from the late nineteenth century to 1970. *Medical History, 40,* 173–196.

Van Alten, D., Eskes, M., and Treffers, P. (1989). Midwifery in the Netherlands. The Wormerveer study; selection, mode of delivery, perinatal mortality and infant morbidity. *British Journal of Obstetrics and Gynaecology, 96,* 656–662.

Van Andel, F.G., and Brinkman, N. (1997). Government policy and cost containment of pharmaceuticals. In A. J. P. Schrijvers (Ed.), *Health and Health Care in the Netherlands* (pp.152–162). Utrecht, the Netherlands: De Tijdstroom.

Van Bavel, M. A. P. (1986). Ingezonden [Letter to the editor]. *Nederlands Tijdschrift voor Geneeskunde* [Dutch Journal of Medicine], *130,* 2141.

Van Crimpen, R. (2000). Nieuwe tijden breken aan [A new day dawns]. *Tijdschrift voor Verloskundigen* [Journal for Midwives], *25*(6), 437.

Van Daalen, R. (1988). De groei van de ziekenhuisbevalling: Nederland en het buitenland. [The growth of hospital birth: The Netherlands and elsewhere]. *Amsterdams Sociologisch Tijdschrift, 15*(3), 414–445.

Van Daalen, R. (1993). Family change and continuity in the Netherlands: Birth and childbed in text and art. In E. Abraham-Van der Mark (Ed.), *Successful Home Birth and Midwifery: The Dutch Model* (pp. 77–94). Westport, CT: Bergin and Garvey.

Van Daalen, R., and van Goor, R. (1993). Interview with Gerrit-Jan Kloosterman. In E. Abraham-Van der Mark (Ed.), *Successful Home Birth and Midwifery: The Dutch Model* (pp. 191–200). Westport, CT: Bergin and Garvey.

Van den berg-Helder, A. F. (1980). Neurological investigation and acid-base equilibrium in umbilical cord blood. Paper presented at the Symposium on Optimalization of Obstetrics in the Netherlands, Free University, Amsterdam.

Van der Borg, H. A. (1992). *Vroedvrouwen: Beeld en Beroep* [Midwives: Image and Profession]. Wageningen: Wageningen Academic Press.

Van der Horst, H. (1996). *The Low Sky: Understanding the Dutch.* Den Haag: Scriptum.

Van der Hulst, L. (1989, November 10). Vroedvrouw en Dekker [Midwife and Dekker]. *Medische Contact, 45.*

Van der Kooij, S. (1990, January 25). Letter to the members of the NVOG.

Van der Lugt, B. J. A. M., Remmink, A. J., Canten, J., Elferink, W., and Kempers, M. (1991, March). Enkele verloskundige resultaten bij selectie volgens de nieuwe midwsche indicatielijst [Some obstetrics results using the selection criteria of the new medical indications list]. *Nederlands Tijdschrift voor Obstetrie en Gynaecologie, 104*, 54–58.

Van der Velden, K. (1999). *General Practice at Work.* Utrecht, the Netherlands: NIVEL.

Van der Velden L. F. J., Bennema-Broos, M., and Hingstman, L. (2001). *Monitor Arbeidsmarkt Obstetrici/Gynaecologen* [Monitor Labor Market Obstetricians/Gynecologists]. Utrecht, the Netherlands: NIVEL.

Van der Velden, L. F. J., and Hingstman, L. (1999). *Behoefteraming Obstetrici/Gynaecologen, 1997–2010: Een Tussenbalans* [Estimate of Need for Obstetricians and Gynecologists, 1997–2010: Finding a Balance]. Utrecht, the Netherlands: NIVEL.

Van der Zee, J. (2000, July 12). Personal communication.

Van Ginkel, R. (1992). Typically Dutch . . . Ruth Benedict on the National Character of Netherlanders. *The Netherlands' Journal of Social Sciences, 28*(1), 50–71.

Van Ginkel, R. (1997). *Notities over Nederlanders* [Notes about the Dutch]. Amsterdam: Boom.

Van Huis, M. (2001). Emoties rondom de thuisbevalling [Emotions around home birth]. *Tijdschrift voor Verloskundigen, 26*(4), 344–345.

Van Lieburg, M. J. (1984). *Memoryboek van de Vrouwens.* Amsterdam: Rodopi.

Van Lieburg, M., and Marland, H. (1989). Midwife regulation, education, and practice in The Netherlands during the nineteenth century. *Medical History, 33,* 296–317.

Van Teijlingen, E. R. (1990). The profession of maternity home care assistant and its significance for the Dutch midwifery profession. *International Journal of Nursing Studies, 27,* 355–366.

Van Teijlingen, E. R. (1993). Maternity home care assistant: A unique occupation. In E. Abraham-Van der Mark (Ed.), *Successful Home Birth and Midwifery: The Dutch Model* (pp. 161–171). Westport, CT: Bergin and Garvey.

Van Teijlingen, E. R. (1994). A social or medical model of childbirth? Comparing the arguments in Grampian (Scotland) and the Netherlands. Ph.D. thesis, University of Aberdeen.

Van Teijlingen, E. (2003). Dutch Midwives: The difference between image and reality (pp. 120–134). In S. Earle and G. Letherby (Eds.), *Gender, Identity and Reproduction: Social Perspectives,* London: Palgrave.

Van Vree, W. (1996). *Nederland als Vergaderland: Opkomst en Verbreiding van een Vergaderregime* [The Netherlands as Meeting Land: The Rise and Spread of the Meeting Regime]. Groningen: Wolters Noordhoff.

Ventura, S. J., Martin, J. A., Curtin, S. C., Mathews, T. J., Park, M. M. (2000). Births: Final data for 1998. *National Vital Statistics Reports, 48*(3). Hyattsville, MD: National Center for Health Statistics.

Verbrugge, H. P. (1968). *Kraamzorg bij Thuisbevalling* [Postpartum Care at Home Birth]. Gronigen, the Netherlands: Wolters Noordhof.

Verdenius, W., and Groeneveld, A. (1986). Ingezonden [Letter to the editor]. *Nederlands Tijdschrift voor Geneeskunde, 130,* 2140.

Viisainen, K., Gissler, M., Hemminki, E. (1994). Birth outcomes by level of obstetric care in Finland: A catchment area-based analysis. *Journal of Epidemiology and Community Medicine, 48,* 400–405.

Viisainen, K., Gissler, M., Hartikainen, A-L, and Hemminki, E. (1999). Accidental out-of-hospital births in Finland: Incidence and geographical distribution, 1963-1995. *Acta Obstetricia et Gynecologica Scandinavica, 78,* 372–378.

Viisainen, K., Gissler, M., Raikkonen, O., Perala, M., and Hemminki E. (1998). Interest in alternative birth settings in Finland. *Acta Obstetrica et Gynecologica Scandinavica, 77,* 729–735.

Volkskrant. (2000, January 3). Met houten toeter en kaarsen wachten op millenniumbaby [Waiting for the millennium baby with candels and a wooden fetoscope].

Vredevoogd, C. B., Wolleswinkel-van den Bosch, J. H., Amelink-verburg, M. P., Verloove-Vanhorick, S. P., and Mackenbach, J. P. (2001, March 10). Perinatale sterfte getoetst: Resultaten van een regionale audit [Perinatal death tested: Results of a regional audit]. *Nederlands Tijdschrift voor Geneeskunde* [Dutch Journal of Medicine], *145*(10), 482–487.

Vuijsje M. (1999, April). Hilda Verwy-Jonker en Marjet van Zuijlen over grote en kleine vrouwenzaken [Hilda Verwey-Jonker and Marjet van Zuijlen on large and small women's issues]. *Opzij,* 60–63.

Wagner, M. (1995, March 13). Don't blame midwives in maternity care crisis. *New York Times,* A18.

Werkgroep Verloskunde 2000. (1996). *Gaat het primaat verschuiven?* [Will the primaat be eliminated?]. *Tijdschrift voor Verloskundigen*, 21(2), 6–10.

Wertz, R., and Wertz, D. (1977). *Lying-in: A History of Childbirth in America*. New York: Free Press.

WHO (World Health Organization). (1989). *Protecting, promoting, and supporting breast feeding. The special role of maternity services*. A joint WHO/UNICEF statement. Geneva, WHO.

WHO (World Health Organization). (1999). *Care in Normal Birth: A Practical Guide*. Geneva: WHO.

Wiegers, T. (1997). Home or hospital birth: A prospective study of midwifery care in the Netherlands. Ph.D. thesis Leiden University. Utrecht, the Netherlands: NIVEL.

Wiegers, T. (2000, September 7). Personal correspondence.

Wiegers, T., and Beaujean, D. (2002). *Kraamzorg: Terreinbeschriving*. Utrecht, the Netherlands: NIVEL.

Wiegers, T., and Coffie, D. (2002). *Monitor Verloskundige Zorgverlening: Rapportage, Eerste Meting, Najaar, 2001* [Monitor Midwifery Care: Report of the First Measures, Fall, 2001]. Utrecht, the Netherlands: NIVEL.

Wiegers, T., and Coffie, D. (2003). *Monitor Verloskundige Zorgverlening: Rapportage Tweede Meting, Najaar 2002.* [Monitor of Midwife Caregiving: Report from the Second Measure, Fall 2002] Utrecht, the Netherlands: NIVEL.

Wiegers, T., and Hingstman, L. (1999a). *Inventarisatie Verloskundig Actieve Huisartsen* [Inventory of Obstetrically Active Huisartsen]. Utrecht, the Netherlands: NIVEL.

Wiegers, T., and Hingstman, L. (1999b). *Uittreden en Herintreden binnen de Beroepsgroep van Verloskundigen* [Departure and Return within the Professional Group of Midwives]. Utrecht, the Netherlands: NIVEL.

Wiegers, T., Calsbeek, H., and Hingstman, L. (1999). *Knelpunten in de Verloskundige Zorgverlening* [Bottlenecks in Midwifery Care]. Utrecht, the Netherlands: NIVEL.

Wiegers, T., Hingstman, L., and van der Zee, J. (2000). Thuisbevalling in gevaar [Home Birth in danger]. *Medisch Contact, 55*(19).

Wiegers, T., Kierse, M., van der Zee, J., and Berghs, G. (1996). Outcomes of planned home and planned hospital births in low risk pregnancies: Prospective study in midwifery practices in the Netherlands. *British Medical Journal, 313*, 1309–1313.

Wiegers, T., van der Velden, L., and Hingstman, L. (2002). *Behoefteraming verloskundigen 2001–2010*. Utrecht, the Netherlands: NIVEL.

Wiegers T. A., and Berghs, G.A.H. (1994). De keuze voor de plaats van bevallen [The choice for the place of birth]. *Tijdschrift voor Verloskundigen*, (19), 392–400.

Wiegers T. A., van der Zee, J., Keirse, M.J.N.C. (1998). Maternity care in the Netherlands: The changing home birth rate. *Birth*, (25), 190–197.

Wiegers, T. A., van der Zee, J., Kerssens, J. J., Keirse, M.J.N.C. (1998). Home birth or short-stay hospital birth in a low risk population in the

Netherlands. *Soc Sci Med,* (46), 1505–1511.

Wilensky, H. L. (2002). *Rich Democracies: Political Economy, Public Policy, and Performance.* Berkeley, CA: University of California Press.

Wilson, A. (1998). *New Gold Standard?* (Comparison of the Ontario & Dutch Model of Midwifery Care). McMaster University Midwifery Education Program.

Wilson, A. (1995). *The Making of Man-Midwifery: Childbirth in England, 1660–1770.* London: UCL Press.

Wilterdink, N. (1994). Images of national character. *Society, 32*(1), 43–51.

Wolf, N. (2001). *Misconceptions: Truth, Lies, and the Unexpected on the Journey to Motherhood.* New York: Doubleday.

Yankauer, A. (1983). The valley of the shadow of birth. *American Journal of Public Health, 73,* 635–638.

Youngson, A. J. (1979). *The Scientific Revolution in Victorian Medicine.* New York: Holmes and Meier Publishers.

Ziekenfondsraad. (1987). *Verloskundige Indicatielijst* [Obstetric Indications List]. Amstelveen, the Netherlands: Ziekenfondsraad.

Ziekenfondsraad. (1991). *Werkgroep Verloskunde: Verloskunde in de Toekomstige Zorgverzekering* [Obstetrics Work Group: Obstetrics and the Future of Health Care Insurance] Amstelveen, the Netherlands: Ziekenfondsraad.

Ziekenfondsraad. (1999, January).*Vademecum Verloskunde: Eindrapport van het Werkoverleg Verloskunde van de Ziekenfondsraad* [Final Report of the Sickness Funds Council Work Group on Obstetrics]. Amstelveen, the Netherlands: Ziekenfondsraad.

Zondervan, K. T., Buitendijk, S. E., Anthony, S., van Rijssel, E.J.C., and Verkerk, P. H. (1995). Frequntie en determinanten van episiotomie in de tweedelijnsverloskunde in Nederland [Frequency and determinants of episiotomy in second line obstetrics in the Netherlands.] *Nederlands Tijdschrift voor Geneeskunde* [Dutch Journal of Medicine], *139*(9): 449–452.

Index

Raymond De Vries is Professor of Sociology at St. Olaf College and Visiting Professor at the Center for Bioethics, University of Minnesota. He is the author and editor of seven previous books including, most recently, *Birth by Design: Pregnancy, Maternity Care, and Midwifery in North America and Europe.*